Liver, Nutrition, and Bile Acids

NATO ASI Series

Advanced Science Institutes Series

A series presenting the results of activities sponsored by the NATO Science Committee, which aims at the dissemination of advanced scientific and technological knowledge, with a view to strengthening links between scientific communities.

The series is published by an international board of publishers in conjunction with the NATO Scientific Affairs Division

A	**Life Sciences**	Plenum Publishing Corporation
B	**Physics**	New York and London
C	**Mathematical and Physical Sciences**	D. Reidel Publishing Company Dordrecht, Boston, and Lancaster
D	**Behavioral and Social Sciences**	Martinus Nijhoff Publishers
E	**Engineering and Materials Sciences**	The Hague, Boston, and Lancaster
F	**Computer and Systems Sciences**	Springer-Verlag
G	**Ecological Sciences**	Berlin, Heidelberg, New York, and Tokyo

Recent Volumes in this Series

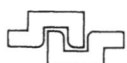

Series A: Life Sciences

Liver, Nutrition, and Bile Acids

Edited by

G. Galli
Institute of Pharmacology and Pharmacognosy
Milan, Italy

and

E. Bosisio
Institute of Pharmacology and Pharmacognosy
Milan, Italy

Plenum Press
New York and London
Published in cooperation with NATO Scientific Affairs Division

Proceedings of a NATO Advanced Study Institute on
Liver, Nutrition, and Bile Acids,
held September 25–October 5, 1983,
in Maratea, Italy

Library of Congress Cataloging in Publication Data

NATO Advanced Study Institute on Liver, Nutrition, and Bile Acids (1983:
    Maratea, Italy)
    Liver, nutrition, and bile acids.

    (NATO ASI series. Series A, Life sciences; v. 90)
    "Proceedings of a NATO Advanced Study Institute on Liver, Nutrition, and Bile
Acids, held September 25–October 5, 1983, in Maratea, Italy"—T.p. verso.
    "Published in cooperation with NATO Scientific Affairs Division."
    Includes bibliographies and index.
    1. Liver—Diseases—Congresses. 2. Biliary tract—Diseases—Congresses. 3.
Gallstones—Congresses. 4. Bile acids—Congresses. 5. Cholesterol—Metab-
olism—Congresses. 6. Nutrition—Congresses. I. Galli, Giovanni. II. Bosisio, E.
(Enrica) III. North Atlantic Treaty Organization. Scientific Affairs Division. IV. Ti-
tle. V. Series. [DNLM: 1. Bile Acids and Salts—physiology—congresses. 2.
Liver—physiology—congresses. 3. Liver—physiopathology—congresses. 4. Nu-
trition—congresses. WI 703 N279L 1983]
RC845.N37   1986   616.3'6   85-9457
ISBN 978-1-4615-9429-1   ISBN 978-1-4615-9427-7 (eBook)
DOI 10.1007/978-1-4615-9427-7

©1985 Plenum Press, New York
Softcover reprint of the hardcover 1st edition 1985
A Division of Plenum Publishing Corporation
233 Spring Street, New York, N.Y. 10013

PREFACE

This volume is a collection of the lectures and commu-
nications presented at the Nato Advanced Study Institute on
"Liver, Nutrition and Bile Acids" held in Maratea, Italy,
September 1983.

The research areas covered by the Meeting are very wide,
having to do with the liver and biliary pathophysiology,
nutrition, gallstone disease and atherosclerosis prevention.
Scientists from the major clinical and basic disciplines
provided an update overview of the complex mechanisms regulating the biosynthesis and catabolism of cholesterol and the
formation and metabolism of bile acids.

The NATO ASI has given the opportunity for thorough
general discussions on problems of growing interest in
medical sciences in the spirit of the NATO Meetings. This
wealth of information is reflected in the present collection.

We are grateful to all the contributors for the presentation of the results of their research.

A particular thanks is addressed to Mrs. Brita Rolander
Chilò of the Nutrition Foundation of Italy for her invaluable
advice and for the organization of the Institute as well as
for the editorial work.

Giovanni Galli
Enrica Bosisio

CONTENTS

COORDINATE REGULATION OF THE THREE ENYMES IN

CHOLESTEROL BIOSYNTHESIS

Ajit Sanghvi

Department of Pathology
University of Pittsburgh School of Medicine
Pittsburgh, PA 15261

It has been observed by several investigators, including Kandutsch et al. (1), and Spector et al. (2), Myant and Mitropoulos (3), and others that it is crucial that the concentration of unesterified, or free cholesterol, within the cell be regulated between very narrow limits. It is known that the unesterified cholesterol which is present in cell membranes functions to modulate fluidity of the phospholipid bilayer. A change in the membrane content of free cholesterol, therefore, may affect fluidity and thereby bring about changes in permeability, which in turn may affect the properties of membrane-bound enzymes and transport systems. It is for this reason that an excess of free cholesterol within the cell may be considered to be toxic to vital cell functions. The storage of cholesterol in the form of cholesterol esters, and in the case of liver cell, the utilization of cholesterol via the bile acid synthesis, provides an elegant means for the control of the amount of unesterified cholesterol present within the cell.

In this article, I will review the evidence which is consistent with the concept that the activities of three enzymes--namely, HMG-CoA reductase, acyl-CoA cholesterol acyltransferase or ACAT, and cholesterol 7 α-hydroxylase--which are intimately concerned with the metabolism of cholesterol are regulated in a coordinate manner by a process of phosphorylation/dephosphorylation of the enzymes. Based on this evidence, Dr. Scallen and our group have formulated the proposal that such regulation provides a short-term mechanism for intracellular unesterified cholesterol homeostasis.

As shown in Fig. 1, the reduction of HMG-CoA to mevalonic acid, which is the commitment step in cholesterol biosynthesis, is catalyzed by HMG-CoA reductase. The first indication that the activity of this enzyme may be regulated by phosphorylation/dephosphorylation was

1

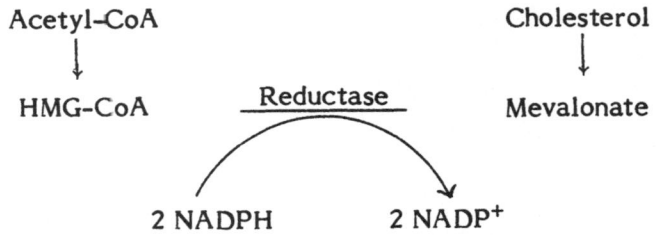

Fig. 1   General outline of formation of cholesterol from acetyl-CoA.

provided by the studies of Beg et al. in 1973 (4). These studies were prompted by an earlier observation of Bricker and Levey in 1972 (5) that cholesterol synthesis was lowered by cAMP. Beg and Gibson showed that reductase activity in rat liver microsomes was severely diminished when they were preincubated in the presence of ATP and magnesium chloride. They also observed that the diminished reductase activity, as a result of ATP magnesium treatment, was restored towards almost normal levels if these treated microsomes were centrifuged and resuspended in a buffer containing a fraction of the cytosol. In turn, this reactivation was blocked by 100 mM sodium fluoride. This was evidence suggesting a reversible modulation of reductase activity possibly brought about by the action of a protein kinase and a phosphoprotein phosphatase. Further studies by Begg, Stonik and Brewer (6) showed that there was progressive inactivation of reductase activity with two different concentrations of ATP and reactivation of the enzyme in the presence of EDTA and a phosphotase. These observations by Beg and others were further confirmed by Brown et al. (7) when they showed a progressive increase in HMG-CoA reductase activity with increasing amounts of alkaline phosphatase in the incubations. These data also indicated a greater activation of reductase activity if the time of preincubation with alkaline phosphatase was increased from 30 minutes to 60 minutes. Their own studies led Brown and Goldstein to speculate that in the live animal, HMG-CoA reductase was almost fully active--that is, dephosphorylated-- to the extent of 85-90%, and that the inactive--that is, phosphorylated-- form of the enzyme observed in vitro may simply represent an artifact at the time the animals are being killed and the liver is being removed or a result of procedural manipulations during microsome preparation. They concluded, correctly, that the long-term alteration in cholesterol synthesis does not involve changes in the state of phosphorylation of reductase, but rather it requires changes in the total amount of enzyme protein.

In contrast, recent studies in Dr. Scallen's laboratory (8, 9) and from Beg and Brewer (10) support the view that short-term changes in reductase activity in the intact animal most likely involve a change in the phosphorylation state of the enzyme. Thus, they have observed that intragastric administration of mevalonolactone to rats produces an inhibition of reductase activity which may be overcome by incubation of microsomes in the presence of different amounts of phosoprotein phosphatase. However, the reactivation of the enzyme was seen only in rats killed 20 minutes following mevalonolactone administration, but not in rats killed 60 minutes following mevalonolactone administration. Again, this reactivation of reductase following 20 minutes of mevalonolactone administration could be brought about only in the absence of potassium fluoride and it could not be observed in the presence of 50 mM potassium fluoride. In other words, the reactivation of reductase required active participation of a phosphatase.

They made similar observations with respect to the effect of short- and long-term cholesterol feeding on the inactivation/reactivation of HMG-CoA reductase. Arebalo et al. (9) observed that rats fed 2% cholesterol and killed 60 minutes later showed the expected inhibition of reductase activity. This inhibition could be overcome with the treatment of microsomes by phosphoprotein phosphatase. But, if the same experiment was carried out two hours or 120 minutes after cholesterol feeding, the inhibition of reductase activity could not be overcome by treatment with phosphoprotein phosphatase. Further support for these data comes from the work of Beg and Brewer (10), who showed that mevalonate and cholesterol feeding produce inactivation of reductase in vivo by phosphorylation. These studies, then, are consistent with the conclusion that phosphorylation of HMG-CoA reductase is the first step in a series of in vivo regulatory events which produce inactivation and ultimately degradation of the enzyme.

The evidence so far from several laboratories with respect to HMG-CoA reductase suggests a cascade system of regulation of its activity, as shown in Fig. 2. A phosphoprotein phosphatase by dephosphorylating the enzyme produces the active form. ATP magnesium, together with a reductase kinase, brings about or produces the inactive form of the enzyme. Reductase kinase, in turn, appears to exist in an active as well as an inactive form. In this instance, reductase kinase-kinase, or a reductase kinase-kinase, together with ATP magnesium, brings about or produces an active reductase kinase; and a phosphatase by removing a phosphate moiety from this enzyme produces an inactive reductase kinase.

The second enzyme which is intimately concerned with the metabolism of cholesterol is acyl-CoA:cholesterol acyltransferase, or ACAT. ACAT is a membrane-bound, microsomal enzyme that catalyzes the formation of long chain fatty-acyl cholesterol esters in rat liver and in other tissues. This enzyme is important in regulating the concentration of unesterified cholesterol in the cell and, thus, it provides a mechanism for the removal of a potentially harmful excess of unesterified cholesterol. I will now present briefly the evidence that the short-term

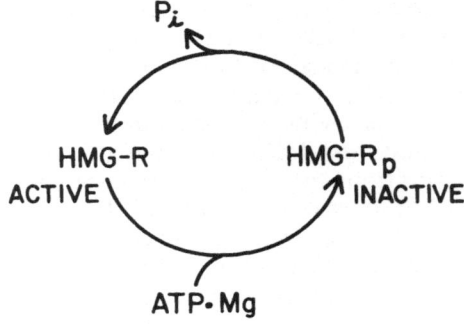

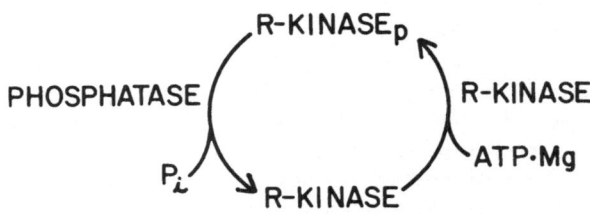

Fig. 2   Activation-inactivation of HMG-CoA reductase and reductase kinase by phosphorylation-dephosphorylation.

regulation of the activity of this enzyme also occurs by way of changes in the phosphorylation state of the enzyme. These studies were all conducted in the laboratory of Dr. Scallen in New Mexico (11).

As shown in Fig. 3, they studied the formation of cholesterol ester with time in rat liver microsomes in imidazole buffer. As can be seen, in the presence of magnesium there was a considerable decline in the amount of cholesterol ester formed, but that it could be completely prevented or blocked if potassium fluoride and EDTA were included in the incubation mixture. In a separate experiment, they studied cholesterol ester formation as a function of magnesium ion concentration in the medium. Again, the ACAT activity declined with increasing magnesium in the medium, whereas inclusion of EDTA together with magnesium, stabilized the enzyme activity. This information is consistent with the data from our laboratory which demonstrates the presence in microsomes of a Mg++ sensitive phosphatase which inactivates 7α-hydroxylase.

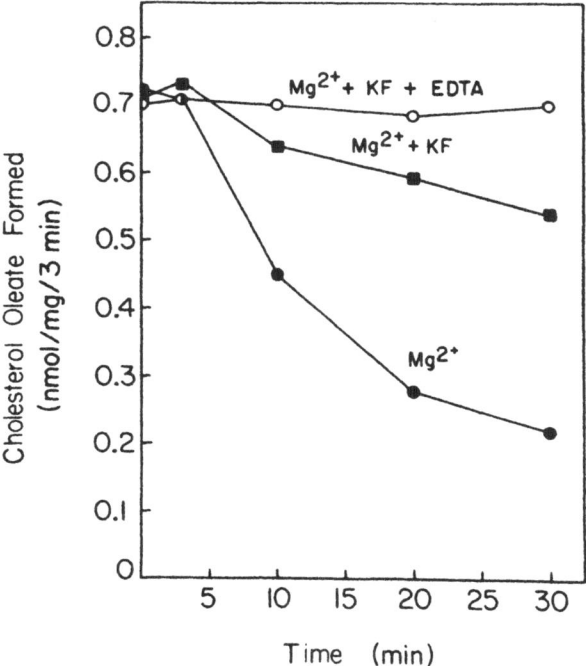

Fig. 3   Effect of preincubation time on the Mg^{2+} inactivation of ACATase in the absence or presence of potassium fluoride and EDTA. Microsomes (6 ml, 1 mg/ml) were preincubated with Mg^{2+} (added as $MgCl_2$, 5 mM) in imidazole buffer, with or without KF (100 mM) or EDTA (5 mM).

In Table 1 is shown the effect of ATP concentration on the reactivation of microsomal ACAT by a partially purified microsomal protein kinase. This data illustrates that cholesterol oleate formation increases with an increase in the amount of ATP added. In Fig. 4 is shown the reversible modulation of ACAT activity where dephosphorylating conditions bring about a decrease in the enzyme activity, which is reactivated in the presence of ATP and protein kinase. These data, taken together, illustrate (Fig. 5) that ACAT is active when phosphorylated-- that is, in the presence of protein kinase and ATP--while it is inactive when it is dephosphorylated or in the presence of protein phosphatase and magnesium.

Table 1.   Effect of ATP Concentration on the Reactivation of Microsomal ACATase by a Partially Purified Microsomal Protein Kinase

ATP added, mM	Cholesterol oleate formed, nmol/mg of protein per 3 min.
None	0.05
0.2	0.11
2.0	0.42
5.0	0.45

Previously published evidence from our laboratory (12, 13) concludes that cholesterol 7α-hydroxylase activity is similarly regulated; that is, the phosphorylated form of the enzyme is active, whereas dephosphorylated form of the enzyme is inactive. Here I will briefly show some of this evidence.

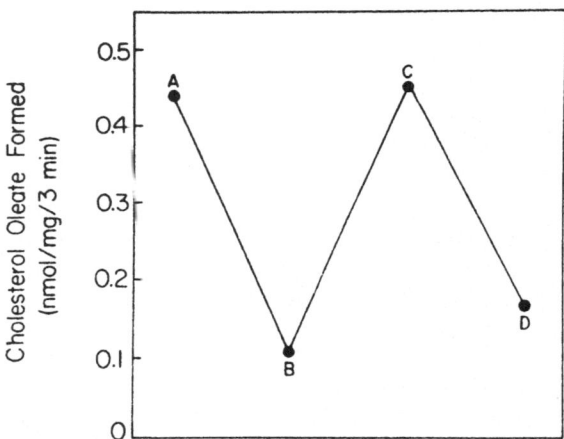

Fig. 4   Cyclic activation/inactivation of ACATase by preincubation conditions favoring phosphorylation (A,C)/dephosphorylation (B,D) of the enzyme.

We may observe in Fig. 6 that cholesterol 7α-hydroxylase activity declines rapidly in microsomes incubated in TRIS or imidazole buffer, whereas the activity is stable in the phosphate buffer. These experiments were our first indication that the loss of 7α-hydroxylase activity may be occurring by a process of dephosphorylation. In Fig 7. it is shown that the decline in cholesterol 7α-hydroxylase activity is proportional to the amount of E. coli alkaline phosphatase present in the medium. Again, the decline in activity is greater the longer the microsomes are in the

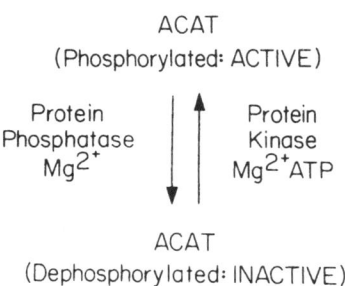

ACAT
(Phosphorylated: ACTIVE)

Protein
Phosphatase
Mg^{2+}

Protein
Kinase
$Mg^{2+}ATP$

ACAT
(Dephosphorylated: INACTIVE)

Fig. 5   Diagram showing activation of ACATase by phosphorylation as well as inactivation of the enzyme by dephosphorylation.

presence of phosphatase. The recovery of 7α-hydroxylase activity is shown in Table 2. There is a loss in 7α-hydroxylase activity in the presence of phosphatase. When phosphatase is removed by centrifugation and microsomes are incubated in the presence of ATP and a cytosolic protein fraction, which is reported to have protein kinase activity, the 7α-hydroxylase activity is almost fully restored.

These data indicate that both the ACAT and 7α-hydroxylase enzymes are active when phosphorylated and inactive when dephosphorylated. The HMG-CoA reductase, on the other hand, is inactive when phosphorylated, but active when dephosphorylated.

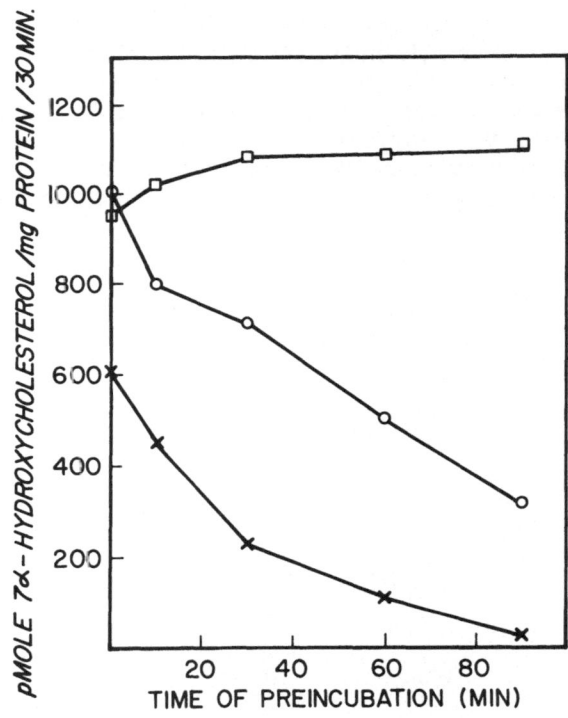

Fig. 6   Effect of preincubation of rat liver microsomes in (i) 0.2 M phosphate buffer, □—□; (ii) 20 mM imidazole·HCl + 5 mM DTT, x—x; and (iii) 20 mM Tris·HCl + 5 mM DTT, O—O; on 7α-hydroxycholesterol production.

The data discussed here so far provides a basis for proposing a mechanism (14) that may regulate the amount of unesterified cholesterol present in the cell (Fig. 8). In the liver cell, the utilization of cholesterol is regulated by ACAT and cholesterol 7α-hydroxylase. Both of these enzymes appear to be active in the phosphorylated state. The enzyme which regulates cholesterol synthesis, that is, HMG-CoA reductase, is active when dephosphorylated. Therefore, synthesis and utilization are oppositely regulated by phosphorylation/dephosphorylation.

Table 2.*   Reactivation of 7α-hydroxylase activity with ATP

Experiment	pmoles/ 7α-hydroxycholesterol/ mg protein/ 30 minutes
Control	1780
+ Alkaline Phosphatase	300
+ ATP Mg + NaF + Cytosolic Protein	1200

*Microsomes (0.3 mg protein) were preincubated for 30 minutes in 0.1 M phosphate buffer (control) followed by a 120-minute preincubation with E. coli alkaline phosphatase. After removal of phosphatase by centrifugation, microsomes were preincubated for 90 minutes in the presence of 2 mM ATP, 4 mM $MgCl_2$, 50 mM NaF, and 500 μg cytosolic protein fraction.

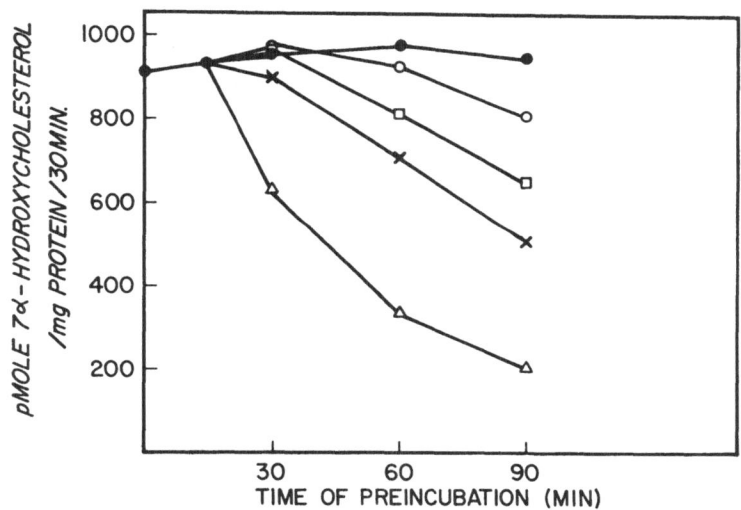

Fig. 7   Effect of E. coli alkaline phosphatase added to microsomes after 15 minutes of preincubation in 0.1 M phosphate buffer on 7α-hydroxycholesterol formation. ●—●, controls; O—O, 5 units; □—□, 10 units; x—x, 20 units; and △—△, 40 units phosphatase.

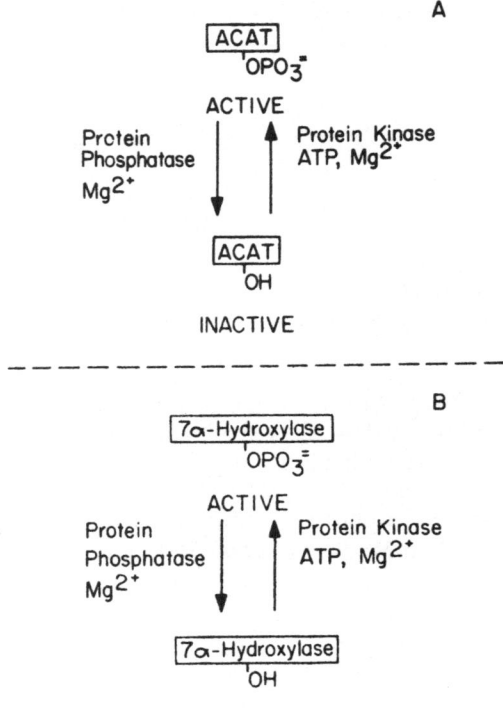

Fig. 8   Diagram showing the phosphorylation/dephosphorylation of
enzymes in rat liver involved in the regulation of cholesterol
utilization.   (A) ACATase (ACAT); (B) cholesterol 7α -
hydroxylase.

The regulatory implication of such a proposal is shown in Fig. 9. In
the event of cholesterol excess, such as dietary cholesterol entering the
cell, the regulatory adjustment would be as follows: HMG-CoA reductase
activity would decline, as a consequence of phosphorylation, whereas the
activities of ACAT and 7α-hydroxylase enzymes would be stimulated. In
the instance of cholesterol deprivation, for example a cholesterol-free
diet or a cultured liver cell grown in lipid-deficient medium, the
regulatory adjustment would be: HMG-CoA reductase activity would
increase as a consequence of dephosphorylation, but ACAT and 7α-
hydroxylase activities would decline under these conditions.

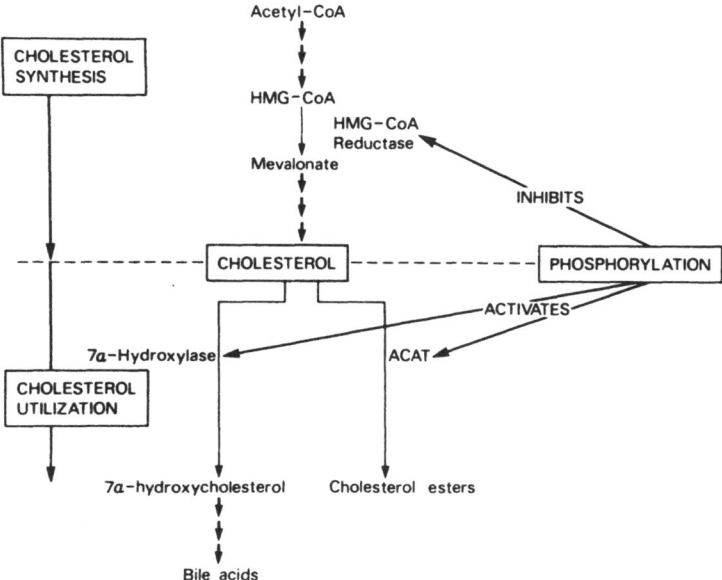

Fig. 9   Diagram of cholesterol synthesis and utilization in rat liver.

In studies conducted in our laboratory, we have observed that in microsomes obtained from rats given mevalonolactone, the 7α-hydroxylase activity increases relative to that in the control animals given only saline, consistent with our proposal. This effect of mevalonolactone on 7α-hydroxylase activity is manifest 20 minutes following mevalonolactone. But there is no further increase in enzyme activity if it is measured 60 minutes after mevalonolactone (Fig. 10).

In conclusion, the regulation of these three key enzymes in cholesterol metabolism by coordinate phosphorylation/dephosphorylation would seem to provide an elegant, short-term mechanism for intracellular cholesterol homeostasis.

Acknowledgement

Participation in these studies of Drs. Diven and Seltman, together with competent technical assistance of Mrs. Marguerite Rizk, is gratefully acknowledged.

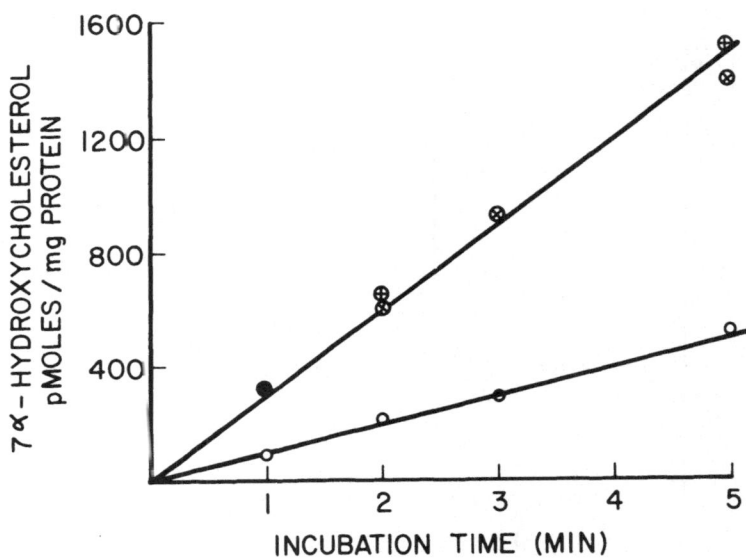

Fig. 10   The open circles (O—O) represent control 7α-hydroxylase activity; (x—x and ⊕—⊕) represent activity at 20 and 60 minutes, respectively, following mevalonolactone.

References

1.   Kandutsch, A.A., Chen, H.W. and Heiniger, H.-J. (1978)   Science **201**:498-501.
2.   Spector, A.A., Mathur, S.N. and Kaduce, T.L. (1979)   Prog. Lipid Res. **18**:31-53.
3.   Myant, N.B. and Mitropoulos, K.A. (1977) J. Lipid Res. **18**:135-153.
4.   Beg, Z.H., Allmann, D.W. and Gibson, D.M. (1973), Biochem. Biophys. Res. Commun. **54**:1362-1369.
5.   Bricker, L.A. and Levey, G.S. (1972) J. Biol. Chem. **247**:4914-4915.
6.   Beg, Z.H., Stonik, J.A. and Brewer, B.H.,Jr. (1978) Proc. Natl. Acad. Sci. USA **75**:3678-3682.
7.   Brown, M.S., Goldstein, J.L., and Dietschy, J.M. (1979) J. Biol. Chem. **254**:5144-5149.
8.   Arebalo, R.E., Hardgrave, J.E., Noland, B.J. and Scallen, T.J. (1980) Proc. Natl. Acad. Sci. USA **77**:6429-6433.
9.   Arebalo, R.E., Hardgrave, J.E. and Scallen, T.J. (1981) J. Biol. Chem. **256**:571-574.

10. Beg, Z.H. and Brewer, H.B. Jr. (1981) Cur. Topics Cell. Reg. **20**:139-184.
11. Gavey, K.L, Trujillo, D.L. and Scallen, T.J. (1983) Proc. Natl. Acad. Sci. USA **80**:2171-2174.
12. Sanghvi, A., Grassi, E., Warty, V., Diven, W., Wight, C. and Lester, R. (1981) Biochem. Biophys. Res. Comm. **103**:886-892.
13. Sanghvi, A., Grassi, E. and Diven, W. (1983) Proc. Natl. Acad. Sci. USA **80**:2175-2178.
14. Scallen, T.J. and Sanghvi, A. (1983) Proc. Natl. Acad. Sci. USA **80**:2477-2480.

MICROSOMAL CHOLESTEROL 7α-HYDROXYLASE PHOSPHATASES

Ajit Sanghvi, Warren Diven, and Joyce Sweeney

Department of Pathology
University of Pittsburgh School of Medicine
Pittsburgh, PA 15261

When rat liver microsomes are incubated at 37° in TRIS buffer, there is a time-dependent loss of the activity of cholesterol 7α-hydroxylase (1). This loss of activity can be prevented if the incubation is carried out in phosphate buffer or if fluoride is added to the TRIS buffer system. These results are consistent with the presence of a protein phosphatase in the microsomal fraction. To determine that this activity was not due to other subcellular fractions, we prepared microsomes by our standard procedure and also by the calcium precipitation technique of Kamath et al. (2) as modified by Goodwin and Margolis (3). These preparations were tested for the presence of enzyme activities considered to be markers for other subcellular fractions. The results of these assays

Table 1. Enzyme Activity (U/mg protein)

Fraction	Gluc-6 Phosphatase	β-Glycerol Phosphate Phosphatase	Esterase	Succinic Dehydrogenase	Arylsulfatase A
Mitochondria	121	521	1.7	15	580
Microsomes	196	73	12.9	3	183
Ca^{2+} prepared microsomes	53	136	4.4	3	156
Cytosol	0	311	2.7	0	140

are shown in Table I. It can be seen that although the mitochondrial fraction is somewhat contaminated with microsomal enzymes, there is less mitochondrial or lysosomal contamination in our microsomal fraction.

To begin the purification and characterization of this enzyme activity, we investigated the use of cholic acid to solubilize the enzyme from microsomes. Microsomes were suspended in 10 mM TRIS buffer, pH 7.0, with 0.1 mM EGTA, 0.1% mercaptoethanol and 2% cholic acid, and stirred for one hour at 4oC. The pellet was centrifuged at 300,000 x g for 20 minutes. About 70% of the activity contained in the microsomal preparation was recovered by this procedure. A second extraction of the pellet did not solubilize any additional enzyme activity. The supernatant was dialyzed against the same TRIS buffer in order to remove the cholic acid. This dialyzed material was again centrifuged at 300,000 x g for 20 minutes and the supernatant applied to a DEAE Sephadex column (1 x 20 cm) equilibrated with the same buffer. The column was washed with 170 ml buffer and then eluted with 300 ml of a 0-0.5 M NaCl gradient in the TRIS buffer. Fractions of 5 ml were collected and analyzed for enzyme activity using the 4 MU assay we have described earlier (4). The results are shown in the figure. Fractions containing activity were combined and assayed for activity and protein. The results of this solubilized and partial purification are indicated in Table II.

Note that there is a small amount of activity remaining in the pellet after cholate extraction. This is only 3% of the total microsomal activity, but the increase in specific activity and the fact that it is not solubilized by this procedure suggests that it may be a separate enzyme. In this experiment only about 2.5% of the recovered activity was retained on the DEAE column and 97% came through in the initial wash. This ratio

Table 2. Solubilization and Partial Purification of Microsomal Phosphatase

	U/ml	Protein	U/mg	Total	% Recov.
Microsomes	36216	14.0	2587	1195128	–
Cholate Suspension	25607	10.5	2439	845031	71
Supernatant	24673	10.1	2443	814209	68
Pellet	1103	0.2	5515	36399	3
Dialyzed Supernatant	18318	9.7	1888	586176	49
DEAE					
Break through	8108	3.1	2615	421616	35
Retained	78	0.2	390	10920	

varies from preparation to preparation but both fractions are always present. The enzyme in the initial wash does not represent overloading of the column since, when the recovered material is applied to a second DEAE Sephadex column, no material is retained. Thus we have preliminary evidence which suggests there are at least three phosphatases associated with rat liver microsomes: two enzymes extracted by cholic acid and one remaining associated with the membrane fraction. We now must test these fractions for their phosphoprotein phosphatase activity and to see which enzyme is active in dephosphorylating cholesterol 7α-hydroxylase.

References

1. Sanghvi, A., Grassi, E., Warty, V., Diven, W., Wight, C., and Lester, R., Biochem. Biophys. Res. Comm. 103:886-892 (1981).
2. Kamath, S.A., and Narayan, K.A., Anal. Biochem. 48:53-61 (1972).
3. Goodwin, C.D., and Margolis, S.J., J. Lipid Res. 17:297-303 (1976).
4. Sanghvi, A., Grassi, E., Bartman, C., and Diven, W.F., Lipids 17:644-649 (1982).

BILE ACIDS AND CHOLESTEROL ABSORPTION

George V. Vahouny and Linda L. Gallo

The George Washington University
School of Medicine and Health Sciences
Washington, DC 20037, USA

The obligatory role of bile acids in the overall efficiency of cholesterol absorption from the intestine has been extensively documented. Prior to 1920, it had already been demonstrated that bile duct ligation[1] or bile diversion[2] in dogs, markedly diminished the capacity of the intestine to absorb cholesterol. In the 1950's several laboratories reported that interruption of the normal entero-hepatic circulation of bile and its contained bile salts, resulted in a decrease in lipids in the thoracic duct lymph of experimental animals[3,4], a marked reduction in the absorbability of oleic acid and of corn oil fatty acids[4], and a complete cessation of cholesterol absorption into lymph[5-7]. Complimentary data has been reported by others in humans with complete biliary obstruction[8], and in animals and humans using bile acid-sequestering anion exchange resins, such as cholestyramine[9,10].

This fundamental role of bile salts in the intestinal absorption of sterols is a reflection of the potential requirements for this cholesterol metabolites in various steps of intraluminal and epithelial cell mechanisms of cholesterol absorption (Figure 1). These include; solubilization of cholesterol in the intestinal lumen by mixed micelles, containing biliary bile salts and phospholipids, and the products of triglyceride digestion; modification of the intestinal surface barriers to cholesterol transfer, including the "unstirred water layer" and the mucin "coat": and the cellular esterification of cholesterol prior to incorporation of the resulting esters into the lipoprotein core lipids.

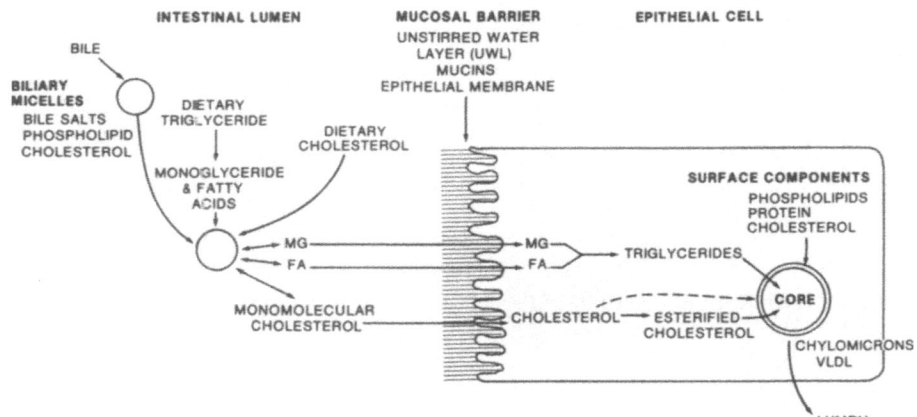

Fig. 1. Schematic representation of the luminal, membrane and
cellular aspects of cholesterol absorption from the
intestine. Abbreviations: MG, monoglycerides; FA,
unesterified fatty acids; VLDL, very low density
lipoproteins.

OVERVIEW OF CHOLESTEROL ABSORPTION[11-15]

As shown in Figure 1, cholesterol entering the lumen is largely
derived from two sources; endogenous, which is primarily biliary
cholesterol; and exogenous, or dietary cholesterol. These sources
are distinguished by the fact that endogenous cholesterol of bile is
already in an efficient state of solubility as a component of the
mixed bile salt-lecithin micelles, which are contained in bile. In
contrast, dietary cholesterol enters the intestine emulsified with
dietary glycerides or in membranes. Efficient absorption requires
its availability, and its solubilization in pre-existing micelles.
However, irrespective of source, the majority if not all of the
luminal cholesterol is unesterified and this is the form which is
ultimately required for translocation across the mucosal surface
barriers[16].

The distribution of cholesterol between the luminal oil phase
(provided largely by dietary fat) and the micellar phase, is therefore a major influence in the efficient absorption of cholesterol,
and can be influenced by both the content and composition of the
dietary fat. As the products of fat digestion (monoglycerides, fatty
acids) are produced, micelles are expanded, increasing the solubility
potential for cholesterol[17,18], and improving overall absorption[19,20]. Thus, it has been clearly demonstrated that cholesterol
absorption is most efficient in the presence of unesterified fatty
acids[19,21] and particularly those which are mono or polyunsaturated[21,22].

A second major influence on overall cholesterol absorption involves the intestinal mucosal surface. In addition to the micro-villar membrane itself, this surface contains a variable amount of mucinous glycoprotein[23] and a resistance to lipid transport referred to as the unstirred water layer[24]. Evidence to support the existence of this unstirred layer is largely-derived from in vitro experimental data[25,26] and from theoretical consider-ations[27], which suggest that this "barrier" is of importance in transport restrictions with large lipoidal-molecules, and can be, in part, overcome by bile salt-containing micelles. More recently, however, greater emphasis has been placed on the role of surface mucins as a transport barrier[28,29], and this layer has been suggested to largely represent the purported unstirred layer.

The mechanisms of intracellular transport of cholesterol have been neglected, largely due to technical difficulties, including isotope exchanges and other problems inherent with broken cell prep-arations. It has been postulated[30] that there is a rapid exchange or transfer of cholesterol among intracellular lipoproteins and organelles of the mucosal cell. However, to date, there is no infor-mation regarding the presence or function of sterol carrier proteins in these cells, as has been described for other tissues with a high turnover of cholesterol (e.g.[31]).

Finally it is clear that, unlike long-chain fatty acids which can appear in portal blood in limited amounts[32], cholesterol is absorbed exclusively into the lymphatic circulation[32,33]. A small amount of unesterified cholesterol can appear in lymph and is largely associated with chylomicron and lipoprotein "coat", or limiting membrane. However, this "coat" has a limited capability for signifi-cant transport, and the mass transport cholesterol (like that of triglycerides) requires esterification and incorporation into the lipoprotein core. Thus, the transfer of significant amounts of cholesterol from intestinal lumen to lymph is associated with exten-sive esterification (70-90%) with fatty acids, and this occurs in the mucosal epithelial cells[11]. There are two intestinal enzymes potentially important in the esterification of unesterified choles-terol: cholesterol esterase, or sterol ester hydrolase (EC. 3.1.1.13); and ACAT, or acyl CoA:cholesterol:acyl transferase (EC 2.3.1.26) (see 14,15).

SPECIFITY OF BILE SALTS IN CHOLESTEROL ABSORPTION

Several lines of evidence suggest that, in addition to a re-quirement for an intact enterohepatic circulation of bile, choles-terol absorption is dependent on the chemical nature of the luminal bile acid. In acute studies on the absorption of cholesterol in thoracic duct lymph of rats, a quantitative relationship between administered cholesterol, fatty acids and sodium taurocholate was established[7]. With these maximized conditions, and measuring the appearance of cholesterol in lymph, it was reported[34] that only cholic acid (3α, 7α, 12α-trihydroxycholanic acid) or its glycine or taurine conjugates, produced a significant increase in cholesterol absorption, while cholanic acid, lithocholic acid (3α) and deoxycholic and (3α, 12α) had no effect. These findings have been confirmed by others[35,36], comparing the free or conjugated forms of cholic acid with either chenodeoxycholic acid (3α, 7α) or ursodeoxycholic acid (3α, 7β). In addition, recent studies in the human under highly controlled conditions[37-39] are compatible with the animal studies, in that administration of cholic and stimulated cholesterol absorption, while no significant effects were observed following administration of either chenodeoxy-, deoxy-, or ursodeoxycholic acid.

This specifity for cholate or its conjugates on cholesterol absorption has also been demonstrated by modification of biliary bile acid composition by hormonal perturbations (see[40]). For example, in hypothyroid rats, there is a diminished biliary output of bile acids[41], and a shift in the ratio of biliary cholate and chenodeoxycholate. This ratio is approximately 3:1 cholate to chenodeoxycholate in normal rats and is shifted dramatically (9:1) in hypothyroid rats[42]. As might be expected, this hormonal deficiency results in multiple alterations in overall physiology, among which are hypercholesterolemia and increased absorbability of cholesterol[40]. Conversely, administration of thyroid hormones (L-thyroxine or triiodothyronine) results in diminished levels of biliary cholate, and proportional increases in chenodeoxycholate. This shift (from a normal 3:1 ratio to a 1:3 ratio of cholate: chenodeoxycholate)[43] is associated with a dramatic decrease in cholesterol absorption into lymph[44].

These varied experimental approaches (Table 1) are consistant with the hypothesis that cholic acid or its conjugates have a unique role in cholesterol absorption.

POTENTIAL SITES OF BILE ACID SPECIFITY FOR CHOLESTEROL ABSORPTION

Intraluminal Phase

The physical chemistry of micellar structure and formation has been reviewed extensively elsewhere[40,45-47], and is only briefly summarized. The concentration at which micellar aggregation of bile salts molecules occurs (critical micellar concentration, CMC) is affected by bile salt structure, pH, temperature and a variety of other factors. Conjugated bile salts have a higher CMC than the unconjugates, and the CMC for trihydroxycholanates (cholic acid) is higher than for the dihydroxy derivatives. Among the latter, deoxycholate forms micelles at a lower CMC than does chenodeoxycholate.

Table 1. Bile Acid Specifity for Cholesterol Absorption.

Experimental Manipulation	Species	Effect on relative biliary cholate pool	Effect on cholesterol absorption(ref)
Oral or gastric administration			
Cholic acid	rat	↗	↗ (34,35)
	man	↗ (Antibiotic administration)	↗ (39)
Dehydrocholate	rat	↘	↘ (34)
Cholanate	rat	↘	↘ (34)
Deoxycholate	rat	↘	↘ (34)
	man	↘	↘ (38)
Chenodeoxycholate	rat	↘	↘ (35)
	man	↘	↘ (36,37)
Ursodeoxycholate	man	↘	↘ (36)
Hypothyroid	rat	↗	↗ (42)
Thyroid hormone administration	rat	↗	↗ (42,44)

In addition to differences in CMC for the bile salts, their aggregation numbers and sizes vary depending on their structure. Sodium taurocholate has an aggregation number of 22 and a radius of 20-24 Å. Thus, trihydroxy bile salts form smaller and presumably more stable micelles than the dihydroxy analogous.

Simple micelles, composed only of bile salts, have a limited capacity to solubilize cholesterol. With taurocholate for example, one molecule of cholesterol is solubilized by 25 molecules of bile salt, while addition of a monoglyceride to the preparation essentially doubles the solubilization of cholesterol[17]. Obviously, the participation of additional amphipaths and amphiphiles, such as phospholipids and fatty acids, in the micellar structure causes dramatic increases in sterol solubility (from 100-1000 fold)[48].

From the available physiochemical and physiological data, therefore, it is unlikely that the dramatic effects of cholate or its conjugates on cholesterol transport can be attributed simply by differences in either solubilization of cholesterol by mixed micelles containing different bile salts in varying ratios, or to the equilibrium of cholesterol between the micellar and the mono-molecular phases in the lumen.

Mucosal Membrane Effects

A second site at which bile salts affect overall cholesterol absorption involves the mucosal cell surface. A variety of evidences clearly demonstrate that translocation of cholesterol across this barrier is initially dependent on solubilization of sterol in micelles containing bile salts, and that the transport occurs by passive diffusion[26]. Studies from this[49] and other laboratories[50] have provided sufficient data to exclude cellular uptake of intact micelles containing cholesterol. Thus, current evidence favors the view that cholesterol absorption occurs from monomolecular phase[26].

A variety of studies have suggested that a major limitation to cholesterol absorption exists at the epithelial cell surface. Also, several lines of evidence (e.g.[24-26]) support the concept of an unstirred water layer (UWL) at the mucosal surface, which provides a major resistance to transport of long-chain fatty acids and cholesterol into the cell. The thickness, and therefore resistance, of this layer is variable and is a function of physical mixing[51]. Based on experimental data and theoretical considerations[25-27], the suggested role of the bile salt micelle is to overcome the "resistance" of the UWL to lipid diffusion across the microvillar membrane. There is, however, little evidence to suggest that this "resistance" is differentially affected by trihydroxy bile salt-containing micelles, as opposed to micelles containing dihydroxy bile salts. Thus, although an (UWL) may limit sterol diffusion at the mucosal cell surface, there does not appear to be a major specifictiy of a unique bile salt structure in modifying the resistance of this barrier.

Recently, the role of the UWL as a major diffusion limitation has been questioned[28,29]. It is known that the mucosal surface is coated with micropolysaccharides (mucins) secreted by goblet cells and epithelial cells[29]. The structural and functional importance of these mucins have been reviewed elsewhere[29]. It has been suggested that this mucin layer may, in fact, represent a major diffusion barrier in the intestine, and can account for the phenomena attributed to the UWL[28]. Our own studies[52] have indicated that cholesterol is extensively bound to an intestinally-derived sialomucin, and this interaction severely limits transmembrane translocation of the sterol. However, in the presence of simple or mixed micelles containing taurocholate, this mucin is solubilized and released from the surface, cholesterol absorption to the surface is diminished, and membrane translocation of the sterol is dramatically increased (Table 2).

Thus, the same conditions described for decreasing the resistance of the UWL also affect the mucin-cholesterol interaction, and improve cholesterol absorption. However, there again, does not

24

Table 2. Surface Adsorption and Cellular Absorption of Cholesterol.

Incubation media for intestinal tissue incubations	Surface adsorption	Cellular uptake
Cholesterol	20	0.02
+ Oleic acid	10	0.01
Oleic acid + lecithin	6	0.01
Oleic acid + taurocholate	4	0.41
+ Oleic acid + taurocholate + lecithin	3	0.50

μmol

Data derived from [52]

appear to be a major difference between bile salt analogues in this regard. Overall, therefore, the importance of bile salts in micellar solubilization and in aspects of membrane diffusibility has been demonstrated, but the effects on these aspects of cholesterol absorption do not adequately describe the apparent specificity for cholic and acid conjugates.

Cellular Phase

The cellular esterification of cholesterol prior to efficient translocation into lymph in the chylomicron and VLDL core[53] has been considered by many to be the limiting step in absorption. This is based on a variety of physiological and pharmacological evidences (see[11-15]. It is at this site that a unique requirement for cholic acid has been demonstrated in the rat (Table 3).

Of the two potentially esterifying enzymes associated with intestinal mucosa, sterol ester hydrolase, also referred to as cholesterol esterase (CE'ase) has been extensively investigated in

Table 3. Effect of Individual Bile Salts on Cholesterol Absorption In Vivo and CE'ase Activity In Vitro.

Bile salt addition	Increase in lymph cholesterol %	Sterol ester hydrolase activity units
None	–	0
Cholanate (dehydroxy)	0	2
Lithocholate (3α-hydroxy)	0	1
Deoxycholate (3α,12α-dihydroxy)	14	4
Triketocholantate	0	5
Cholate (3α,7α,12α-trihydroxy)	90	30

From 34,59,61,62

our laboratories. Our interest was based on the observations that pancreatectomy in experimental animals[54,55] or humans[56], or diversion or pancreatic juice in rats[57,58], resulted in a complete inability to absorb significant amounts of cholesterol from the intestine. Oral administration of pancreas preparations[54,56] or reintroduction of pancreatic juice[57,58] reestablished intestinal absorption and esterification of the sterol.

CE'ase has been purified from rat pancreatic juice[59] and rat pancreas[60,61] by a variety of techniques, including immunoaffinity chromatography. The enzyme protein is elaborated in pancreas as a 69,000 MW species which is inactive in synthesizing cholesterol esters[59,61]. However, cholic acid or its conjugates bind specifically to this monomer[61] producing an aggregation of 6 subunits to form the enzymatically - active species[59,61]. Although certain other bile salt analogues have differential binding and aggregating ability, in no case is an enzymatically-active species produced (Table 3). Other studies have demonstrated substrate specificity[59], resistance to proteolytic and temperature inactivation [61,62], and active site characteristics of the cholic acid-enzyme complex[59,61].

The transfer of luminal pancreatic CE'ase into mucosal cells has been demonstrated by both biochemical and immunological[63,64] techniques and our current studies suggest specific receptor sites on the microvillar membrane for the enzyme. Although not generally recognized, the phenomenon of intact protein absorption has been previously reported (e.g.[65,66]. Furthermore, although active absorption of bile salts occurs in the distal ileum, significant amounts of bile salts, including taurocholate, are absorbed throughout the intestine, including the sites of cholesterol absorption (see[40]). Thus, currently, available physiological and biochemical evidence clearly indicates that intestinal CE'ase of the intestine can account entirely for the cholesterol esters appearing in lymph, and that this phase of cholesterol absorption is regulated by the cholate content of bile.

The second cholesterol esterifying activity in intestine, is ACAT (see[15]), a microsomal enzyme[67,68] which is not well characterized. Unlike CE'ase the ACAT system requires high energy intermediates of the fatty acid, which suggests that overall absorption and esterification of sterols is an energy-dependent transport. This activity is inhibited by bile salts[68] and the lack of specificity for sterol esterification has recently been suggested.

Recent studies in our laboratories[70] have evaluated the role of each of these enzyme systems in the regulation of luminal cholesterol absorption in the rat. Rats were surgically prepared to contain a mesenteric lymph duct catheter, drainage of common bile (bile + pancreatic juice) and an indwelling infusion catheter in the duodenum. Animals received a constant duodenal infusion (3 ml/h) of a saline maintenance solution, containing 10 mM sodium taurocholte to replenish bile acids. During the 36 h diversion of pancreatic juice, the mucosa has been shown to be deficient in CE'ase[58]. At this time, infusions were continued with either (a) no further additions; (b) donor pancreatic juice; (c) pancreatic juice plus control rabbit serum IgG. After an additional 12 h of infusion, animals were given a lipid test meal, and cholesterol absorption was assessed over 6 h. In addition, the mucosal activities of CE'ase and ACAT were assayed after six-hour lymph collection period.

As shown in Table 4, control animals (no enzyme infusion) absorbed essentially none of the administered cholesterol (0.9 mol), while those given fresh pancreatic juice absorbed 5.2 mol of the administered (65 mol) dose. In addition, mucosal CE'ase activity was markedly increased during pancreatic infusion, while ACAT was unchanged. Similarly, infusion of pancreatic juice treated with control IgG resulted in increased levels of mucosal CE'ase and increased absorption of cholesterol, while again, ACAT was unchanged. Finally, when fresh pancreatic juice was pretreated with anti-CE'ase antibodies; its infusion was neither effective in "restoring" mucosal CE'ase levels nor improving cholesterol absorption.

These data provide convincing evidence that, at least in the rat, pancreatic CE'ase, a cholic acid-dependent enzyme, is responsible for regulation of cholesterol absorption into lymph. It nevertheless remains possible, although unlikely, that CE'ase regulates cellular uptake of the sterol, while ACAT is responsible for the esterification reaction[71].

Table 4. Relationship between Cholesterol Absorption and Activities of Intestinal Sterol Ester Hydrolase (SEH) and ACAT.

Additions to maintenance infusion (10 mM Taurocholate)	Absorption of [4^{14}C] Cholesterol	Enzyme activities	
		CE'ase	ACAT
(a) None	0.9 ± 0.1	2.2 ± 0.2	2.6 ± 0.3
(b) Fresh pancreatic juice	5.2 ± 1.6	8.3 ± 1.8	3.1 ± 0.3
(c) Juice treated w/ control IgG	6.8 ± 1.4	6.0 ± 1.5	2.6 ± 0.5
(d) Juice treated w/ anti-SEH IgG	1.1 ± 0.2	1.5 ± 0.04	2.9 ± 0.8

Taken from [70]

SUMMARY

The obligatory role of bile salts for intestinal absorption of cholesterol can be accounted for by multifaceted functions in the luminal, translocation and cellular phases of absorption. Micellar solubilization of unesterified cholesterol is a requisite for overall absorption of cholesterol into lymph. This increases by many-fold, the monomolecular form of sterol, and allows for efficient membrane translocation.

The luminal requirements for bile salts are general, and do not adequately describe the known specifity for cholate and its conjugates which has been demonstrated in several species including man. This specifity appears to be a function, at least in part, of a cholic acid – dependent enzyme, sterol ester hydrolase (cholesterol esterase).

Acknowledgements

The author respectively acknowledges the major contributions of many coworkers, and particularly, Dr. C R Treadwell. Supported in part by Grants USPHS HL-02033 AM 17269, AM-26346 and USDA 82-CRCR 1001.

REFERENCES

1. M. A. Rothschild, The relationship of the liver to the cholesterin metabolism, Proc.NY Pathol.Soc., 14:229 (1914).
2. J. H. Mueller, The assimulation of cholesterol and its esters, J.Biol.Chem., 22:1 (1915).
3. B. Borgstrom, On the mechanism of the intestinal fat absorption. V. The effect of bile diversion on fat absorption in the rat, Acta Physiol.Scand., 28:279 (1953).
4. K. S. Kim and J. L. Bollman, Absorption of fat in the absence of both bile and pancreatic juice, Arch.Surg., 69:247 (1954).
5. M. D. Siperstein, I. L. Chaikoff, and W. L. Reinhardt, C^{14}-cholesterol: V. Obligatory function of bile in intestinal absorption of cholesterol, J.Biol.Chem., 198:111 (1952).
6. A. C. Ivy, R. Suzuki, C. R. Prasad, Obligatory function of a continuous flow of normal bile for cholesterol absorption, Am.J.Physiol., 193:521 (1958).
7. G. V. Vahouny, C. H. Woo, and C. R. Treadwell, Quantitative effects of bile salt and fatty acid on cholesterol absorption in the rat, Am.J. Physiol., 193:41 (1958).
8. E. Quintao, S. M. Grundy, and E. H. Ahrens, Jr., An evaluation of four methods for measuring cholesterol absorption by the intestine in man, J.Lipid Res., 12:221 (1971).

9. S. R. Hyun, G. V. Vahouny, and C. R. Treadwell, Effect of hypo-cholestrolemic agents on intestinal cholesterol absorption, Proc.Soc.Exp.Biol.Med., 112:496 (1963).
10. G. V. Vahouny, T. Roy, L. L. Gallo, J. A. Story, D. Kritchevsky, and M. M. Cassidy, Dietary Fibers, III. Effect of chronic intake on cholesterol absorption and metabolism in the rat, Am.J.Clin.Nutr., 33:2182 (1980).
11. C. R. Treadwell and G. V. Vahouny, Cholesterol absorption, in: "Handbook of Physiology - The Alimentary Canal," American Physiological Society, Bethesda, MD, pp. 1438 (1968).
12. J. M. Dietschy and J. D. Wilson, Regulation of sterol metab-olism, N.Engl.J.Med., 282:1128,1179,1241 (1970).
13. A. B. R. Thomson and J. M. Dietschy, Intestinal lipid absorp-tion: Major extracellular and intracellular events, in: "Physiology of the Gastrointestinal Tract," L.R. Johnson, ed., Raven Press, New York, pp.1147 (1981).
14. G. V. Vahouny and D. Kritchevsky, Plant and marine sterols and cholesterol metabolism, in: "Nutritional Pharmacology," G.A. Spiller, ed., Alan R. Liss, New York, pp.31 (1981).
15. L. L. Gallo, Cholesterol and other sterols:-Absorption, metab-olism and roles in atherogenesis, in: "Nutrition and Heart Disease," E.B. Feldman, ed., Churchill Livingston, New York, p.83 (1983).
16. G. V. Vahouny and C. R. Treadwell, Absolute requirement for free sterol for absorption by rat intestinal mucosa, Proc.Soc.Exp. Biol.Med., 116:496 (1964).
17. F. P. Woodford, Enlargement of taurocholate micelles by added cholesterol and monolein: Self-diffusion measurements, J.Lipid Res., 10:539 (1969).
18. J. D. Wilson, The role of bile acids in the overall regulation of steroid metabolism, Arch.Int.Med., 130:493 (1973).
19. K. S. Kim and A. G. Ivy, Factors influencing cholesterol absorp-tion, Am.J.Physiol., 171:302 (1952).
20. G. V. Vahouny, L. Fawal, and C. R. Treadwell, Factors facilitat-ing cholesterol absorption from the intestine via lymphatic pathways, Am.J.Physiol., 188:342 (1957).
21. G. V. Vahouny and C. R. Treadwell, Comparative effects of dietary fatty acids and triglycerides on lymph lipids in the rat, Am.J.Physiol., 196:881 (1959).
22. C. Sylven and B. Borgstrom, Intestinal absorption and transport in the rat: Influence of the fatty acid chain length of the carrier triglyceride, J.Lip.Res., 10:351 (1969).
23. G. Forstner, J. Sturgess, and J. Forstner, Malfunction of intestinal mucus and mucus production, Adv.Exp.Med.Biol., 89:349 (1977).
24. J. M. Dietschy, V. L. Sallee, and F. A. Wilson, Unstirred water layers and absorption across the intestinal mucosa, Gastro-enterology, 61:932 (1971).
25. V. L. Sallee and J. M. Dietschy, Determinants of intestinal mucosal uptake of short and medium-chain fatty acids and alcohols, J.Lip.Res., 14:475 (1973).

26. H. Westergaard and J. M. Dietschy, The mechanism whereby bile acid micelles increase the rate of fatty acid and cholesterol uptake into the intestinal mucosal cell, J.Clin.Invest., 58:97 (1976).

27. J. M. Diamond and E. M. Wright, Biological membranes: The physical basis of ion and nonelectrolyte selectivity, Ann.Rev.Physiol., 31:581 (1969).

28. F. Nimmerfall and J. Rosenthaler, Significance of the Goblet-cell mucin layer, the outermost barrier to passage through the gut wall, Biochem.Biophys.Res.Commun., 94:960 (1980).

29. K. W. Smithson, D. B. Millar, L. R. Jacobs, and G. M. Gray, Intestinal diffusion barrier: Unstirred water layer or membrane surface mucous coat, Science, 214:1241 (1981).

30. P. Favarger and E. F. Metzger, La resorption intestinale du deuterocholesterol et sa repartition dans l'organisme animal sous forme libre et esterifiée, Helv.Chem.Acta, 35:1811 (1952).

31. R. Chanderbhan, B. J. Noland, T. J. Scallen, and G. V. Vahouny, Sterol carrier protein$_2$: Delivery of cholesterol from adrenal lipid droplets to mitochondria for pregenenolone synthesis, J.Biol.Chem., 257:8928 (1982).

32. S. Hyun, G. V. Vahouny, and C. R. Treadwell, Portal absorption of long-chain fatty acids in the rat, Biochim.Biophys.Acta, 137:296 (1967).

33. M. W. Biggs, M. Friedman, and S. O. Byers, Intestinal lymphatic transport of absorbed cholesterol, Proc.Soc.Exp.Biol.Med., 78:641 (1951).

34. G. V. Vahouny, H. M. Gregorian, and C. R. Treadwell, Comparative effects of bile acids on intestinal absorption of choles-terol, Proc.Soc.Exp.Biol.Med., 101:538 (1959).

35. R. F. Raicht, B. I. Cohen, and E. H. Mosbach, Effects of sodium taurochenodeoxycholate and sodium taurocholate on cholesterol absorption in the rat, Gastroenterology, 67:1155 (1974).

36. M. O. Reynier, J. C. Montet, A. Gerolami, C. Marteau, C. Crotte, A. M. Montent, and S. Mathieu, Comparative effects of cholic, chenodeoxycholic, and ursodeoxycholic acids on micellar solubilization and intestinal absorption of cholesterol, J.Lipid Res., 22:467 (1981).

37. M. Ponz de Leon, N. Carulli, P. Noria, R. Lora, and F. Zironi, The effect of chenodeoxycholic acid (CDCA) on cholesterol absorption, Gastroenterology, 77:223 (1979).

38. M. Ponz de Leon, N. Carulli, P. Loria, R. Lora, and F. Zironi, Cholesterol absorption during bile acid feeding: Effect of ursodeoxycholic (UDCA) administration, Gastroenterology, 78:214 (1980).

39. M. Ponz de Leon and N. Carulli, The influence of bile acid pool composition on the regulation of cholesterol absorption, inI: "Falk Symposium 24," G. Paumgartner, A. Stiehl, and W. Gerok, eds., MTP Press Ltd., p.133 (1981).

40. W. T. Beher, Chemistry and physiology of bile acids and their influence on atherosclerosis, in: "Monographs on Athero-

sclerosis," D. Kritchevsky, O.J. Pollak, and H.S. Simms, eds., S. Karger, Basel (1976).

41. S. Eriksson, Influence of thyroid activity on excretion of bile acid and cholesterol in the rat, Proc.Soc.Exp.Biol.Med., 94:582 (1957).

42. O. Strand, Influence of propylthiouracil and D- and L-tri-iodothyronine on excretion of bile acids in bile fistula rats, Proc.Soc.Exp.Biol.Med., 109:668 (1962).

43. K. Ushida, Y. Nomura, M. Kadowaki, K. Myata, and T. Miyake, Effects of dietary cholesterol and L-thyroxine on biliary bile acid composition and secretory rate, and on plasma, liver and bile cholesterol levels in rats, Endocrin.Jap., 17:107 (1970).

44. T. H. Lin, R. Rubinstein, and W. L. Holmes, A study of the effect of D- and L-triiodothyronine on bile acid excretion of rats, J.Lipid Res., 4:63-67 (1963).

45. A. F. Hofmann and D. M. Small, Detergent properties of bile salts. Correlation with physiological function, Ann.Med.Rev., 18:333 (1967).

46. D. M. Small, Size and structure of bile salts nucelles. Influence of structure, concentration, counterion concentration, PH, and temperature, Adv.Chem., 8:31 (1968).

47. M. C. Carey and D. M. Small, Micelle formation by bile salts. Physical-chemical and thermodynamic considerations, Arch. Intern.Med., 130:506 (1972).

48. A. F. Hofmann, Fat digestion. The interaction of lipid digestion products with micellar bile acid solution, in: "Lipid Absorption: Biochemical and Clinical Aspects," K. Rommel et al., eds., University Park Press, Baltimore, P.3 (1976).

49. A. G. Thornton, G. V. Vahouny, and C. R. Treadwell, Absorption of lipids from mixed micellar bile salt solutions, Proc.Soc. Exp.Biol.Med., 127:629 (1968).

50. A. F. Hofmann and V. J. Yeoh, The relationship between concentration and uptake by rat small intestine in vitro, for two micellar solutes, Biochim.Biophys.Acta, 233:49 (1971).

51. F. A. Wilson, V. L. Sallee, and D. M. Dietschy, Unstirred water layers in intestine: Rate determinant of fatty acid absorption from micellar solutions, Science, 174:1031 (1971).

52. R. M. Mayer, C. R. Treadwell, L. L. Gallo, and G. V. Vahouny, Intestinal mucin and cholesterol absorption in vitro, Biochim.Biophys.Acta, in press (1984).

53. G. V. Vahouny, E. M. Blendermann, L. L. Gallo, and C. R. Treadwell, Differential transport of cholesterol and oleic acid in lymph lipoproteins, J.Lipid Res., 21:415 (1980).

54. I. L. Chaikoff and A. Kaplan, The influence of the ingestion of raw pancreas upon the blood lipids of completely depancreat-ized dogs maintained with insulin, J.Biol.Chem., 112:155 (1935).

55. W. J. Lossow, R. H. Migliorini, N. Brot, and I. L. Chaikoff, Effect of total exclusions of the exocrine pancreas in the

rat upon _in vitro_ esterification of C^{14}-labeled cholesterol by the intestine and upon lymphatic absorption of C^{14}-labeled cholesterol, J.Lipid Res., 5:198 (1964).

56. C. C. Bell and L. Swell, Effect of total pancreatectomy on cholesterol absorption and the serum cholesterol level in man, Proc.Soc.Exp.Biol.Med., 128:575 (1968).

57. H. H. Hernandez, I. L. Chaikoff, and J. Y. Kiyasu, Role of pancreatic juice in cholesterol absorption, Am.J.Physiol., 181:523 (1955).

58. C. R. Borja, G. V. Vahouny, and C. R. Treadwell, Role of pancreatic juice in cholesterol absorption, Am.J.Physiol., 206:233 (1964).

59. J. Hyun, H. Kothari, E. Herm, J. Mortensen, C. R. Treadwell, and G. V. Vahouny, Purification and properties of pancreatic juice cholesterol esterase, J.Biol.Chem., 244:1937 (1969).

60. H. H. Hernandez and I. L. Chaikoff, Purification and properties of pancreatic cholesterol esterase, J.Biol.Chem., 228:447 (1957).

61. K. B. Calame, L. Gallo, E. Cheriathundam, G. V. Vahouny, and C. R. Treadwell, Purification and properties of subunits of sterol ester hydrolase from the rat pancreas, Arch.Biochem. Biophys., 168:57 (1975).

62. G. V. Vahouny, H. Kothari, and C. R. Treadwell, Specificity of bile salt protection of cholesterol esterase against proteolytic inactivation, Arch.Biochem,Biophys., 121:242 (1967).

63. L. L. Gallo, T. Newbill, J. Hyun, G. V. Vahouny, and C. R. Treadwell, Role of pancreatic cholesterol esterase in the uptake and esterification of cholesterol by isolated intestinal cells, Proc.Soc.Exp.Biol.Med., 156:277 (1977).

64. L. L. Gallo, Y. Chiang, G. V. Vahouny, and C. R. Treadwell, Localization and origin of rat intestinal cholesterol esterase determined by immunocytochemistry, J.Lipid Res., 21:537 (1980).

65. W. A. Walker, K. J. Isselbacher, and K. J. Bloch, Intestinal uptake of macromolecules II. Effect of parenteral immunization, J.Immunol., 111:221 (1973).

66. A. L. Warshaw, W. A. Walker, and K. J. Isselbacher, Protein uptake by the intestine: Evidence for absorption of intact macromolecules, Gastroenterology, 66:987 (1974).

67. R. Haugen and K. R. Norum, Coenzyme A-dependent esterification of cholesterol in rat intestinal mucosa, Scand.J.Gastroent., 11:615 (1976).

68. K. R. Norum, P. Helgerud, and A. C. Lilljeqvist, Enzyme esterification of cholesterol in rat intestinal mucosa catalyzed by acyl CoA: Cholesterol acyltransferase, Scand.J.Gastroent., 16:401 (1981).

69. F. J. Field and S. N. Mathur, β-sitosterol: Esterification by intestinal acylcoenzyme A: Cholesterol acyltransferase (ACAT) and its effects on cholesterol absorption, J.Lipid Res., 24:409 (1983).

70. L. L. Gallo, S. B. Clark, S. Myers, and G. V. Vahouny, Choles-
    terol absorption in rat intestine: Role of cholesterol
    esterase and acyl CoA: Cholesterol acyltransferase, <u>Biochim.
    Biophys.Acta,</u> submitted.
71. S. G. Bhat and H. L. Brockman, The role of cholesterol ester
    hydrolysis and synthesis in cholesterol transport across
    intestinal mucosal membrane. A new concept, <u>Biochem.Biophys.
    Res.Comm.,</u> 109:486 (1982).

REGULATION OF CHOLESTEROL ABSORPTION IN HUMANS

Maurizio Ponz de Leon

Semeiotica Medica and Clinica Medica 2
Università di Modena
41100 Modena, Italy

INTRODUCTION

Cholesterol is undoubtedly the most abundant sterol present in the mammalian species; it has been estimated that cholesterol represents 0.2% of body weight, that in an average man of 70 Kg means 145g, 8 of which contained in the blood[1]. Cholesterol is virtually insoluble in water, however, having a hydroxyl group is soluble at the surface and can form monolayers[2].

It can reasonably be calculated that a normal diet, in a western country, contains 0.3-2.0g of cholesterol per day (Table 1) most as free sterol (80-90%)[3,4]. Cholesterol is not an essential dietary component since its endogenous biosynthesis can supply a sufficient amount of cholesterol for a normal cellular function[5]. Apart from the diet, cholesterol may enter the gastrointestinal lumen by endogenous sources, mainly bile but also from degraded enteric cells and intestinal secretions[6,7]. At variance with other nutrients, the clinical interest is elucidating the various aspects of cholesterol absorption is directed more to the inhibition than to the promotion of this process. In fact, absorption from the intestine is one of the ways by which the body enriches of cholesterol, and this excess of cholesterol may contribute to the development of atherosclerosis. Similarly, the reduction of cholesterol absorption might be a useful instrument for the clinician in preventing this disease.

The main purpose of this review is to consider and evaluate all the factors which can influence or regulate cholesterol absorption with particular regard to the human physiology.

Table 1. Cholesterol Content of Common Foods.

	Cholesterol (mg/100g)
1. High cholesterol content	
Brain	2,500
Egg yolk	1,500
Butter	250
2. Medium cholesterol content	
Meats	60-90
Fishes	30-80
Cheeses	10-100
Clams	50
3. Low cholesterol content	
Milk	15
Yoghurt	8
Vegetable margarine	Trace
Olive oil	"
Safflower oil	"
Bread	"
Egg white	"
Vegetables and fruits	"

CLINICAL METHODS IN THE STUDY OF CHOLESTEROL ABSORPTION

As shown in Table 1, most of the cholesterol ingested with a normal diet comes from dairy products, eggs, meats and animal fat. Approximately an equivalent amount of cholesterol (0.5-2.0g) comes from bile and other endogenous sources. It is usually assumed that endogenous and exogenous cholesterol mix completely during digestion so that their absorption should be identical[5,8]. This point, however, has been recently questioned.

At variance with the rat and other animal models, where cholesterol absorption can accurately be estimated by canulating the thoracic duct and by measuring the appearance of luminal cholesterol into the lymph, all the methods used in humans are relatively indirect and, in addition, involve the use of labeled cholesterol. Furthermore, evidence has been provided indicating that there are considerable losses of luminal cholesterol in the gastrointestinal tract, possibly due to the degradation of the sterol nucleus by bacteria[9], especially when liquid formula diets are used[10]. Because of this drawback, Ahrens and colleagues have repeatedly suggested that sitosterol - an unabsorbable plant sterol which undergoes the same metabolic degradation of cholesterol - should always be used in cholesterol absorption studies to correct losses of cholesterol not due to absorption[11].

Recently Sodhi et al. subdivided the various methods for studying cholesterol absorption into two groups[12]. In one of them balance studies and a metabolic steady-state condition are required so that the possibility of error due to the isotopic exchange between cholesterol in the lumen and in the intestinal wall are minimized. These studies, however, take a very long time before a metabolic steady-state is reached, consequently they can hardly be applied to measure changes of cholesterol absorption due to different experimental conditions[13,14,15]. In the second group measurements of cholesterol absorption are made after a single or a few administrations of labeled sterols, so that the possible error due to isotopic exchange cannot be excluded "a priori". However, these methods permit a rapid estimation of cholesterol absorption and are probably the most suitable in evaluating the effect of different dietary regimens, metabolic conditions or drugs on cholesterol absorption[16, 17,18,19,20]. A third group of methods has recently been developed by Grundy and coworkers; these methods are based on the intubation of patients with polymumen tubes - positioned under fluoroscopic control in the duodeno-jejunal region - and on the infusion of mixtures containing different amounts of cholesterol together with bile acids and other solvents. The main drawback of these techniques is the discomfort to the patient; in addition, unless fecal neutral sterols are also studied, they can only give an estimate of segmental absorption [21,22].

Recently Samuel and McNamara showed - with a triple-lumen intubation technique in sic volunteers - that isotopic exchange between luminal and mucosal (newly synthesized) cholesterol did not occur [23]. In addition this careful study indicated the possibility of a differential absorption of endogenous and exogenous cholesterol over a 100-200 cm segment of small bowel.

PROCESSES OF CHOLESTEROL ABSORPTION

Endoluminal Phase

Cholesterol reaches the small bowel both from endogenous and exogenous source. Approximately 85% of dietary cholesterol is in free form and 10-15% is esterified with fatty acids[3,5]. In the stomach dietary fat and cholesterol are emulsified, the process being favored by the products of digestion and by the movements of the stomach. As the stomach empties little lipid droplets appear in the duodenum and mix with endogenous biliary lipids. Borgstrom, in 1960, showed that dietary cholesterol and endogenous cholesterol were completely mixed during digestion, so that absorption took place from a unique pool[8]. At variance with this view, Lutton and Brot-Laroche found that dietary cholesterol was not homogeneously mixed with endogenous cholesterol; thus, in bile fistula rats, the absorption of biliary cholesterol is slightly higher than that of dietary cholesterol. In addition, the absorption of biliary cholesterol is virtually complete in the proximal small bowel whereas dietary cholesterol - at least in the rat - seems to be absorbed also more distally[24]. More recently Dulery and Reisser collected further evidence of the existence of a non homogeneous mixture of cholesterol from different sources in the rat intestinal lumen; in this study, however, exogenous cholesterol was transported across the mucosa more rapidly than biliary cholesterol[25]. The existence of different pools of cholesterol available for absorption in the intestinal lumen, in humans, has yet to be proven; however, as already mentioned, evidence for a differential absorption of endogenous and exogenous cholesterol has recently been provided[23].

The cholesterol esters present in the intestinal lumen during digestion are rapidly hydrolyzed to the free alcohol and fatty acids[5]. Vahouny et al. showed that a pancreatic enzyme - cholesterol esterase or cholesterol esters hydrolase - is responsible for both the hydrolysis of cholesterol esters in the intestinal lumen and the esterification of the absorbed cholesterol in the intestinal mucosa[6,26]. Because of the pH, the nature of the substrate and other undefined factors the reaction is directed towards hydrolysis in the lumen and towards esterification in the mucosa[5]. Although the ideal substrate for hydrolysis seems to be micellar cholesterol [27], an action of the enzyme at the oil-water interface of the lipid droplets cannot be excluded. The pancreatic origin of the rat cholesterol esterase has been repeatedly suggested, since in absence of pancreatic juice both hydrolysis of cholesterol esters and cholesterol absorption are significantly lower[28].

Rat cholesterol esterase activity is closely dependent on the presence of bile acids; though both trihydroxy and dihydroxy bile acids effectively solubilize cholesterol esters, the hydrolytic reaction is significantly higher with cholic acid and its conjugates[5]. Purification of the rat pancreatic juice cholesterol esterase showed crude subunits of 70,000 molecular weight by Sephadex G 200 gel filtration[26]; these subunits-in presence of cholic acid - aggregate to a 400,000 molecular weight form which seems to be the active enzyme.

The mechanisms whereby cholesterol and the lipolytic products are solubilized in the intestinal lumen in form of mixed micelles have been extensively reviewed in the last few years[2,4,7]. Although at the present most of the available evidence indicates that the formation of micelles provides the most plausible mechanism by which fat and cholesterol are solubilized and brought in contact with the absorptive cells, alternative hypotheses have recently been suggested which deserve further investigations[29,30].

From 1916 it was known that animals with ligated bile duct did not absorb cholesterol, however, only in 1952 Siperstein et al.

clearly demonstrated that bile acids were an obligatory requirement for cholesterol absorption[31,32]. Bile acids are powerful detergent molecules whose main functions are to keep cholesterol in soluble form in bile and to promote fat and cholesterol absorption in the intestine. During digestion, bile (i.e. a mixed micellar solution of bile acids, lecithin and cholesterol) and gastric chyme (i.e. an emulsion of all droplets, partially stabilized by proteins, constituted by triglycerides, cholesterol, cholesterol esters, phospholipids and flat soluble vitamins) mix in the proximal small bowel. At the same time the pancreatic enzymes start the cleavage of triglycerides (to mono, diglycerides and fatty acids), of cholesterol esters and of lecithin (to lysolecithin and fatty acids). As the digestion progresses bile is diluted and micelles enlarge since they include the products of lipolysis; thus, intestinal micelles are markedly different, in size and composition, from biliary micelles.

The importance of bile acids and of the lipolytic products for cholesterol absorption in humans has been clearly shown by Simmonds et al.[33]: a micellar solution of bile acids, cholesterol and monoglycerides was infused introuodenally to volunteers; sampling intestinal juice along the small bowel showed that as the lipolytic products were absorbed and their micellar concentration was markedly reduced cholesterol tended to precipitate out of solution and was recovered in large amounts in the sediment fraction after ultracentrifugation. In contrast, the mass of bile acids does not fall appreciably until the distal ileum is reached (where a specific site for active absorption is placed), thus remaining available to bring subsequent molecules of cholesterol in solution for absorption.

Cell Surface Events

Once cholesterol has been solubilized into mixed micelles it is theoretically ready for uptake. However, before moving from the micellar phase of the luminal content to the mucosal cell interior cholesterol must pass through two biological barriers: the first is the unstirred water layer adjacent to all biological membranes, the second is the lipid-protein microvillus membrane. The unstirred layer can be conceived as a series of water lamellae extending outwards from the cell membrane to the bulk luminal phase, and so becoming progressively more stirred. Those lamellae which are closer to the microvillus membrane and that are virtually unstirred may be considered not in equilibrium with the bulk phase so representing a true resistance to uptake[34,35].

Experimental data indicate that the diffusion of micelles through the unstirred water layer is the rate limiting step among the cell surface events of cholesterol absorption. Wilson et al. firstly showed that the reduction of thickness of the unstirred layer, obtained by vigorous stirring, increased the rate of absorption of relatively insoluble molecules like long chain fatty acids[36]. In contrast, the uptake of more soluble compounds, such as medium chain fatty acids and bile acids, was unaffected by stirring.

When the micelles crossing through the unstirred water layer reach the cell membrane, cholesterol and the other lipids are taken up and transferred into the cell interior. The intimate mechanism of this process is still unclear, although several hypotheses have been raised. First, micelles could be taken up intact with all their constituents; though simple, this possibility seems unlikely, since the individual components of micelles are taken up at different rates[6,7]. Secondly, it has been suggested that mixed micelles bring cholesterol to the brush border and that after "collision" with the cell membrane the micelle disaggregates and the individual components are taken up[37]. According to this mechanism the micelles seem to interact with the membrane and because of this interaction cholesterol and other poorly soluble lipids could be taken up. Westergaards and Dietschy, however, showed that the rate of cholesterol uptake from a micellar solution was linearly related to the concentration of cholesterol in the bulk phase when the concentration of bile acids was constant, but the rate of uptake was reduced when the concentration of bile acids was increased relatively to that of cholesterol and of fatty acids[38]. These findings cannot be explained with a simple interaction between micelles and cell membrane and make this second possibility unlikely.

The third and most likely possibility is that cholesterol and the other insoluble lipids are taken up from a monomer aqueous phase in dynamic equilibrium with micellar lipids[38]. In a recent review Thomson and Dietschy compared micelles to a "reservoir" from which cholesterol has to partition into an aqueous monomeric phase before being taken up into the epithelial cell[7].

In summary, the cell surface events include the overcoming of the resistance to diffusion due to the unstirred layer and the maintenance of a maximal monomeric concentration at the aqueous microvillus membrane interface. Because of their physicochemical characteristics mixed bile acid micelles represent the most suitable tool for both these purposes[39].

Intramucosal Events

The small intestine plays an active role in cholesterol synthesis[40]; thus, as luminal cholesterol is taken up by the enterocytes it mixes with the newly synthesized cholesterol and probably with the cholesterol which enters into the mucosal cells from serum lipoproteins. Cholesterol in the mucosal cell - either from the lumen or newly synthesized - can be disposed in three main ways: First, it may be lost in the lumen with esfoliation of enterocytes or with enteric secretions. Second, it may be incorporated into structural component of the cellular membrane or of organelles. Finally, cholesterol, together with proteins and other lipids, can be assembled in form of chylomicrons or VLDL and transferred to the lymph[5,7]. The relative contribution of luminal cholesterol and of newly synthesized cholesterol to these three events is virtually unknown. The cholesterol control of the intestinal mucosa is in the order of 10-20 µg/mg of proteins, of this more than 70% is located in the microsomal and in the soluble fractions[41]. Furthermore, most of the cholesterol in the intestinal mucosa is in the free form while some 50-80% of lymph cholesterol is esterified[5]. These data suggest that esterification occurs immediately before the transfer of cholesterol from the mucosa to the lymph and point out the importance of the formation of esters in the overall process of cholesterol absorption.

Among the various intracellular processes the one aspect that has been best studied concerns the formation of cholesterol esters. Many types of evidence suggest that the formation of esters is important, if not essential, for the transport of the mucosal cholesterol into the lymph and the general circulation. First, although the percentage of cholesterol esters in the mucosa is small (10-20%) the great majority of cholesterol appearing in the lymph is in form of esters[5]. Secondly, studies in rats have shown that sterols such as epicholesterol, which do not form esters, are absorbed much more slowly and at a lower extent than cholesterol[42,43]. Finally, Ito et al. reported that cholestane-3β,5α,6β-triol, a compound capable of inhibiting the formation of cholesterol esters, acts as an inhibitor of cholesterol absorption[44]. At variance with these observations, Gallo-Torres et al. suggested that esterification is not obligatory for cholesterol absorption[45].

Mucosal esterification of cholesterol is due to the activity of at least two enzymes: Cholesterol Esterase and Acyl-CoA Cholesterol Acyltransferase (ACAT).

Some thirty years ago Swell et al. showed that the rat intestinal mucosa possesses an enzymatic activity which catalyzes the formation of cholesterol esters[46,47]. The enzyme was called "Cholesterol Esterase" and its properties were similar to those of the pancreatic cholesterol esterase. Over the past three decades Vahouny and colleagues extensively studied the properties of this enzyme, its subcellular localization, the possible sources and finally they proceeded to the purification of the enzyme[5,26,28,48]. The authors' hypothesize that the pancreas secretes subunits of cholesterol esterase. In the intestinal lumen the subunits, in presence of trihydroxy bile acids, aggregate to the active enzyme which catalyzes the hydrolysis of cholesterol esters from a micellar substrate and at the optimal pH of 6.6. The enzyme is then absorbed and localizes mostly in the supernatant of the mucosal cells; here, at the optimal pH of 6.2, cholesterol esterase operates in reverse inducing the esterification of cholesterol and speeding up its transport in the lymph. Other studies do not support this view, thus, it has been recently shown, in lymph fistula rats, that the transport of cholesterol from the intestinal lumen to the lymph was unaffected by the absence of pancreatic cholesterol esterase and that there was no relationship between mucosal cholesterol esterase activity and cholesterol esters output in lymph, so suggesting that the enzyme was not rate-limiting for cholesterol esterification[49]. Preliminary studies on the human cholesterol esterase activity showed that the enzyme possesses some general characteristics of the rat enzyme, such as time-activity relationship, subcellular distribution and optimal pH. However (at variance with the rat enzyme) the human cholesterol esterase activity does not seem to be enhanced by trihydroxy bile acids[50].

Haugen and Norum firstly showed that the rat intestinal mucosa contains a CoA-dependent enzyme which catalyzes the esterification of cholesterol[51]. This enzyme is strictly CoA dependent and its maximal activity is obtained in presence of an acyl-CoA generating system requiring acyl-carnitine, CoA and hepatic acyl carnitine transferase. The enzyme is mostly located in the microsomal fraction and the optimal pH ranges between 6.4 and 7.2. ACAT activity is higher in the proximal jejunum than in the rest of the digestive tract and oleic acid appears to be the preferred acyl group[52]. The human ACAT has an optimal pH of 7.2-8.2 and its specific activity, in normal young men, was 3.6 ± 1.37 nmol of esters formed/hour/mg of protein, an activity which can account for all the cholesterol esters appearing in the lymph during the digestion of a cholesterol rich diet[53]. Normal activity was found in two pancreasectomized patients, suggesting that the enzyme is not of pancreatic origin[54].

The relative role of either cholesterol esterase or ACAT in cholesterol absorption is unclear. Probably both these enzymatic activities are of importance and might operate in parallel promoting cholesterol esterification and absorption; this contention, however, is still unproved and further studies are needed.

The actual knowledge of the mechanisms whereby cholesterol esters leave the mucosal cells and enter the lymphatic circulation is still incomplete. The fact, however, that the cholesterol esters do not accumulate in the mucosal cells suggests a rapid disposition of the absorbed and esterified cholesterol[6]. Cholesterol does not leave the intestine alone but incorporated into chylomicrons and VLDL; this implies the simultaneous transfer into lymph of proteins, triglycerides, phospholipids and carbohydrates. Proteins, phospho-lipids and free cholesterol are arranged at the surface of the lipo-protein, whereas triglycerides and cholesterol esters form the core of the particle.

Although the rate-limiting step in cholesterol and triglycerides absorption has not been clearly identified, a number of experimental models suggests that the final assembly and the exocytosis of chylomicrons are of fundamental importance in this process. Thus, in the rat, the inhibition of protein synthesis by puromicin results in impairment of chylomicrons secretion and intracellular lipid accumulation[55,56]. Similarly, in abetalipoproteinemia, a hereditary absence of lipoproteins, the secretion of chylomicrons is impaired, with consequent accumulation of lipids in the mucosal cells[57]. Moreover, it has been suggested that microtubules are of importance in the transport of newly synthesized products - including intestinal lipoproteins - out of the cells[58].

GENERAL ASPECTS OF CHOLESTEROL ABSORPTION

Quantitative Aspects in Humans

Dietary cholesterol intake varies considerably depending on the foods which are eaten (Table 1). In the United States the average cholesterol intake ranges between 0.3 and 1.5g/day[1,2]; these figures are presumably similar to those of many European countries and of Australia.

Endogenous cholesterol comes predominantly from bile and, to a much lesser extent, from the intestinal cell esfoliation and bacteria [6]. The output of biliary cholesterol has been studied by mean of marker dilution techniques employing duodenal intubation with polylumen tubes. The values observed in non-obese normal subjects range between 27 and 59 mg/h, i.e. 650-1400 mg/day[59,60]. These data are similar to those estimated by measuring fecal neutral sterols of endogenous origin (in which cholesterol from endogenous sources other than bile was included)[61] indicating that in quantitative terms the contribution of the mucosal cells and of bacteria to the endoluminal cholesterol pool is probably negligible. Thus, the endoluminal cholesterol pool is in the order of 0.5-3.0g/day of this a fraction of 20-60% is absorbed, though, as already mentioned it is not yet clear if endogenous and exogenous cholesterol are absorbed at the same rate and extent[23,24,25].

The unabsorbed cholesterol is excreted with the feces; colonic bacteria, however, convert part of the unabsorbed cholesterol either to coprostanol (in which the double bond between C-5 and C-6 of the sterol ring is saturated) or to coprostanone (in which the β hydroxyl group is oxidized to a ketonic group).

Sites of Cholesterol Absorption

The intestinal site where cholesterol is absorbed has not been precisely determined. Intubation studies in humans showed that cholesterol was absorbed over the length of the small bowel but absorption was maximal in the jejunum[62]. A further confirm of this was obtained in the above mentioned study of Simmonds et al.[33]: as fatty acids and the other lipolytic products were absorbed (leaving the micellar phase) cholesterol tended to precipitate out of the solution, thus becoming less available for absorption. The fact that cholesterol absorption presumably takes place in the proximal small bowel is in keeping with the fact that both cholesterol esterase and ACAT activities are maximal in the proximal intestine[48,54].

Kinetics of Cholesterol Absorption

It is generally assumed that cholesterol absorption has the characteristics of a passive process. Chow and Hollander studied cholesterol absorption by everted sacs of rat small bowel and found that this was linearly related to both time and concentration; in addition, cholesterol uptake was completely independent on changes of temperature[64]. Moreover, the fact that cholesterol absorption is usually fractional and not complete has been interpreted as suggestive of a passive diffusion process. At variance with this view, Sylven suggested that the absorption of either cholesterol or fatty acids might be an energy dependent active process[65]. In their experimental model when the blood supply to an intestinal segment was interrupted the rate of cholesterol absorption decreased markedly and became similar to that of sitosterol. The injection of the respiratory inhibitor KCN induced a decrease of cholesterol uptake similar to that produced by the exclusion of blood flow. The authors interpreted these results as due to damage of the cell membrane induced by exclusion of blood supply or by respiratory inhibition.

Fate of the Absorbed Cholesterol and the Interaction Between Absorption, Synthesis, Degradation and Excretion

The absorbed cholesterol leaves the intestine in form of chylomicrons and VLDL. Once entered the general circulation the catabolism of these lipoproteins initially takes place in the capillary bed; here, owing to the activation of lipoprotein lipase, the major portion of triglycerides is removed[66]. The products of this peripheric lipolysis are called "remnants" and are removed by the liver[67]. Cholesterol from the remnants seems to be the major modulator of cholesterol synthesis in the liver[68].

Thus, through these events the absorbed cholesterol enters the total body cholesterol pools and becomes indistinguishable from the cholesterol synthesized in the body tissues. The interaction between cholesterol absorption and cholesterol synthesis has been extensively studied both in animals and humans, though the results are extremely variable from species to species. In rabbit, for instance, cholesterol feeding causes a sharp increase of cholesterol in the blood and in the body tissues with generalized atherosclerosis[69,70]. This animal apparently has a great capacity to absorb cholesterol which is not fully compensated by the decrease of cholesterol synthesis and by the increased conversion of cholesterol in bile acids. On the other hand, in the rat there is only a minor increase of cholesterol in the body tissues after feeding large amounts of cholesterol[71]. This animal responds to an increased cholesterol absorption by switching off cholesterol synthesis and by enhancing the excretion of bile acids.

The interplay between absorption, synthesis and excretion of cholesterol has also been extensively studied in humans. Bhattathiry and Siperstein, in 1963, showed that feeding large amounts of cholesterol almost entirely suppressed the synthesis of cholesterol by the liver and suggested that humans possess a hepatic feedback mechanism for regulating cholesterol synthesis similar to that of other animals[72]. These findings are in keeping with more recent observations on the role of chylomicron remnants in the regulation of hepatic cholesterogenesis[68]. In human studies, Gamel and Dietschy showed that intestinal cholesterol synthesis was unaffected by the absorbed cholesterol while bile acids appeared to be the major modulators of this process[73]. This has been further supported by other studies where conditions like external biliary drainage, cholestyramine feeding or ileal bypass surgery - all causing a marked decrease of bile acid concentrated in the mucosal cells - were followed by a sharp rise of intestinal cholesterogenesis[73,74,75].

The interaction between absorption, synthesis and excretion has also been investigated by balance studies but with conflicting results. Grundy et al. found that feeding large amounts of cholesterol led to an expansion of cholesterol body pools and that only after 5-6 weeks of continuous feeding the excretion of fecalneutral sterols increased to come into balance with the absorbed cholesterol[76]. The authors' found no apparent decrease of cholesterol synthesis nor any compensatory increase of fecal bile acid output. Similar studies were repeated by the same group in hyperlipidemic patients[77]. Again the most important compensatory mechanism to the increased cholesterol absorption was the excretion of fecal neutral sterols, whereas no increase of bile acid output was detected; cholesterol synthesis was unchanged in one patient, slightly reduced in three and completely suppressed in two. The authors gave particular emphasis to the great variability from patient to patient of the interaction between absorption, synthesis and excretion of neutral sterols and to the differences of the adaptive response to the absorbed cholesterol between humans and other animal species.

Long term balance studies (25 weeks) have recently been performed by Lin and Connor in two patients, one of whom was hypercholesterolemic[78]. The patients were kept for 5 weeks to a diet very poor of cholesterol (37 mg/day) and subsequently changed to a cholesterol rich diet (1109 mg/day) for the following weeks. The results of their study are somewhat at variance with the above mentioned investigations and can be summarized as follows: First, the mass of cholesterol which was absorbed increased markedly in both subjects when passing to the cholesterol rich diet. Second, during the high cholesterol dietary period endogenous cholesterol production was markedly reduced but not totally suppressed. Third, changing to a high cholesterol regimen was followed by an increased bile acid excretion without any parallel increase of endogenous neutral sterol excretion. Finally, the various compensatory mechanisms did not prevent cholesterol overaccumulation in both subjects, though this was much smaller in the normocholesterolemic patient.

From the above mentioned studies it can be said that the cholesterol absorbed from the gut evokes several defensive mechanisms (i.e. partial inhibition of cholesterol synthesis, increased conversion of cholesterol to bile acids, increased excretion of endogenous cholesterol) which enables the body to compensate for the ingested cholesterol. However, these compensatory mechanisms often do not prevent the accumulation of cholesterol in the body pools, especially in hypercholesterolemic patients.

Relation Between Dietary Cholesterol and Serum Cholesterol Levels

The complexity and the variability from subject to subject of the interaction between cholesterol absorption, synthesis, degradation and excretion are undoubtedly the main reason of the controversies still existing upon the effect of dietary cholesterol on serum cholesterol levels. Many controlled studies have clearly shown that when large amounts of cholesterol are given with the diet (usually as egg yolk) a significant elevation of serum cholesterol levels is observed[79,80]. However, many other studies failed to show any significant change of serum cholesterol after adding one or more eggs (or other cholesterol rich food) to a normal diet[81,82]. It is worth noting that the importance of the relationship between dietary and serum cholesterol is due to the so-called "Lipid (or heart-diet) Hypothesis". This hypothesis is mainly based on two proposals: the first is that total serum cholesterol - and in particular low density lipoprotein cholesterol - represents one of the major risk-factors of atherosclerosis; the second is that the serum lipoprotein pattern can be influenced by changes of dietary habits.

FACTORS INFLUENCING AND REGULATING CHOLESTEROL ABSORPTION

Several factors are known to influence and in some way to regulate cholesterol absorption; they will be discussed with particular regard to the human physiology.

Amount of Cholesterol in the Diet.

The effect of the amount of cholesterol in the diet on the extent of cholesterol absorption is still debatable. In some animal species the relationship between dietary cholesterol and the absorption values has been clearly established. In rats, for instance, by increasing the exogenous load of cholesterol the absorbed fraction tended to decrease but, in the range of values of these experiments, the actual mass of cholesterol transported into the lymph was increased[83].

Karvinen et al. studied the capacity of the human intestine to absorb cholesterol with the balance technique[84]. Cholesterol was added - in increasing amounts from 1 to 9g - to a basal mixed diet containing 380 mg of cholesterol per day. The authors found that the absorbed fraction tended to decrease (from 60 to 20%) with increasing loads of cholesterol, whereas the average maximal capacity to absorb cholesterol was in the order of 2g/day. In contrast, the results of other studies (with the isotope steady state technique) showed a maximal absorption of no more than 200-400 mg/day[15]. Borgstrom et al. were able to perform cholesterol absorption studies in humans by canulating the left thoracic duct and measuring the appearance of cholesterol in the lymph after feeding diets containing different amounts of cholesterol[85]. The number of patients was limited (six) and one of them had gastrointestinal troubles, thus the results should be interpreted with caution. When the patients were turned from a high-fat low-cholesterol (0.3g) to a high-fat high-cholesterol (1.6g) test meal, in only two of them there was a consistent increase of the cholesterol transport in the lymph, whereas in the remaining four there was no appreciable change. The authors speculated that when cholesterol is given with a fat-rich meal the increase of biliary lipid secretion leads to a large pool of endogenous cholesterol that in some individuals may actually saturate the absorption capacity of the intestine for cholesterol.

Three studies at least have clearly indicated that the extent of cholesterol absorption in humans, is closely related to the amount of dietary cholesterol[16,86,87]. In these studies either crystalline or egg yolk cholesterol have been given in single doses ranging from 100 to 2,000 mg; in all instances as the amount of the fed cholesterol was increased the absorbed fraction tended to decrease. In spite of this - and in keeping with the above mentioned studies - the actual mass of cholesterol which was absorbed increased linearly with increasing exogenous loads. According to these studies no upper ceiling of the amount absorbed was seen, even for quantities of cholesterol which should be close to the maximum available in a western diet.

There is no proper explanation for the contrasting results observed in the aforementioned human studies. No doubt, however, that the various methodologies used may actually contribute in explaining the observed results. Indeed, it is worth nothing that the last three studies - carried out virtually with the same method - gave very similar results.

Presence of Bile Acids in the Upper Intestine

The obligatory role of bile acids in the overall process of cholesterol absorption has been largely documented both in animals and in humans. In 1952 Siperstein et al. showed that when labeled cholesterol was given to bile fistula rats virtually no radioactivity was recovered in the thoracic duct lymph in the following 24 hours [32]. In keeping with these animal studies Quintao et al. reported that when one patient with primary biliary cirrhosis and complete biliary obstruction was given 1g of cholesterol/day - dissolved in a liquid formula fatty diet - no cholesterol was absorbed[77]. Similarly, dietary cholesterol absorption was significantly lower than normal in patients with advanced liver cirrhosis, who had a marked reduction of total bile acid pool size[88].

It is worth noting that bile acids are not indispensable for the absorption of dietary triglycerides (though they probably speed up this process) indeed, Porter et al. showed that patients with external biliary fistula may absorb more than 70% of dietary fats[89]. Thus, providing that the intestinal mucosa is integral and the activity of the pancreatic lipase normal, bile acids are not essential for fat absorption but their presence is crucially important for cholesterol absorption. As already discussed the reason of this probably lies in the fundamental role played by bile acids in the various steps of cholesterol absorption.

Role of Individual Bile Acids

Up to a few years ago relatively little was known about the role of each individual bile acid on cholesterol absorption, especially in humans. Vahouny et al. studied the effect of feeding different bile acids to lymph fistula rats. The authors measured the appearance of cholesterol in the lymph and found that trihydroxy bile acids feeding produced a significant increase of total lymph cholesterol; in contrast, no increase was seen with cholanic, lithocholic and deoxycholic acid[90]. In similar studies, Gallo-Torres et al., failed to show any clear cut difference between trihydroxy and dihydroxy bile acids regarding their effect on cholesterol absorption[45]. In contrast, Raicht et al. found much higher cholesterol absorption during taurocholic than during taurochenodeoxycholic acid feeding in rats studied with the balance technique. Similar results were subsequently reported by Reynier et al., who found cholic acid (CA) superior to both chenodeoxycholic (CDCA) and ursodeoxycholic (UDCA) acid in promoting cholesterol absorption[91,92].

Adler et al. studied the effect of individual bile acids on cholesterol absorption in humans but with inconclusive results[93]. Two other studies, executed with different techniques, showed that CDCA feeding (i.e. CDCA pool expansion) did not appreciably change cholesterol absorption[94,95]. It should be noted, however, that the amount of cholesterol which was given when the measurements of absorption were done was very small (21 mg)[95] or unfixed[94]. At variance with these results Ponz de Leon et al., using the fecal isotope ratio method, reported a significant decrease (50% on average) of cholesterol absorption after feeding 15 mg/kg/day of CDCA for 3 weeks[96]. In this study the patients were kept under metabolic control and had a constant daily intake of cholesterol (500 mg). In addition, the labeled sterols were given with a fixed dose of cold cholesterol. Similar results were observed by the same group after feeding UDCA or deoxycholic (DCA) acid[97,98]. In all these studies the fed bile acid became the most abundant in bile, suggesting the selective expansion of its pool size. A reduction of cholesterol absorption after DCA feeding, in humans, has also been recently reported by Gallo-Torres et al. using a different technique[99]. Moreover, Von Bergmann and Leiss recently reported a reduction of both the mass and the percentage of cholesterol absorption after UDCA or DCA feeding to normal volunteers[100]; while Leijd and Angelin - using the serum isotope ratio method - found a significant decrease of cholesterol absorption in seven hyperlipidemic patients who were given therapeutically effective doses of CDCA[101].

Many studies failed to show any consistent effect of CA on cholesterol absorption[93,95,101]. However, as already mentioned, the feeding of CA alone leads to an increase of both CA and DCA pools. When CA was given together with broad spectrum antibiotics - in order to suppress colonic bacterial flora and so to prevent DCA formation and to achieve a selective expansion of CA pool - a significant increase of cholesterol absorption was observed[98].

The controversies about the effect of individual bile acids on cholesterol absorption in humans may be related to several factors, including the dose of the given bile acid, the length of the treatment, the method used to measure the absorption values and, most important, the mass of cholesterol given to the patient during each study. However, it seems to us that most of available data indicate that when dihydroxy bile acids are given (and their pool is expanded) cholesterol absorption tends to decline, whereas the selective expansion of trihydroxy bile acid pool leads to an increase of the absorption values. Thus, it is likely that the ratio between dihydroxy and trihydroxy bile acids represents an important regulatory factor of cholesterol absorption. This contention is further supported by two observations: First, many animal studies have shown that the administration of CA and its conjugates lead to an increase of cholesterol absorption, whereas this effect is much less apparent with dihydroxy bile acids[90,91,92]. Second, in a recent study cholesterol absorption and bile acid pool size have been studied in a large group of patients with liver cirrhosis of various degree of severity[88]. A close linear relationship was found between the percentage of cholesterol which was absorbed and the size of CA pool, in the sense that advanced cirrhosis was usually associated with small CA pool size and very low values of cholesterol absorption, whereas in well compensated patients both parameters were in the normal range.

Dietary Fat and Other Nutrients

It is generally accepted that dietary fats increase the rate and the extent of cholesterol absorption; this view is based upon animal studies[102] but the experimental evidence in humans is scanty and indirect[33]. Dietary fats probably facilitate cholesterol absorption by providing monoglycerides, fatty acids and phospholipids necessary for cholesterol solubilization in mixed micelles[6]; in addition, fats stimulate gallbladder contraction and provide fatty acids necessary for the mucosal esterification of cholesterol. The type of triglyceride may also be important; Sylven and Borgstrom[102] studied - in lymph fistula rats - the absorption of cholesterol dissolved in triglycerides containing fatty acids of different chain length. They found that the extent of the lymphatic transport of cholesterol increased proportionally with the chain length of fatty acid component within the range 6 to 18 carbon atoms.

The degree of saturation of fatty acids might also be somewhat related to cholesterol absorption, especially in relation to the well known hypocholesterolemic effect of polyunsaturated fatty acids[103, 104]. Human studies, however, showed that polyunsaturated fat feeding caused an increased excretion of both acidic sterols and endogenous neutral sterols but had no apparent effect on cholesterol absorption[105,106].

Rampone showed that lecithin decreased cholesterol absorption in the rat intestine in vitro[107]; this observation has subsequently been confirmed by other studies both in animals and humans. In contrast lysolecithin - which is normally produced in the intestinal lumen by the action of phospholipase A on lecithin - did not show any consistent effect on cholesterol absorption[108]. Synthetic diether phosphatidylcholine, which is not split by the pancreatic enzymes, significantly inhibited cholesterol absorption in rats without affecting the enterohepatic circulation of bile acids[109]. The mechanisms whereby lecithin and its synthetic diether analogue inhibit cholesterol absorption are unclear. Recent studies gave no support to the possibility that lecithin inhibits cholesterol absorption by interacting with mixed micelles, by increasing their sizes or by showing their diffusion rate through the unstirred water layer [110]. As alternative hypotheses the authors speculated that lecithin might "encapsulate" cholesterol into mixed micelles preventing its absorption or that lecithin interacts with the enterocyte cell membrane in some way to reduce the permeability to cholesterol.

Role of Dietary Fiber and Other Indigestible Compounds

Over the last 20 years many studies have shown that dietary fiber may have a hypocholesterolemic effect[111,112]. However, the largely held public belief that all fibers are hypolipidemic is not supported by the experimental data. Bran, for instance, which is mainly constituted by cellulose and hemicellulose, does not seem to have any effect on serum lipids[113], whereas it has been shown that pectin, guar-gum and alfa-alfa saponins have a definite hypocholesterolemic effect[114,115,116].

Since fiber is not absorbed and acts within the gastrointestinal lumen, its effect on cholesterol absorption has been extensively investigated. Two recent human studies indicated that the administration of 15-45g of pectin per day was associated with a significant increase of fecal acidic sterol excretion but with only a minor increase of fecal neutral sterols[114,117]. It was suggested that pectin, like cholestyramine, impairs bile acid more than cholesterol absorption, though the final result is an increase of cholesterol elimination and a reduction of serum cholesterol levels. Very similar results have recently been reported by feeding 100g/day of oat bran[118]. In contrast, the addition of large amounts of bran (mainly cellulose, hemicellulose and lignin) to a normal diet did not modify appreciably the levels of serum cholesterol, nor the excretion of acidic and neutral sterols, nor the absorption of cholesterol [113]. A similar lack of inhibition of cholesterol absorption was observed in rats fed a high residue semisynthetic diet[119].

In summary, it is unlikely that the relatively small amount of fiber present in a normal western diet may affect cholesterol absorption, it is by contrast well documented that the administration of large amounts of certain unabsorbable plant materials may actually decrease cholesterol absorption and might have a role as hypocholesterolemic agents.

Small Bowel Transit Time and Cholesterol Absorption

Traber and Ostwald recently showed that in certain guinea pigs that are "resistant" to the accumulation of cholesterol in the various body tissues during high cholesterol diet feeding. Intestinal transit time is more rapid than in the other guinea pigs that become hypercholesterolemic and develop atherosclerosis[120]. The authors suggested that in the resistant group the more rapid intestinal transit time allows less absorption of cholesterol, thus limiting the expansion of cholesterol body pools. This observation prompted Ponz de Leon et al. to investigate the relation between cholesterol absorption and small bowel transit time in humans by studying the effect of acute changes of small bowel transit on the values of the absorbed cholesterol[121]. Intravenous metoclopramide and intramuscular atropins were used respectively to accelerate and to slow down small bowel transit in a group of patients without gastrointestinal and hepatic troubles. Metochlopramide significantly accelerated intestinal transit and this was associated with a marked reduction of cholesterol absorption in each patient. In contrast, though atropine significantly slowed transit time this effect was not associated with any consistent change of cholesterol absorption. The authors suggested that the rate of transit through the small bowel could be one of the physiological factors regulating the extent of cholesterol absorption in humans. The fact that prolongation of transit time was not followed by any change of absorption may suggest that the rate limiting step of this process in not influenced by a longer permanence of cholesterol in the intestinal lumen.

These findings might have practical implications; thus, dietary fiber is known to decrease intestinal transit[122] and, as already discussed, some dietary fiber seems to have a hypocholesterolemic effect. Moreover, Wald et al. recently reported that gastrointestinal transit time was prolonged in the luteal phase of menstrual cycle when compared to the follicular phase[123]; finally, many gastrointestinal hormones have a definite effect on small bowel motility [124].

Hormones and Cholesterol Absorption

The role of hormones in the regulation of cholesterol absorption has been poorly explored; there is no doubt, however, that thyroid hormones are those which received more attention. Rosenmann and Friedman did not find any significant difference of cholesterol absorption between pharmacologically induced hyper or hypothyroid rats[125]. In contrast, two more recent studies in the same animal indicated that L-thyroxin feeding caused a marked decrease of both biliary and exogenous cholesterol absorption[126]. Moreover thyroidectomy enhanced the absorption and transport of cholesterol.

Abrams and Grundy found that hypothyroid patients had a virtually normal cholesterol absorption, but that the absorbed fraction was lowered after treatment with thyroxin[127]. The authors speculated that the accelerated transit time induced by hyperthyroidism could be responsible for the reduced cholesterol absorption. To similar conclusions came Carulli et al. who studied cholesterol absorption and small bowel transit both in hyper and in hypothyroid patients[128]. The authors found that thyroid hyperfunction was associated with a very rapid intestinal transit and with a cholesterol absorption significantly lower than normal; in contrast, hypothyroid patients had a very slow transit time and in 3 out of 5 cholesterol absorption was at the upper limits of normal. Furthermore, in 4 hyperthyroid patients with a low cholesterol absorption the absorbed fraction rose sharply after antithyroid therapy[129]. The authors suggested that besides transit time bile acid pool composition might also have influenced cholesterol absorption; in fact, hypothyroid patients tended to have larger total bile acid pools, mainly constituted by CA, whereas in hyperthyroid patients pool size was smaller and bile enriched with dihydroxy bile acids.

Drugs and Cholesterol Absorption

Although there are tens of hypocholesterolemic agents, the effect of these drugs on cholesterol absorption has been critically evaluated only for a few of them. Sedaghat et al. with the balance technique reported that cholesterol absorption was markedly reduced in 3 out of 4 patients treated with 2g/day of neomycin[130]. In keeping with these findings, Thompson et al. found that neomycin interferes with the endoluminal events of fat absorption, causing an increased precipitation of bile acids and fatty acids out of mixed micelles[131]. In contrast, Hardison and Rosemberg did not report any reduced concentration of micellar bile acids (or fatty acids) during neomycin feeding[132]. Two studies at least have shown that nicotinic acid feeding does not induce any change of cholesterol absorption[133,134]. Clofibrate seems to have a slight, though significant, effect on cholesterol absorption; this has been observed both with the balance technique[135] and with the serum isotope ratio method[136].

Plant sterols – especially β-sitosterol, given at the dose of 10-15g/day – are known to reduce serum cholesterol levels by inhibiting cholesterol absorption[137,138]. This effect could be due either to competitive inhibition for mucosal uptake or to crystallization and coprecipitation of the sterols or to other unknown mechanisms. Mattson et al. recently showed that when β-sitosterol was dissolved in the test meal together with cholesterol – so that both the sterols were presented simultaneously to the intestinal mucosa a much smaller amount of the plant sterol (1g) was sufficient to induce a significant (42% on average) decrease of cholesterol absorption[139]. If confirmed, these findings might render much easier the use of phytosterols in the treatment of hypercholesterolemia.

CONCLUSIONS

It has been our attempt to present the most important and recent aspects of cholesterol absorption with special regards to the human physiology. In spite of the numerous studies, there are still many unsettled problems – such as the development of an ideal method for studying cholesterol absorption, the possible different metabolic fats of exogenous and endogenous cholesterol or the clarification of the rat-limiting step in the overall process of absorption – which represent a stimulus and a challenge for further studies. Finally, much has to be done on the regulation of cholesterol absorption and on the pharmacological ways by which we can interfere with this process.

Acknowledgements

The author wishes to thank Prof. Nicola Carulli (Clinica Medica 1°, University of Modena) and Prof. Sebastiano Calandra (Patologia Generale, University of Modena) for helpful discussions and for their constructive criticism. Thanks are also due to Dr. Francesca Carubbi and Dr. Paola Di Donato for their help in searching the many References, and to Mrs. Chris Kieran for her help in preparing and correcting the manuscript.

This work is dedicated to Mario Coppo, Professor of Internal Medicine at the University of Modena from 1947 to 1978, and now Professor Emeritus. It was my privilege to work with Professor Coppo.

REFERENCES

1. J. R. Sabina, "Cholesterol," M. Dekker, ed., Inc., New York and Basel, pp.489 (1977).
2. M. C. Carey and D. M. Small, Micelle, formation by bile salts; physical, chemical and thermodynamic considerations, Arch. Int.Med., 130:506-527 (1972).
3. N. McIntyre, Cholesterol absorption, in: "Lipid Absorption: Biochemical and Clinical Aspects," K. Rommel and H. Goebell, eds., pp. 73-84 (1976).
4. P. R. Holt, The role of bile acids during the process of normal fat and cholesterol absorption, Arch.Int.Med., 130:574-582 (1972).
5. C. R. Treadwell and G. V. Vahouny, Cholesterol absorption, in: "Handbook of Physiology," C.F. Code and W. Heidel, eds., American Physiology Society, Washington DC, Vol V, pp. 2391-2407 (1976).
6. J. D. Wilson, The role of bile acids in the overall regulation of steroid metabolism, Arch.Int.Med., 130:493-505 (1972).
7. A. B. R. Thomson and J. M. Dietschy, Intestinal lipid absorption: Major extracellular and intracellular events, in: "Physiology of the Gastrointestinal Tract," L.R. Johnson, ed., Raven Press, New York, pp. 1147-1220 (1981).
8. B. Borgstrom, Studies on the intestinal cholesterol absorption in the human, J.Clin.Invest., 39:809-815 (1960).
9. B. A. Kottle and M. T. R. Subbiah, Sterol balance studies in patients on solid diets: Comparison of two non absorbable markers, J.Lab.Clin.Med., 86:530-538 (1972).
10. L. DenBesten, W. E. Connor, T. H. Kent, and D. Lin, Effect of cellulose in the diet on the recovery of dietary plant sterols from the feces, J.Lipid Res., 11:341-345 (1970).
11. S. M. Grundy and E. H. Ahrens, jr., Dietary sitosterol as an internal standard to correct for cholesterol losses in sterol balance studies, J.Lipid Res., 9:374-387 (1968).

12. H. S. Sodhi, B. J. Kudchodkar, and D. T. Mason, "Clinical Methods in the Study of Cholesterol Metabolism," D. Kritchevsky and D.J. Pollak, eds., S. Karger AG, pp. 43-56 (1979).

13. E. Quintao, S. M. Grundy, and E. H. Ahrens, jr., An evaluation of four methods for measuring cholesterol absorption by the intestine in man, J.Lipid Res., 12:221-232 (1971).

14. T. A. Miettinen, E. H. Ahrens, jr, and S. M. Grundy, Quantitative isolation and GLC analysis of total dietary and fecal neutral steroids, J.Lipid Res., 6:411-424 (1965).

15. J. D. Wilson and C. A. Lindset, jr., Studies on the influence of dietary cholesterol on cholesterol metabolism in the isotopic steady state in man, J.Clin.Invest., 44:1805-1814 (1965).

16. B. Borgstrom, Quantification of cholesterol absorption in man by fecal analysis after the feeding of a single isotope-labeled meal, J.Lipid Res., 10:331-337 (1969).

17. H. S. Sodhi, L. Horlick, D. J. Nazir, and B. J. Kudchodkar, A simple method for calculating absorption of dietary cholesterol in man (35560), Proc.Soc.Exp.Biol.Med., 137:277-279 (1971).

18. J. R. Crouse and S. M. Grundy, Evaluation of a continuous isotope feeding method for measurement of cholesterol absorption in man, J.Lipid Res., 19:967-971 (1978).

19. D. B. Zilversmit, A model for cholesterol absorption: Isotope versus mass, single dose vs constant infusion, J.Lipid Res., 24:297-302 (1983).

20. P. Samuel, D. J. McNamara, E. H. Ahrens, jr., J. R. Crouse, and T. Parker, Further validation of the plasma isotope ratio method for measurement of cholesterol absorption in man, J.Lipid Res., 23:480-489 (1982).

21. S. M. Grundy and H. Y. I. Mok, Deterination of cholesterol absorption in man by intestinal perfusion, J.Lipid Res., 18:263-271 (1977).

22. H. Y. I. Mok and S. M. Grundy, Cholesterol and bile acid absorption during bile acid therapy in obese subjects undergoing weight reduction, Gastroenterology, 78:62-67 (1980).

23. P. Samuel and D. J. McNamara, Differential absorption of exogenous and endogenous cholesterol in man, J.Lipid Res., 24:265-276 (1983).

24. C. Lutton and E. Brut-Laroche, Biliary cholesterol absorption in normal and L-thyroxin-fed rats, Lipids, 14:441-446 (1978).

25. C. Dulery and D. Reisser, Intestinal absorption of biliary and exogenous cholesterol in the rat, Biochim.Biophys.Acta, 710:164-171 (1982).

26. K. B. Calame, L. Gallo, E. Cheriathundam, G. V. Vahouny, and C. R. Treadwell, Purification and properties of subunits of sterol esters hydrolase from rat pancreas, Arch.Biochem.Biophys., 168:57-65 (1975).

27. G. V. Vahouny, S. Weersing, and C. R. Treadwell, Micellar-solubilized substrates and cholesterol esterase activity in vitro, Arch.Biochem.Biophys., 107:7-15 (1964).

28. C. R. Boria, G. V. Vahouny, and C. R. Treadwell, Role of bile and pancreatic juice in cholesterol absorption and esterification, Am.J.Physiol., 206:223-228 (1964).

29. M. C. Carey, The enterohepatic circulation, in: "The Liver: Biology and Pathobiology," J. Arias, H. Popper, D. Schachter, and D.A. Shafritz, eds, Raven Press, New York, pp.429-465 (1982).

30. J. S. Patton, and M. C. Carey, Watching fat digestion: The formation of visible product phases by pancreatic lipase is described, Science, 204:145-148 (1979).

31. J. H. Mueller, The mechanism of cholesterol absorption, J.Biol. Chem., 27:463-480 (1916).

32. M. D. Siperstein, I. L. Chaikoff, and W. O. Reinhardt, ^{14}C-cholesterol: V. Obligatory role of bile in intestinal absorption of cholesterol, J.Biol.Chem., 198:111-114 (1952).

33. W. J. Simmonds, A. F. Hofmann, and E. Theodor, Absorption of cholesterol from a micellar solution: Intestinal perfusion studies in man, J.Clin.Invest., 45:874-890 (1967).

34. J. M. Dietschy, V. L. Sallee, and F. A. Wilson, Unstirred water layers and absorption across the intestinal mucosa, Gastroenterology, 61:932-934 (1971).

35. B. E. Lukie, H. Westergaard, and J. M. Dietschy, Validation of a chamber that allows measurement of both tissue uptake rates and unstirred layer thickness in the intestine under conditions of controlled stirring, Gastroenterology, 67:652-661 (1974).

36. F. A. Wilson, V. L. Sallee, and J. M. Dietschy, Unstirred water layers in intestine: Rate determinant of fatty acid absorption from micellar solutions, Science, 174:1031-1033 (1971).

37. S. G. Schultz and C. K. Strecker, Cholesterol and bile salts influxes across brush border of rabbit jejunum, Am.J. Physiol., 220:59-65 (1971).

38. H. Westergaard and J. M. Dietschy, The mechanism whereby bile acid micelles increase the rate of fatty acid and cholesterol uptake into the intestinal mucosal cell, J.Clin.Invest., 58:97-108 (1976).

39. A. B. R. Thomson, Unidirectional flux rate of cholesterol and fatty acids into the intestine of rats with drug-induced diabetes mellitus: Effect of variations of the effective resistance of the unstirred water layer and the bile acid micelle, J.Lipid Res., 21:687-698 (1980).

40. A. Gangl and R. K. Ockner, Intestinal metabolism of lipids and lipoproteins, Gastroenterology, 68:167-186 (1975).

41. J. L. Merchant and R. A. Heller, 3-hydroxy-3-methyl-glutaryl coenzyme A reductase in villus and crypt cells of the rat ileum, J.Lipid Res., 18:722-733 (1977).

42. H. H. Hernandez, I. L. Chaikoff, W. G. Dauben, and S. Abraham, The absorption of 14-C-labeled epicholesterol in the rat, J.Biol.Chem., 206:757-765 (1954).

43. L. Swell, E. Stutzman, M. D. Law, and C. R. Treadwell, Intestinal metabolism of epicholesterol-4-C-14, Arch.Biochem. Biophys., 97:411-416 (1962).

44. M. Ito, W. E. Connor, E. J. Blanchette, C. R. Treadwell, and G. V. Vahouny, Inhibition of lymphatic absorption of cholesterol by cholestane-3β-5α,6β-triol, J.Lipid Res., 10:694-702 (1969).

45. H. E. Gallo-Torres, O. N. Miller, and J. G. Hamilton, A comparison of the effect of bile salts on the absorption of cholesterol from the intestine of the rat, Biochem.Biophys.Acta., 176;605-615 (1969).

46. L. Swell, J. E. Byron, and C. R. Treadwell, Cholesterol esterase. IV. Cholesterol esterase of the rat intestinal mucosa, J.Biol.Chem., 186:543-548 (1950).

47. L. Swell and C. R. Treadwell, Cholesterol esterase. VI. Relative specificity and activity of pancreatic cholesterol esterase, J.Biol.Chem., 212:141-150 (1955).

48. L. L. Gallo, Y. Chiang, G. V. Vahouny, and C. R. Treadwell, Localization and origin of the rat intestinal cholesterol esterase determined by immunocytochemistry, J.Lipid Res., 21:537-545 (1980).

49. S. M. Watt and W. J. Simmonds, The effect of pancreatic diversion on lymphatic absorption and esterification of cholesterol in the rat, J.Lipid Res., 22:157-165 (1981).

50. F. Carubbi, M. Ponz de Leon, P. Di Donato, and N. Carulli, Cholesterol esterase activity of human intestinal mucosa: Properties of the enzyme and effect of different bile acids, Gut, 23:A887 (abstract) (1982).

51. R. Haugen and K. R. Norum, Coenzyme A dependent esterification of cholesterol in rat intestinal mucosa, Scand.J.Gastroenterol., 11:615-621 (1976).

52. K. R. Norum, P. Helgerund, and A. C. Lillijeqvist, Enzymic esterification of cholesterol in rat intestinal mucosa catalyzed by ACAT, Scand.J.Gastroenterol., 16:401-410 (1981).

53. P. Helgerund, K. Saarem, and K. R. Norum, ACAT in human intestine: Its activity and some properties of the enzymic reaction, J.Lipid Res., 22:271-277 (1981).

54. K. R. Norum, A. C. Lillijeqvist, P. Helgerund, E. R. Normann, Mo A., and B. Selbekk, Esterification of cholesterol in human small intestine: The importance of ACAT, Eur.J.Clin.Invest., 9:55-62 (1979).

55. H. I. Friedman and R. R. Cardell, jr., Effect of puromycin on the structure of rat intestinal epithelial cells during fat absorption, J.Cell Biol., 52:15-40 (1972).

56. R. M. Glickman and K. Kirsch, Lymph chylomicron formation during the inhibition of protein synthesis, J.Clin.Invest., 52:2910-2920 (1973).

57. R. E. Levy, D. S. Frederickson, and L. Lebster, The lipoprotein and lipid transport in abetalipoproteinemia, J.Clin.Invest., 45:531-541 (1966).

58. R. M. Glickman, J. L. Perrotto, and K. Kirsch, Intestinal lipo-protein formation: Effect of colchicine, Gastroenterology, 70:347-352 (1976).

59. R. D. Adler, A. L. Metzger, and S. M. Grundy, Biliary lipid secretion before and after cholecystectomy in American indians with cholesterol gallstones, Gastroenterology, 66: 1212-1217 (1974).

60. E. A. Shaffer and D. M. Small, Biliary lipid secretion in cholesterol gallstone disease: The effect of cholecystectomy and obesity, J.Clin.Invest., 59:823-840 (1977).

61. L. J. Bennion and S. M. Grundy, Effects of obesity and caloric intake on biliary lipid metabolism in man, J.Clin.Invest., 56:996-1011 (1975).

62. B. Arnesjo, A. Nilsson, J. Barrowman, and B. Borgstrom, Intes-tinal digestion and absorption of cholesterol and lecithin in humans, Scand.J.Gastroenterol., 4:653-665 (1969).

63. E. R. Schiff, N. C. Small, and J. M. Dietschy, Characterization of the passive and active transport mechanism for bile acid absorption in the small intestine and colon of the rat, J.Clin.Invest., 51:1351-1362 (1972).

64. S. L. Chow and D. Hollander, Initial cholesterol uptake by everted sacs of rat small intestine: Kinetics and thermo-dynamic aspects, Lipids, 13:239-245 (1978).

65. C. Sylven, Influence of blood supply on lipid uptake from micellar solutions by the rat small intestine, Biochim. Biophys.Acta, 203:365-375 (1970).

66. E. N. Bergman, R. J. Havel, B. M. Wolfe, and T. Bohmer, Quanti-tative studies of the metabolism of chylomicron triglycerides and cholesterol by liver and extrahepatic tissues of sheep and dogs, J.Clin.Invest., 50:1831-1839 (1971).

67. T. G. Redgrave, Formation of cholesteryl ester-rich particulate lipid during metabolism of chylomicrons, J.Clin.Invest., 49:465-471 (1970).

68. A. D. Cooper, The regulation of 3-hydroxy-3-methylglutaryl coenzyme A reductase in the isolated perfused rat liver, J.Clin.Invest., 57:1461-1470 (1976).

69. K. J. Ho., G. B. Taylor, Comparative studies on tissue choles-terol, Arch.Pathol., 85:585-594 (1968).

70. J. M. Andersen, S. D. Turley, and J. M. Dietschy, Relative rates of sterol synthesis in the liver and various extrahepatic tissues of normal and cholesterol-fed rabbits, Biochim. Biophys.Acta, 711:421-430 (1982).

71. W. T. Beher, K. K. Casazza, M. E. Beher, A. M. Filus, and J. Bertasius, Effect of cholesterol on bile acid metabolism in the rat, Proc.Soc.Exp.Biol.Med., 134:595-602 (1970).

72. E. P. M. Bhattathiry and M. D. Siperstein, Feedback control of cholesterol synthesis in man, J.Clin.Invest., 42:1613-1618 (1963).

73. J. M. Dietschy and W. G. Gamel, Cholesterol synthesis in the intestine of man: Regional differences and control mechan-isms, J.Clin.Invest., 50:872-880 (1971).

74. C. J. Packars and J. Shepherd, The hepatobiliary axis and lipo-protein metabolism: Effects of bile acid sequestrants and ileal bypass surgery, J.Lipid Res., 23:1081-1098 (1982).
75. E. F. Stange, K. E. Suckling, and J. M. Dietschy, Synthesis of coenzyme A dependent esterification of cholesterol in rat intestinal epithelium, J.Biol.Chem., 258:12868-12875 (1983).
76. S. M. Grundy, E. H. Ahrens, jr., and J. Davignon, The inter-action of cholesterol absorption and cholesterol synthesis in man, J.Lipid Res., 10:304-315 (1969).
77. E. Quintao, S. M. Grundy, and E. H. Ahrens, jr., Effects of dietary cholesterol on the regulation of total body choles-terol in man, J.Lipid Res., 12:233-247 (1971).
78. D. S. Lin and W. E. Connor, The long term effect of dietary cholesterol upon the plasma lipids, lipoproteins, cholesterol absorption, and the sterol balance in man, J.Lipid Res., 21:1042-1052 (1980).
79. W. E. Connor, R. E. Hodges, and R. E. Bleier, Effect of dietary cholesterol upon serum lipids in man, J.Lab.Clin.Med., 57: 331-342 (1961).
80. A. Keys, J. T. Anderson, and F. Grande, Serum cholesterol response to changes in the diet, II. The effect of choles-terol in the diet, Metabolism, 14:759-765 (1965).
81. G. Slater, J. Head, G. Dhopeshwarkar, S. Robinson, and R. B. Alfin-Slater, Plasma cholesterol and triglyceride in men with added eggs in the diet, Nutr.Rept.Int., 14:249-260 (1976).
82. M. W. Porter, W. Yamanaka, S. Carlson, and N. Flynn, Effect of dietary egg on serum cholesterol and triglyceride of human males, Am.J.Clin.Nutr., 32:490-495 (1977).
83. G. V. Vahouny, W. E. Connor, T. Roy, D. S. Lin, and L. L. Gallo, Lymphatic absorption of shellfish sterols and their effect on cholesterol absorption, Am.J.Clin.Nutr., 34:507-513 (1981).
84. E. Karvinen and T. M. Lin, Capacity of human intestine to absorb exogenous cholesterol, J.Appl.Physiol., 11:143-147 (1957).
85. B. Borgstrom, S. Radner, and B. Werner, Lymphatic transport of cholesterol in the human being: Effect of dietary choles-terol, Scand.J.Clin.Lab.Invest., 26:227-235 (1970).
86. B. J. Kudchodkar, H. S. Sodhi, and L. Horlick, Absorption of dietary cholesterol in man, Metabolism, 22:155-163 (1973).
87. W. E. Connor and D. S. Lin, The intestinal absorption of dietary cholesterol by hypercholesterolemic (type II) and normo-cholesterolemic humans, J.Clin.Invest., 53:1062-1070 (1974).
88. M. Ponz de Leon, P. Loria, R. Iori, and N. Carulli, Cholesterol absorption in cirrhosis: The role of total and individual bile acid size, Gastroenterology, 80:1428-1437 (1981).
89. H. P. Porter, D. R. Saunders, G. Tytgat, O. Brunser, and C. E. Rubin, Fat absorption in bile fistula man, A. Morphological and biolchemical study, Gastroenterology, 60:1008-1019 (1971).
90. G. V. Vahouny, H. M. Gregorian, and C. R. Treadwell, Comparative effects of bile acids on intestinal absorption of choles-terol, Proc.Soc.Exp.Biol.Med., 101:538-540 (1959).

91. R. F. Raicht, B. I. Cohen, and E. H. Mosbach, Effect of sodium taurochenodeoxycholate and sodium taurocholate on cholesterol absorption in the rat, Gastroenterology, 67:1155-1161 (1974).

92. M. O. Reynier, J. C. Montet, A. Gerolami, C. Marteau, C. Crotte, A. M. Montet, and S. Mathieu, Comparative effect of cholic, chenodeoxycholic, and ursodeoxycholic acids on micellar solubilization and intestinal absorption of cholesterol, J.Lipid Res., 22:467-473 (1981).

93. R. D. Adler, L. J. Bennion, W. C. Duane, and S. M. Grundy, Effects of low dose chenodeoxycholic acid feeding on biliary lipid metabolism, Gastroenterology, 68:326-334 (1975).

94. T. N. Tangedahl, J. L. Thistle, A. F. Hofmann, and J. W. Matseshe, Effect of β-sitosterol alone or in combination with chenic acid on cholesterol saturation of bile and cholesterol absorption in gallstone patients, Gastroenterology, 76:1341-1346 (1979).

95. K. Einarsson and S. M. Grundy, Effect of feeding cholic acid and chenodeoxycholic acid on cholesterol absorption and hepatic secretion of biliary lipids in man, J.Lipid Res., 21:23-34 (1980).

96. M. Ponz de Leon, N. Carulli, P. Loria, R. Iori, and F. Zironi, The effect of chenodeoxycholic acid (CDCA) on cholesterol absorption, Gastroenterology, 77:223-230 (1979).

97. M. Ponz de Leon, N. Carulli, P. Loria, R. Iori, and F. Zironi, Cholesterol absorption during bile acid feeding: Effect of ursodeoxycholic acid (UDCA) administration, Gastroenterology, 78:214-219 (1980).

98. M. Ponz de Leon, N. Carulli, R. Iori, P. Loria, and M. Romani, Regulation of cholesterol absorption by bile acids: Role of deoxycholic and cholic acid pool expansion on dietary cholesterol absorption, Ital.J.Gastroenterol., 15:86-93 (1983).

99. H. E. Gallo-Torres, O. N. Miller, and J. C. Hamilton, Some effects of deoxycholate administration on the metabolism of cholesterol in man, Am.J.Clin.Nutr., 32:1363-1375 (1979).

100. K. Von Bergmann and D. Leiss, Effect of various bile acids on cholesterol absorption in humans, in: "Bile Acids and Cholesterol in Health and Disease," G. Paumgartner, A. Stiehl and W. Gerok, eds., MTP Press Ltd., pp.203-212 (1983).

101. B. Leijd and B. Angelin, Effect of chenodeoxycholic and cholic acid feeding on plasma lipoprotein and cholesterol absorption in hyperlipoproteinemia: A cross-over study, in: "Bile Acids and Cholesterol in Health and Disease," G. Paumgartner, A. Stiehl and W. Gerok, eds., MTP Press Ltd., pp.191-202 (1983).

102. C. Sylven and B. Borgstrom, Intestinal absorption and lymphatic transport of cholesterol in the rat: Influence of the fatty acid chain length of the carrier triglyceride, J.Lipid Res., 10:351-355 (1969).

103. A. Kuksis, J. J. Myher, K. Geher, G. J. L. Jones, J. Shepherd, C. J. Packard, J. D. Morrisett, O. D. Taunton, and A. M. Gotto, Effect of saturated and unsaturated fat diets on lipid

profiles of plasma lipoproteins, Atherosclerosis, 41:221–240 (1982).

104. D. K. Bloomfield, Cholesterol metabolism. III. Enhancement of cholesterol absorption and accumulation in safflower oil-fed rats, J.Lab.Clin.Med., 64:613–623 (1964).

105. S. M. Grundy, Effect of polyunsaturated fats on lipid metabolism in patients with hypertriglyceridemia, J.Clin.Invest., 55:269–282 (1975).

106. P. J. Nestel, N. Havenstein, Y. Homma, T. W. Scott, and L. J. Cook, Increased sterol excretion with polyunsaturated-fat high-cholesterol diets, Metabolism, 24:189–198 (1975).

107. J. A. Rampone, The effect of lecithin on intestinal cholesterol uptake by rat intestine in vitro, J.Physiol., 229:505–514 (1973).

108. J. A. Rampone and L. R. Long, The effect of phosphatidylcholine and lysophosphatidylcholine on the absorption and mucosal metabolism of oleic acid and cholesterol in vitro, Biochim. Biophys.Acta., 486:500–510 (1977).

109. P. J. O'Connor and J. B. Rodgers, The effect of diether phosphotidylcholine on the enterohepatic circulation of biliary sterols, Biochim.Biophys.Acta., 450:402–409 (1976).

110. J. A. Rampone and C. M. Machida, Mode of action of lecithin in suppressing cholesterol absorption, J.Lipid Res., 22:744–752 (1981).

111. D. Kritchevschy, Food product and hyperlipidemia, Arch.Surg., 113:52–54 (1978).

112. D. Kritchevschy, Metabolic effect of dietary fiber, West.J.Med., 130:123–127 (1979).

113. T. C. Raymond, W. E. Connor, D. S. Lin, S. Warner, M. M. Fry, and S. L. Connor, The interaction of dietary fiber and cholesterol upon the plasma lipids and lipoproteins, sterol balance, and bowel function in humans, J.Clin.Invest., 60:1429–1437 (1977).

114. A. Miettinen and S. Tarpila, Effect of pectin on serum cholesterol fecal bile acids and biliary lipids in normolipidemic and hyperlipidemic individuals, Clin.Chim.Acta, 79:471–477 (1977).

115. D. J. A. Jenkins, A. R. Leeds, C. Newton, and J. H. Cummings, Effect of pectin, guar gum and wheat fiber on serum cholesterol, Lancet, I:1116–1117 (1975).

116. M. R. Malinow, P. McLaughlin, L. Papworth, C. Stafford, B. S. G. Kohler, A. L. Livington, and P. R. Cheeke, Effect of alfaalfa saponins on intestinal cholesterol absorption in rats, Am.J. Clin.Nutr., 30:2061–2067 (1977).

117. M. Kay and A. S. Truswell, Effects of citrus pectin on blood lipids and fecal steroid excretion in man, Am.J.Clin.Nutr., 30:171–175 (1977).

118. R. W. Kirby, J. W. Anderson, B. Sieling, E. D. Rees, W. J. Lin Chen, R. E. Miller, and R. M. Kay, Oat-bran intake selectively lowers serum low-density lipoprotein cholesterol con-

centration of hypercholesterolemic men, <u>Am.J.Clin.Nutr.</u>, 34:824-829 (1981).

119. J. Balmer and D. B. Zilversmit, Effect of dietary roughage on cholesterol absorption, Cholesterol turnover and steroid excretion in the rat, <u>J.Nutr.</u>, 104:1319-1328 (1974).

120. M. G. Traber and R. Ostwald, Cholesterol absorption and steroid excretion in cholesterol-fed guinea pigs, <u>J.Lipid Res.</u>, 19:448-456 (1978).

121. M. Ponz de Leon, R. Iori, G. Barbolini, G. Pompei, P. Zaniol, and N. Carulli, Influence of small-bowel transit time on dietary cholesterol absorption in human beings, <u>New Eng. J.Med.</u>, 307:102-103 (1982).

122. D. K. Payler, E. W. Pomare, K. W. Heaton, and R. F. Harvey, The effect of wheat bran on intestinal transit, <u>Gut</u>, 16:209-213 (1975).

123. A. Wald, D. H. Van Thiel, L. Hoechstetter, J. S. Gavaler, K. M. Egler, R. Verm, L. Scott, and R. Lester, Gastrointestinal transit: The effect of menstrual cycle, <u>Gastroenterology</u>, 80:1497-1500 (1981).

124. J. E. McGuigan, Gastrointestinal hormones, <u>Ann.Rev.Med.</u>, 29:307-318 (1978).

125. R. H. Rosenman and M. Friedman, Effect of hyper and hypothyroidism on intestinal absorption of cholesterol in rats, <u>Am.J. Physiol.</u>, 187:381-392 (1956).

126. D. Mathè and F. Chevallier, Effects of the thyroid state on cholesterol metabolism in the rat, <u>Biochim.Biophys.Acta</u>, 441:155-164 (1976).

127. J. J. Abrams and S. M. Grundy, Cholesterol metabolism in hypothyroidism and hyperthyroidism in man, <u>J.Lipid Res.</u>, 22:323-328 (1981).

128. N. Carulli, P. Loria, M. Ponz de Leon, R. Iori, F. Pignatti, and B. Bonati, Thyroid function and sterol metabolism in man, <u>in</u>: "The Endocrines and the Liver," M. Langher, L. Chiandussi, I.J. Chopra, and L. Martini, eds., Academic Press, London and New York, pp.195-204 (1982).

129. P. Loria, M. Bertolotti, R. Iori, M. Ponz de Leon, and N. Carulli, Effect of thyroid function on hepatic sterol metabolism in man, Proceedings of the 7° International meeting on "Bile acids and cholesterol in health and disease", Basel (1982).

130. A. Sedaghat, P. Samuel, J. R. Crouse, E. H. Ahrens, jr., Effects of neomycin on absorption, synthesis and/or flux of cholesterol in man, <u>J.Clin.Invest.</u>, 55:12-21 (1975).

131. G. R. Thompson, J. Barrowman, L. Gutierrez, and R. H. Dowling, Action of neomycin on the intraluminal phase of lipid absorption, <u>J.Clin.Invest.</u>, 50:319-323 (1971).

132. W. G. M. Hardison and I. H. Rosemberg, The effect of neomycin on bile salt metabolism and fat digestion in man, <u>J.Lab.Clin. Med.</u>, 74:564-573 (1969).

133. B. J. Kudchodkar, S. Harbhajan, S. Sodhi, L. Horlick, and D. T. Mason, Mechanism of hypolipidemic action of nicotinic acid, Clin.Pharmacol.Ther., 24: 354-373 (1978).
134. S. M. Grundy, H. Y. I. Mok, L. Zech, and M. Berman, Influence of nicotinic acid on metabolism of cholesterol and triglycerides in man, J.Lipid Res., 22:24-36 (1981).
135. S. M. Grundy, E. H. Ahrens, jr., G. Salen, P. H. Schreibman, and P. J. Nestel, Mechanism of action of clofibrate on cholesterol metabolism in patients with hyperlipidemia, J.Lipid Res., 13:531-551 (1972).
136. D. J. McNamara, N. O. Davidson, P. Samuel, and E. H. Ahrens, jr., Cholesterol absorption in man: Effect of administration of clofibrate and/or cholestyramine, J.Lipid Res., 21:1058-1063 (1980).
137. J. W. Farquhar, R. E. Smith, and M. E. Dempsey, The effect of beta-sitosterol on serum lipids of young men with atherosclerotic heart disease, Circulation, 14:77-82 (1956).
138. S. M. Grundy and H. H. I. Mok, Cholestipol, clofibrate and phytosterols in combined therapy of hyperlipidemia, J.Lab. Clin.Med., 89:354-366 (1977).
139. F. H. Mattson, S. M. Grundy, and J. R. Crouse, Optimizing the effect of plant sterol on cholesterol absorption in man, Am.J.Clin.Nutr., 35:697-700 (1982).

BIOCHEMICAL METHODS FOR SERUM BILE ACID ANALYSIS

A. Roda, S. Girotti, P. Filippetti, A. Piacentini and
P. Simoni

Istituto Scienze Chimiche - Università di Bologna
Via S. Donato, 15, I-40127, Bologna, Italy

INTRODUCTION

Bile acids (BA) are a group of acidic steroids synthesized
in the liver from cholesterol. After conjugation with glycine or
taurine, BA are secreted into the bile and enter the enterohepatic circulation since they are efficiently reabsorbed by the
intestine[1].

Although it is well known that serum bile acids (SBA)
increase in liver disease[2,3] and decrease, especially after
meals, in ileal disfunction, the clinical utility of SBA measurements has not yet been fully established. Variations in SBA
levels are often small[4] while the fractional clearance of BA is
very high and peripheral blood contains BA at very low concentrations (micromolar levels) compared with that of bile (milli-
molar levels).

The qualitative pattern of SBA is very complex, because of
the two primary and three secondary BA exist in both unconjugated
as well as conjugated forms. In addition, lithocholyl conjugates
are mostly sulphated[5]. Several methods have been so far developed
based on different principle; the analytical informations are
different and a complete bile acid pattern is still undefined. In
view of this, the following need to be taken into account in proposing the SBA as a "test": which bile acid a group of bile acids
most closely reflects liver or intestinal function? what sensitivity is required and what other test are already available? The
lack of standardization of the current available methods makes
any comparison difficult and limits the diagnostic value of such
measurement.

We want here to review the most important and recent biochemical methods for SBA analysis, with emphasis on factors such as sensitivity, simplicity, cost and rapidity of execution of the assay.

RADIOIMMUNOASSAY

Since the first RIA for bile acids was described in 1973 by Simmonds et al.[6], several different procedures have been reported[7,25] in the literature, the main characteristics of which are summarized in Table 1. All methods utilize polyclonal antibodies produced in rabbits immunized with a bile acid coupled to a protein. The carrier protein generally bovine serum albumin, has been covalently linked by a peptide bond on a C_{24} carboxy group.

As a consequence, the side chain is completely masked by the protein and the antibodies so produced are specific only for the steroid skeletron[26]. In addition the low titre of the antibody produced could depend on the low molar ratio BA/BSA or on the high metabolic biotransformation of the immunogen. A more specific and higher affinity antibodies and consequently a greater accuracy and sensitivity of RIA may be achieved with new bile acid-antigen complexes in which the carrier protein is bound far from the hydroxy groups and to the side chain.

The method generally used for the preparation of the bile acid-protein conjugate is the "mixed anhydride" technique described by Erlanger et al.[27] or the carbodiimide method. Some authors[20] have used thyroglobulin instead of bovine serum albumin as carrier protein of the immunogen because of the higher molecular weight.

As far as the method is concerned, a higher affinity constant of the antibody vs the bile acids compared with that of the bile acid with albumin (100-1000 times) allows us to measure the bile acids direct on serum without any preliminary extraction of bile acids or protein denaturation. Two radioisotopes were commonly utilized to label bile acids: the ^{3}H and the ^{125}I. The first isotope has been extensively used by many authors: it has the advantage of being introduced into steroid molecules and it does not modify the structure (usually at 11-12 position). The main disadvantage is its low specific activity. The specific activity of ^{3}H-labeled bile acid is 3-5Ci/mmoles which limits the lowest amount of labeled antigen competing with antiserum. The mass of the labeled BA in the assay tube is in the order of 0.1 pmol/tube. The use of tracers such as the ^{125}I with a potential higher specific activity reduces the cost of the assay (no liquid scintillation counting) but it has a short half-life and can modify the antigen's immunogenicity and stability. The separation of the antigen is carried out using different methods

Table 1.   Characteristics of the RIA Methods

BA Measured	Acts Direct on Serum	Labeled Antigen	Separation of B/F	Sensitivity (pmol/tube)	Normal Values (μmol/l)	Reference
CCA	Yes	^{3}H	PEG	5	0.54 ± 0.04	6
CCA	No	^{3}H	$(NH_4)_2SO_4$	-	0.55 ± 1.8	7
CCA/CCDCA	Yes	^{3}H	$(NH_4)_2SO_4$	10	0.27/070 ± 0.03	8
SLCA/DCA	Yes	^{3}H	$(NH_4)_2SO_4$	10	0.06 ± 0.01	8
CCA	Yes	^{3}H	Solid phase	-	1.4 ± 0.3	9
CCA	Yes	^{3}H	$(NH_4)_2SO_4$	5	0.45 ± 0.12	10
CCDCA	Yes	^{3}H	$(NH_4)_2SO_4$	5	1.05 ± 0.35	10
CCDCA	Yes	^{3}H	$(NH_4)_2SO_4$	2	0.3 ± 3.8	11
CCA+CCDCA	Yes	^{125}I	Charcoal	0.5	3.47 ± 2.16	12
CCA	Yes	^{3}H	PEG	-	0.62 ± 0.4	13
DCA	Yes	^{3}H	PEG	7.5	0.18 ± 0.92	14
LCA	Yes	^{3}H	PEG	20	0.25 ± 0.016	15
SLCA	Yes	^{3}H	$(NH_4)_2SO_4$	10	1.56 ± 0.11	16
CLCA	Yes	^{3}H	$(NH_4)_2SO_4$	5	0.085 ± 0.04	17
UDCA	Yes	^{3}H	PEG	10	0.15 ± 0.11	18
CCA+free	No	^{125}I	PEG	2	0.43 ± 0.17	19
CCDCA+free	No	^{125}I	PEG	0.5	0.47 ± 0.23	19
DCA+free	No	^{125}I	Charcoal	2	0.33 ± 0.11	19
CCA	Yes	^{125}I	Charcoal	9.5	0.4 ± 1.9	20
CCA	Yes	^{125}I	Charcoal	-		21
3choleic	No	^{125}I	$(NH_4)_2SO_4$	0.6	0.08 ± 0.45	22
CCA	Yes	^{3}H	$(NH_4)_2SO_4$	5	0.49 ± 1.32	23
CCDCA	Yes	^{3}H	$(NH_4)_2SO_4$	2	0.55 ± 2.02	23
CCDCA	Yes	^{125}I	$(NH_4)_2SO_4$	1	1.0 ± 0.6	24
CUDCA	Yes	^{125}I	$(NH_4)_2SO_4$	1	0.19 ± 0.19	25

CCA=Conjugated cholic acid; CCDCA=conjugated chenodeoxycholic acid; DCA=deoxycholic acid; CLCA=conjugated lithocholic acid; SLCA=sulpholithocholic acid; UDCA=ursodeoxycholic acid; CUDCA=conjugated ursodeoxycholic acid

(Table 1). It is also interesting the use of the "solid phase" method in which the antibody is absorbed on a solid bead. At the present time, ammonium sulphate is the most commonly precipitating agent of the antigen-antibody complex. When different RIA methods are intercompared a good agreement has been found suggesting that differences in the antibody specificity or in analytical methodology play a major role in the accuracy and reliability of the method.

The main problem of the bile acids RIA is antibody production. The different methods reported mainly determine conjugated bile acids but not the free forms. Moreover each assay, is specific only for a class of bile acids: this causes some difficulties in comparing the results obtained by different authors. Despite high sensitivity and simplicity the RIA methods are still expensive (radioactive counting, licence and disposal), so that they are limited to a few specialized laboratories.

ENZYME IMMUNOASSAY

Enzyme immunoassay (EIA) is an alternative analytical procedure to radioimmunoassay which takes full advantage of the specificity and sensitivity that result from the use of an antibody but does not employ a radioactive isotope.

Recently many established radioimmunoassay have been changed to enzyme immunoassays to benefit from the increased speed of analysis and reduced costs afforded by this technique. Enzyme immunoassays have also been developed for the determination of serum bile acids (SBA)[28-32]. Two different EIAs have been reported in the literature: based on an "heterogeneous" and "homogeneous" principle.

The principle of the first type of assay is similar to that of RIA: a bile acid covalently linked with an enzyme (peroxidase, -galactosidase) is used a tracer instead of a radioisotope. The enzymatic activity of the tracer is recorded spectrophotometrically (after antigen-antibody complex separation) by measuring specific colour-producing substrates. Matern[28] developed this method for cholic acid conjugates and Maeda[29] for ursodeoxycholic acid. The sensitivity of these methods is quite similar to corresponding RIA as previously reported (see above). This model of enzyme immunoassay could be extended to other bile acids and this may be used on a large scale in medical laboratories.

Baquir et al.[30] developed an "homogeneous" enzyme immunoassay for the determination of conjugate chenodeoxycholate. The procedure does not require extraction of serum and separation of antibody-bound from free antigen, hence, the term "homogeneous". It is not based on the same principle as the common competitive or non-competitive immunoassay but on the principle that when a bile acid-enzyme interacts with the specific antibody the enzymatic activity is drastically reduced. The "homogeneous" method is in principle less sensitive than the "heterogeneous" one but adequate for serum bile acid analysis; the sensitivity is around 10 times less than similar RIA.

Recently in our laboratory we have developed a sensitive enzyme immunoassay for the determination of conjugated chenodeoxycholic acid. The method is based on a competitive principle and the antibody is immobilized on a plastic beads (polystyrene plastic balls). As a "tracer" we use a horseradish-peroxidase-chenodeoxycholylglycine conjugate, prepared by a slight modification of the mixed anhydride reaction. Using an appropriate amount of reagents we obtained a "tracer" with an elevated specific activity. At a working dilution (1 μg/ml) the mass of enzyme labeled- BA is on the order of 1 pg. This leads to ad improvement in the specific activity when compared with a titriated chenodeoxycholic acid (s.a. $\sim$ 3 Ci/mmol). The antibody was purified by salt precipitation; the immunoglobulin rich fraction was diluted to a final concentration of 5 μg/ml with carbonate buffer and adsorbed on the plastic beads. The immobilized antibody is stable for at least 4 months if stored at 4 °C. The procedure used is direct on serum sample (5-10 μl) and requires 1 hour incubation of the antibody with the "tracer" and sample. After that the plastic beads are washed and the substrate (H_2O_2, o-phe-

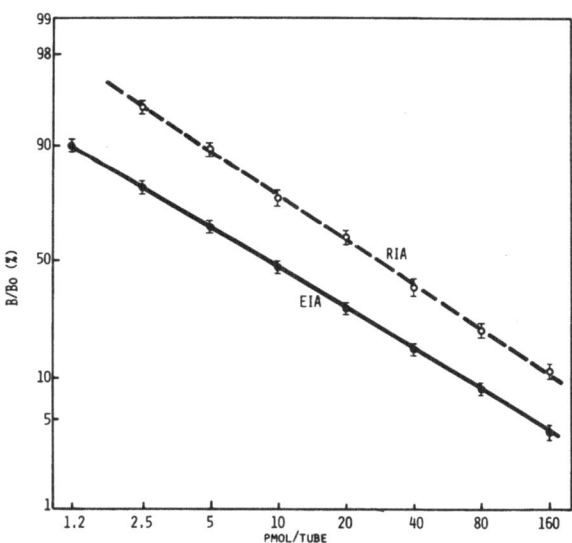

Fig. 1. - Standard curves for the EIA method and a similar RIA procedure

Table 2. Characteristics of EIA for Serum Bile Acids

Specificity	Acts Direct on Serum	Label	Principle of the Method	Sensitivity	Precision (CV %)	Reference
CHL-GLY CHL-TAU	Yes	Peroxydase	Competitive	0.05 μmol/l	18-22	28
CHL-GLY CHN-TAU	Yes	Peroxidase	Homogeneous	50 pmol	8.6	30
URS	Yes	Galactosidase	Competitive	0.08 pmol		29
CHL-GLY CHL-TAU	Yes	Alkaline Phosphatase	Competitive	0.12 μg/ml	6-12.8	32
URS	Yes	Alkaline Phospatase	Elisa	20 pmol	3.22 $\pm$ 1.28	31
CHN-GLY CHN-TAU	Yes	Peroxidase	Solid phase Competitive	0.5 pmol	8-12	A. Roda (in press)

CHL-GLY = Cholylglycine; CHL-TAU = Cholyltaurine; CHN-GLY = Chenodeoxycholylglycine; CHM-TAU = Chenodeoxycholyltayurine; URS = Ursodeoxycholic acid; CV = Coefficient of Variation nylendiamine) is added. The adsorbance (490 nm) is recordered after 30 min of incubation. Fig. 1 reports a typical standard curve for the above method and a similar RIA procedure. The sensitivity is higher for EIA as shown by the mid-range of the curve (Fig. 1). In conclusion the EIA methods for bile acids may have a sensitivity greater than the corresponding RIA due to the higher specific activity of the tracer. In addition, this method presents the advantage of higher stability of the reagent and safety for the operator. The characteristics of published EIA methods are reported in Table 2.

ENZYMATIC ASSAY

The method is based upon the oxidation by a specific hydroxysteroid-dehydrogenase (in particular the 3α-HSD) of the bile acid OH group, with steichiometric generation of NADH from NAD$^+$:

$$\text{STEROID-OH} + \text{NAD}^+ \rightleftharpoons \text{STEROID=O} + \text{NADH} + \text{H}^+$$

The NADH produced is subsequently measured by spectrophotometric or fluorimetric detection. The characteristics of the main enzymatic assays are reported in Table 3. The first application of this principle to serum 3α-hydroxy bile acids was reported by Iwata et al.[33] in 1964. Using spectrophotometric determination of NADH at 340 nm, they found the lowest practical limit of detection to be approximately 0.01 μmol in the final reaction mixture (3 ml). This implied that at least 20 ml of serum were needed for the analysis, introducing a high background and clinical impraticability.

The sensitivity was increased several times by the use of fluorimetric determination of NADH[34-38]. However the preliminary extraction of BA from serum was still required. In 1976 Mashige et al.[39] reported the first direct enzymatic-fluorimetric assay, based upon the use of the 3α-HSD in combination with a resazurine-diaphorase system. The hydrogen of the generated NADH is transferred by diaphorase to resazurine, to yeld the fluorophore, resorfin. The fluorescence of resorfin is then measured at 580 nm with excitation at 560 nm. This method introduced a significant improvement in sensitivity (0.5 μmol/l) and clinical usefulness, since no preliminary extraction was required.

More recently[42] the same group reported a further improvement using the same enzymatic system (3α-HSD/diaphorase) in combination with nitrotetrazolium blue and spectrophotometric detection of the generated diformazan. The lowest point of the curve was 5 μmol/l (200 μl serum sample). More recently, Nicolas et al.[41] have developed an extremely sensitive enzyme "cycling" method. BA are oxidized by 3α-HSD and after selective destruction of NAD excess, the NADH is determined by an enzymatic

Table 3.   Characteristics of the More Recent Enzymatic Methods for Serum Bile Acids

Enzyme	Volume of Serum Required (ml)	Act Direct	NADH Detection	Sensitivity (pmol/tube)	Normal Values (μmol/l)	Reference
3α-HSD	3	No	F	1500	0-8.2	34
3α-HSD	2	No	F	1	0.3-9.3	35
3α-HSD	1-3	No	F	630	0.9-6.3	36
3α-HSD	0.8	Yes	F	1	3-6	37
7α-HSD	1-5	No	F	1000	1.2-6.3	38
3α-HSD	0.1	Yes	F	0.5	6.3 $\pm$ 2.9	39
3α-HSD	0.2	Yes	S	2000	1-7	40
3α-HSD	0.05	Yes	S	0.3	3.03 $\pm$ 1.13	41
3α-HSD	0.2	Yes	S	2.5	3.2 $\pm$ 1.3	40
3α-HSD	0.1	No	S	0.1	-	43

F = fluorimetry; S = spectrophotometry

cycling reaction. The amplifying steps use a 3β - or 17β -HSD to reduce dehydroepiandrosterone to 5-testosterone; then a 3-keto-steroid-5 isomerase enzyme catalyzes the formation of testosterone which is measured spectrophotometrically at 248 nm. This method is highly sensitive (0.3 pmol/tube) but requires long incubation (an overnight incubation is needed to obtain the highest sensitivity), two determinations of absorbance and an UV spectrophotometer.

For further application[43] in clinical practice a spectro-photometric continuous flow-ystem has recently been developed by coimmobilization of 3α -HSD and diaphorase on Sepharose beads. The method is sensitive (0.1 pmol/tube) and economical, allowing assays of 10-15 samples per hour, though a preliminary extraction of bile acids from serum is required.

A specific enzymatic-fluorimetric method based upon the use of 7α -HSD has also been described[38]. The sensitivity of this method is poor, but it allows quantitative measurements of the primary SBA alone (7α -hydroxy bile acids), which may be more useful than total SBA detection in liver disease diagnosis[2,44].

In general enzymatic assays have a lower sensitivity in comparison with other methods such as RIA or EIA (requiring time-consuming cycling reactions, in order to obtain a higher sensitivity). Yet the enzymatic methods have been widely applied in clinical laboratories, since they provide good assay speed combined with low cost, and simple instruments and procedures. However these methods cannot be applied for the evaluation of BA malabsorption syndrome, in which a reduction of BA has been observed.

BIOLUMINESCENT METHODS

Sensitive methods for SBA based on bioluminescence measurement have recently been developed using hydroxysteroid dehydrogenase (3α or 12α or 7α -HSD)[45,49]. The HSD catalyzes the conversion of the bile acid hydroxy group (3α or 7α or 12α) to a keto-group in the presence of $NAD(P)^+$. The resulting $NAD(P)H$, in presence of $NAD(P)H$: FMN oxydoreductase (OXRED), converts FMN to its reduced form ($FMNH_2$). This in turn reacts with decanal and oxygen in the presence of bacterial luciferase to produce light. The intensity of the light emitted is proportional to the amount of bile acids in the initial raction. The overall scheme, for 7α -HSD for instance, is this:

$$\text{Bile acid - } 7\alpha \text{ -OH+NAD}^+ \xrightarrow{7\alpha \text{ -HSD}} \text{bile acid-7-oxo+NADH+H}^+ \qquad (1)$$

$$\text{H}^+ + \text{NADH} + \text{FMN} \xrightarrow{\text{NADH:FMN oxred}} \text{NAD}^+ + \text{FMNH}_2 \qquad (2)$$

$$\text{FMNH}_2 + \text{decanal} + \text{O}_2 \xrightarrow{\text{luciferase}} \text{FMN+decanoic acid+light+H}_2\text{O} \qquad (3)$$

Table 4. Characteristics of the Enzymatic Bioluminescent Methods for Serum Bile Acids with Bacterial Luciferase

Enzyme	Act Direct	Solid Support	Sensitivity (pmol/tube)	CV (%)	Volume of Serum Required (ml)	Samples/h (only flow systems)	Reference
7α-HSD	Yes	Sepharose 4B	0.5	8-10	0.01	-	45
3α-HSD	Yes	-	4	7-14	0.02	-	46
12α-HSD	Yes	Sepharose 4B	4	7.8-8.2	0.01	-	47
7α-HSD	Yes	Sepharose 4B	4	2-5	0.01	30	48
7α-HSD	Yes	Nylon	10	5-10	0.01	20	49

The characteristics of published bioluminescent methods are reported in Table 4.

The first assay developed by one of us was for primary bile acids using 7α -HSD and bioluminescent enzymes immobilized on Sepharose 4B[45] (Table 4). A linear response in the range 1.5 to 50 μmol/l was obtained for SBA on serum heated at 70 °C for 15 min. The use of a Sepharose-immobilized enzyme system increases the catalytic activity per unit enzyme and gives more stable analytical reagents.

The total SBA can be determined by the bioluminescent method for Styrelius et al.[46] using 3α -HSD. The assay utilizes enzymes in solution and is linear for BA concentrations up to 300 μmol/l. The serum samples were treated with trichloroacetic acid directly in the test tube, before the assay, without sub-sampling. No interference was detected, because the sample size analyzed was small (20 μl).

The 12α -HSD, a $NADP^+$ dependent enzyme, was also coimmobilized with bioluminescent enzymes on Sepharose 4B[47]. To improve sensitivity bacterial diaphorase was sometimes used instead NADPH:FMN oxidoreductase, since background is less. The diaphorase containing systems are very sensitive to differences in mixing and shaking. However with an injection method the inter-assay precision is good (8%) and the standard curve is linear from 0.4 to 200 μmol/l.

Comparable sensitive assays have been performed using flow cells[48,49] thereby proving the sensitivity of the immobilized enzymes. This automated version of the assay is possible. The results obtained for serum primary bile acids using the bioluminescent flow assay of Kricka et al.[48] were in good agreement with independent measurements utilizing gas-liquid chromatography, but the factor limiting the continued use of flow cell was bacterial contamination of the Sepharose. This was overcome by our flow system[49] that uses enzymes coimmobilized on nylon. Nylon tubes are ideal for a continuous flow system, presenting no problems such as carryover, packing or distruption of gel matrix. The analysis is carried out directly on serum samples without a pre-incubation step. The detector used is much less expensive than a spectrophotometer or flurometer, while the analysis is rapid and gives a high quantum yield of bioluminescent reactions. These factors, together with the advantage of not being subject to quenching effects, good sensitivity and wide linear range of concentrations, as well as possible use in automatic systems, make these bioluminescent techniques very applicable for SBA analysis. The sensitivity is superior to all end-point enzymatic methods.

In particular the bioluminescent assay shows the same sensitivity as RIA, without dangerous manipulations with radionuclides and cheaper instrumentations and reagents. Moreover the use of 3α, 7α and 12α -HSD makes it possible to determine all the SBA, both conjugated and unconjugated. The unconjugated BA present in serum[30] are not determined by RIA. Thus the bioluminescent methods are economical, rapid and extremely sensitive for measurements of BA concentrations in serum.

CONCLUSION

Sensitive and biochemical methods for SBA are now currently available. The problem of its usefulness in diagnosis is still unsolved and a large-scale prospective studies on SBA related to disease are needed. A quality control study has been performed: 11 laboratories located in different parts of Italy have analyzed SBA by different techniques[51]. The results obtained suggest that at the present time the analysis of serum bile acid requires further standardization, due to different analytical information obtained using various techniques. One of the more sensitive method for SBA seems to be the immunological procedure and several kits are commercially available, but for the above reasons none of them measures the same acid. On the other hand, the enzymatic method measures total bile acid with low sensitivity.

More recently, amplified methods and bioluminescent methods including 3α -HSD, 7α -HSD and more recently 12α -HSD have improved the sensitivity of the latest technique, with small samples and without preseparation or preincubation. Such enzymatic methods, with sensitivity similar or greater than RIA, offer a series of advantages compared with the latest techniques in terms of automation, already realized, cost and safety.

REFERENCES

1. A. F. Hofmann, The enterohepatic circulation of bile acids in man, Clin. Gastroenterol. 6:3 (1977).
2. L. Barbara, A. Roda and E. Roda, Diurnal variations of serum primary bile acids in healthy subjects and hepatobiliary disease patients, Rendic. Gastroenterol. 8:194 (1976).
3. S. Skrede, H.E. Solberg, J.P. Blomhoff and E. Gjone, Bile acid measured in serum during fasting as a test for linear disease, Clin. Chem. 24:1095 (1978).
4. J. C. Glusinovich, M. Dumont, M. Duval and S. Erlinger, Hepatocellular uptake of taurocholate in the dog, J. Clin. Invest. 55:419 (1975).
5. J. M. Dietshy, Mechanism for the intestinal absorption of bile acids, J. Lipid. Res. 91:297 (1968).

6. W. J. Simmonds, M.G. Korman, V.L.W. Go, A.F. Hofmann, Radio-immunoassay of conjugated cholyl bile acids in serum. Gastroenterology 65:705 (1973).

7. G. M. Murphy, S.M. Edkins, J.W. Williams, D. Catty, The preparation and properties of an antiserum for the radioimmunoassay of serum conjugated cholic acid, Clin. Chim. 54:81 (1974).

8. L. M. Demers and G. Hepner, Radioimmunoassay of bile acids in serum, Clin. Chem. 22:602 (1976).

9. J. W. O. Van Den Berg, M. Van Blankenstein, E.P. Bosman-Jacobs, M. Frenkel, P. Hörchner, O.I. Oost-Harwing and I.H.P. Wilson, Solid phase radioimmunoassay for determination of conjugated cholic acid in serum, Clin. Chim. Acta 73:277 (1976).

10. A. Roda, E. Roda, R. Aldini, D. Festi, G. Mazzella, C. Sama and L. Barbara, Development, validation, and application of a single-tube radioimmunoassay for cholic and chenodeoxycholic conjugated bile acids in human serum, Clin. Chem. 23:2107 (1977).

11. S. W. Schalm, G.P. Van Berge-Henegouwen, A.F. Hofmann, A.E. Cowen and J. Turcotte, Radioimmunoassay of bile acids: development, validation, and preliminary application of an assay for conjugates of chenodeoxycholic acid. Gastroenterology 73:285 (1977).

12. J. G. Spenney, B.J. Johnson, B.I. Hirschowitz, A.A. Mihas and R. Gibson, An ^{125}I-radioimmunoassay for primary conjugated bile salts. Gastroenterology 72:305 (1977).

13. A. A. Mihas, J.G. Spenney, B.I. Hirschowitz and R. Gibson, A critical evaluation of a procedure for measurement of serum bile acids by radioimmunoassay, Clin. Chim. Acta 76:389 (1977).

14. S. Matern, R. Krieger, C. Hans and W. Gerok, Radioimmunoassay of serum-conjugated deoxycholic acid, Scand. J. Gastroent. 12:641 (1977)

15. A. E. Cowen, M.G. Korman, A.F. Hofmann, J. Turcotte and J.A. Carter, Radioimmunoassay of unsulfated lithocholates, J. Lipid. Res. 18:692 (1977).

16. A. E. Cowen, M.G. Korman, A.F. Hofmann, J. Turcotte and J.A. Carter, Radioimmunoassay of sulfated lithocholates, J. Lipid. Res. 18:698 (1977).

17. A. Roda, E. Roda, D. Festi, R. Aldini, G. Mazzella, C. Sama and L. Barbara, A radioimmunoassay for lithocholic acid conjugates in human serum and liver tissue, Steroids 32:13 (1978).

18. I. Makino, A. Tashiro, H. Hashimoto, S. Nakagawa and I. Yoshizawa, Radioimmunoassay of ursodeoxycholic acid in serum, J. Lipid. Res. 19:443 (1978).

19. O. Mäentausta and O. Jänne, Radioimmunoassay of conjugated cholic acid, chenodeoxycholic acid and deoxycholic acid

from human serum, with use of ^{125}I-labelled ligands, <u>Clin. Chem.</u> 25:264 (1979).

20. E. Minder, G. Karlaganis, U. Schmied, P. Vitins and G. Paumgartner, A higly specific ^{125}I-radioimmunoassay for cholic acid conjugates, <u>Clin. Chim. Acta</u> 92:177 (1979).

21. P. Miller, S. Weiss, M. Cornell and J. Dockery, Specific ^{125}I-radioimmunoassay for cholylglycine, a bile acid, in serum, <u>Clin. Chem.</u> 27:1698 (1981).

22. E. Minder, Radioimmunoassay determination of serum 3α-hydroxy-5-cholenoic acid in normal subjects and patients with liver disease, <u>J. Lipid. Res.</u> 20:986 (1978).

23. Y. A. Baqir, J. Murison, P.E. Ross and I.A.D. Bouchier, Radioimmunoassay of primary bile salts in serum, <u>J. Clin. Pathol.</u> 32:560 (1979).

24. G. J. Beckett, J.E.T. Corrie and I.W. Percy-Robb, The preparation of ^{125}I-labeled bile acids ligands for use in the radioimmunoassay of bile acids, <u>Clin. Chim. Acta</u> 93:145 (1979).

25. A. Hill, P.E. Ross and I.A.D. Bouchier, ^{125}I-radioimmunoassay of serum ursodeoxycholyl conjugates, <u>Clin. Chim. Acta</u> 127: 327 (1983).

26. A. Roda, E. Roda, R. Aldini, M. Cappelli, D. Festi, C. Sama, G. Mazzella, A.M. Morselli and L. Barbara, Results with six "kit" radioimmunoassays for primary bile acids in human serum intercompared, <u>Clin. Chem.</u> 26:1677 (1980).

27. B. F. Erlanger, F. Borek, S.M. Beiser and S. Lieberman, Steroid-protein conjugates. Preparation and characterization of conjugates of bovine serum albumin with testosterone and with cortisone, <u>J. Biol. Chem.</u> 228:713 (1957).

28. S. Matern, K. Tietjen, H. Matern and W. Gerok, Enzyme labelled immunoassay for a bile acid in human serum, <u>in</u>: "Enzyme labelled immunoassay of hormones and drugs", S.B. Pal. ed., Walter De Gruyter e Co., Berlin, 457 (1978).

29. Y. Maeda, T. Setoguchi, T. Katsuki and E. Ishikawa, Development of a solid-phase immunoassay for ursodeoxycholic acid: application to plasma disappearance of injected ursodeoxycholic acid in the rabbit, <u>J. Lipid. Res.</u> 20:960 (1979).

30. Y. A. Baqir, P.E. Ross and I.A.D. Bouchier, Homogeneous enzyme immunoassay of chenodeoxycholate conjugates in serum, <u>Anal. Biochem.</u> 93:361 (1979).

31. S. Ozaki, A. Tashiro, J. Makino, S. Nakagawa and I. Yoshizawa, Enzyme linked immunoassay of ursodeoxycholic acid in serum, <u>J. Lipid. Res.</u> 20:240 (1979).

32. Immunotechnical Corporation Cambridge, MA; Enbad Cholylglycine EIA kit.

33. T. Ywata and K. Yamasaki, Enzymatic determination and thin-layer chromatography of bile acid in blood, <u>J. Biochem.</u> 56:424 (1969).

34. G. M. Murphy, B.H. Billing and D.N. Baron, A fluorimetric and

enzymatic method for the estimation of serum total bile acids, J. Clin. Path. 23:594 (1970).

35. H. P. Schwartz, K.V. Bergman and G. Paumgartner, A simple method for the estimation of bile acids in serum, Clin. Chim. Acta 50:197 (1974).

36. O. Fausa, Quantitative determination of serum bile acids using a purified 3-alpha-hydroxysteroid dehydrogenase, Scand. J. Gastroenterol. 10:747 (1975).

37. P. A. Siskos, P.T. Cahill and N.B. Javitt, Serum bile acids analysis: a rapid direct enzymatic method using dual beam spectrophotometry, J. Lipid. Res. 18:666 (1977).

38. O. Fausa and B.A. Skalhegg, Quantitative determination of serum bile acids using a 7-alpha-hydroxysteroid dehydrogenase, Scand. J. Gastroenterol. 12:44 (1977).

39. F. Mashige, K. Imai and T. Osuga, A simple and sensitive assay of total serum bile acids, Clin. Chim. Acta, 70:79 (1976).

40. H. Steensland, An automated method for the determination of total bile acids in serum, Scand. J. Clin. Lab. Invest. 38:447 (1978).

41. J. C. Nicolas, J. Chaintreuil, B. Descomps and A. Crastes de Paulet, Enzymatic microassay of serum bile acids: an increased sensitivity with an enzyme amplification technique, Anal. Biochem. 103:170 (1980).

42. F. Mashige, N. Tanaka, A. Maki, S. Kamei and M. Yamanata, Direct spectrophotometry of total bile acids in serum, Clin. Chem. 27:1352 (1981).

43. R. Bovara, G. Carrera, P. Cremonesi and G. Mazzola, Continuous-flow analysis of 3α-hydroxysteroids using immobilized 3α-hydroxysteroid dehydrogenase, Anal. Biochem. 112:239 (1981).

44. M. G. Korman, A.F. Hofmann and W.H.J. Summerskill, Assessment of activity in chronic active liver disease. Serum bile acids compared with conventional tests and histology, N. Engl. J. Med. 290:1399 (1974).

45. A. Roda, L.J. Kricka, M. DeLuca and A.F. Hofmann, Bioluminescence measurement of primary bile acids using immobilized 7α-hydroxysteroid dehydrogenase: application to serum bile acids, J. Lipid. Res. 23:1354 (1982).

46. I. Styrélius, A. Thore and I. Bjorkhem, Bioluminescent assay for total bile acids in serum with use of bacterial luciferase, Clin. Chem. 29:1123 (1983).

47. J. Schoelmerich, J.E. Hinkley, I.A. MacDonald, A.F. Hofmann and M. DeLuca, A bioluminescent assay for 12α-hydroxy bile acids using immobilized enzymes, Anal. Biochem. 133:244 (1983).

48. L. J. Kricka, G.K. Wienhausen, J.E. Hinkley and M. DeLuca, Automated bioluminescent assay for NADH, glucose 6-phosphate, primary bile acids and ATP, Anal. Biochem. 129:392 (1983).

49. A. Roda, S. Girotti, S. Ghini, B. Grigolo, G. Carrea and R. Bovara, Continuous-flow determination of primary bile acids, by bioluminescence with use of nylon-immobilized bacterial enzymes, Clin. Chem. 30:206 (1984).
50. K. D. R. Setchell, A.M. Lawson, E.J. Blackstock and G.M. Murphy, Diurnal changes in serum unconjugated bile acids in normal man, Gut 23:637 (1982).
51. A. Attili (Roma), C. Baccini (Ravenna), L. Cenciotti (Cesena), R. Galeazzi (Ancona), F. Fiaccadori (Parma), A. Morselli, M. Capelli, A. Roda (Bologna), F. Narducci (Perugia), M. Sanguneti (Genova), R. Ruggeri (Forlì), C. Salvioli (Modena), E. Spaccesi (Macerata), Controllo di qualità del dosaggio degli acidi biliari sierici (dati in corso di pubblicazione).

DIAGNOSTIC USEFULNESS OF SERUM BILE ACID DETERMINATION

IN LIVER DISEASES

L. Barbara in collaboration with
D. Festi, A. Roda, A.M. Morselli Labate,
B. Grigolo, R. Frabboni, and S. Vicari

Clinica Medica 3, University of Bologna

Although it has been recognized for many years that elevated concentrations of bile acids (ba) in serum are markers of liver disease (1), only the considerable progress that has been made in the last ten years in the methodology of ba measurement and in elucidating the physiological determinants of serum bile acid (SBA) levels has made it feasible to propose SBA determination in clinical routine. From a technical point of view, the earliest methods (2, 3) (fluorimetric, enzymatic, ecc.) had a low sensitivity and, consequently, the results obtained were often contradictory and incomplete.

The development of a radioimmunoassay for cholylconjugates by the Mayo Clinic group (4) was the first step in establishing sensitive and reliable methods for SBA evaluation. Up to now, other sensitive analytical methods have been developed (gas liquid chromatography, enzyme immunoassay, inverse-isotope dilution-mass spectrometry, ecc.). However each of them gives different information (total bile acid pattern, classes of bile acids, ecc.) and requires different analysis time (5). In 1977 we developed sensitive radioimmunoassays for cholic, chenodeoxycholic and lithocholic acid conjugates (7). According to the data accumulated in our laboratory during the last six years and to the data published in the literature, radioimmunoassay method should be, both for practical and technical reasons, the method of choice for an useful evaluation of SBA in health and disease.

In normal subject, the predominant ba in serum is chnodeoxycholic acid, followed by cholic acid, with a ratio of about 2:1; lithocholic and deoxycholic acid concentrations are lower.

The results of several studies (8), performed both in the experimental animal and in man, have clearly demonstrated that SBA concentrations are determined by the instantaneous balance between input of ba from the intestine and clearance of ba by the liver. Furthermore, SBA closely reflect the dynamics of the enterohepatic circulation (9, 10).

In man, the pool is efficiently conserved within the enterohepatic circulation, being the fecal loss compensated by the hepatic de novo synthesis. Ba pool undergoes to accelerations and decelerations in response to meal and fasting, regulated by the two mechanical pumps (gallbladder and intestinal motility) and the two chemical pumps (hepatocyte and enterocyte absorption) of the enterohepatic circulation (11). SBA reflect this dynamics; in fact they increase after meal and decrease during fasting (9, 10). Several lines of evidence suggest that intestinal input, rather than hepatic uptake, is the main determinant of SBA. In fact experimental studies have shown that, owing to its enormous Vmax, the hepatic clearance is independent of load and that the ba first pass elimination is constant (12, 13). For this reason, when in postprandial state the ba portal concentrations increase, also the ba spillover in the peripheral blood increases.

In patients with liver disease, the concentrations of SBA are frequently higher than in healthy subjects. The factors influencing this elevation are not clearly identified; only in patients with chronic liver disease the mechanism of increased SBA are partially elucidated (14, 15). It has been shown that also in these patients the major determinant of SBA is the intestinal input and that the differences between normal subjects and liver disease patients are the consequence of a reduced hepatic clearance. The latter results not only from a reduced liver blood flow and from portosystemic shunting, but also, and mainly, from a reduced inherent capacity of the liver to remove ba from the blood.

However it is important to note that hepatic uptake operates below saturation also in patients with mild to moderate liver disease and, therefore, the fractional hepatic clearance remains constant, as in normal subjects.

Studies evaluating the possibility to use SBA in the diagnostic approach of liver disease have been performed in the last few years, in concomitance with the improving knowledge of their determinants in health and disease. The definition of timing of the measurement (fasting or postprandial or both) and the evaluation of its accuracy have been the main problems to be overcome.

Postprandial determination was firstly proposed because considered more sensitive than the fasting one, being the former

able to reveal defective uptake by a diseased liver of the endogenous ba load (16).

However, the subsequent observation that hepatic uptake in
liver disease patients, although reduced, is far below its Vmax
and therefore, as in normal subject, the fractional hepatic
clearance is constant in fasting and postprandial conditions,
rouled out the rationale of postprandial determination. An alternative approach, different from fasting determination, was the
administration of a known ba load, either per s or intravenously
(17, 18).

Also in these cases, several problems are still unsolved,
since the evaluation after oral ba load is influenced by gastric
emptying and by dissolution kinetics of the ba preparation and
the evaluation after i.v. administration depends on liver blood
flow (19).

Up to recently, also the definition of the diagnostic effectiveness of SBA has been imprecise and insufficient, since the
most tudies SBA were compared with routine liver function tests
(LFT) only in terms of percent of abnormality.

To overcome these problems, we carried out a study (20)
aimed to determine the sensitivity and discrimination capacity of
both fasting and postprandial SBA measurement and to compare results with those of LFT.

In liver disease patients and in control subjects we evaluated fasting and postprandial serum levels of cholic, chenodeoxycholic and lithocholic acid conjugates and LFT. For the above
mentioned problems, data were subjected to variance and discriminant analyses.

Fasting and postprandial SBA were higher in patients when
compared to controls and were significantly higher in severe than
in mild liver disease. The statistical analyses of our data
showed that SBA determination is more sensitive and discriminant
when obtained fasting than postprandial, and that the most useful
determination is the combination of a primary bile acid (cholic
acid) with lithocholic acid.

As far as the comparison between SBA and LFT is concerned,
our results demonstrated that SBA determination plays an ad-
junctive, rather than substitutive, role with respect to LFT,
since the percent of correct allocation was 75.4% for LFT, 70.1%
for SBA, and increased to 79.6% when LFT plus SBA were considered.

To further improve our methodology for the study of SBA, we are developing other techniques, particularly in order to simplify the analysis and to propose a wider application of ba measurement.

Indeed, recently we developed an enzymatic bioluminescent assay for SBA (21) with a sensitivity comparable to that of immunological methods.

This technique appears a valid alternative to the conventional methods for SBA measurement thanks to its extremely high sensitivity and precision, and to the relative low cost.

Furthermore, since ba concentrations in saliva are independent from flow rate and reflect those in the free fraction in plasma, we have evaluated salivary ba concentrations in patients with liver disease and control subjects. Our preliminary results showed that in patients with liver disease the salivary ba increase and the increment parallels that of serum (22). Salivary ba determination (both by radioimmunoassay and bioluminescence) could be therefore an useful and easy test for wide screening studies.

REFERENCES

1. S. Sherlock, V. Walse, Blood cholates in normal subjects and in liver disease. Clin. Sci. 6:223 (1948).
2. T. Iwata, K. Yamasaki, Enzymatic determination and thin layer chromatography of bile acids in blood. J. Biochem 56:424 (1964).
3. G.M. Murphy, B.H. Billing, D.N. Baron, A fluorimetric and enzymatic method for the estimation of total serum bile acids. J. Clin. Pathol. 23:594 (1970).
4. W.J. Simmonds, M.G. Korman, V.L.M. Go, et al, Radioimmunoassay of conjugated cholyl-bile acids in serum. Gastroenterology 65:705 (1973).
5. A. Roda (1983), Sensitive methods for serum bile acid analysis. In: "Bile Acids in Gastroenterology". L. Barbara, R.H. Dowling, A.F. Hofmann, E. Roda, Eds., MTP Press, Lancaster, pp. 57.
6. A. Roda, E. Roda, R. Aldini, et al, Development, validation, and application of a single-tube radioimmunoassay for cholic and chenodeoxycholic conjugated bile acids in human serum. Clin. Chem. 23:2107 (1977).
7. A. Roda, E. Roda, R. Aldini, et al, A radioimmunoassay for lithocholic acid conjugates in human serum and liver tissue. Steroids 32:13 (1978).
8. N.F. LaRusso, N.E. Hoffman, M.G. Korman, et al, Determinants

of fasting and postprandial serum bile acid leves in healthy man. <u>Am. J. Dig. Dis.</u> 23:391 (1978).

9. N.F. LaRusso, M.G. Korman, N.E. Hoffman, et al, Dynamics of the enterohepatic ciruclation of bile acids. Postprandial serum concentrations of conjugates of cholic acid in health, cholecystectomized patients, and patients with bile acid malabsorption. <u>N. Engl. J. Med.</u> 291:689 (1974).

10. L. Barbara, A. Roda, E. Roda, et al, Diurnal variations of serum primary bile acids in healthy subjects and hepatobiliary disease patients. <u>Rendic. Gastroenterol.</u> 8:194 (1976).

11. A.F. Hofmann, The enterohepatic circulation of bile acids in man. <u>Clin. Gastroenterol.</u> 6:3 (1977).

12. J. Reichen, G. Paumgartner, Uptake of bile acids by the perfused rat liver. <u>Am. J. Physiol.</u> 231:734 (1976).

13. J.C. Glasinovic, M. Dumont, M. Duval, et al, Hepatocellular uptake of taurocholate in the dog. <u>J. Clin. Invest.</u> 55:419 (1975).

14. P. Paré, J.C. Hoefs, M. Ashcavai, Determinants of serum bile acids in chronic liver disease. <u>Gastroenterology</u> 81:959 (1981).

15. R.Y. Poupon, R.E. Poupon, D. Lebrec, et al, Mechanisms for reduced hepatic clearance and elevated plasma levels of bile acids in cirrhosis. <u>Gastroenterology</u> 80:1438 (1981).

16. N. Kaplowitz, E. Kok, N.B. Javitt, Postprandial serum bile acid for the detection of hepatobiliary disease. <u>JAMA</u> 225:292 (1973).

17. H. Tashiro, Oral ursodeoxycholic acid tolerance test for patients with hepatobiliary disease. <u>Acta Hepatol. Jap.</u> 20:369 (1979).

18. N.F. LaRusso, N.E. Hoffman, A.F. Hofmann, et al, Validity and sensitivity of an intravenous bile acid tolerance test in patients with liver disease. <u>N. Engl. J. Med.</u> 292:1209 (1974).

19. A.F. Hofmann, The aminopyrine demethylation breath test and serum bile acid level: nominated but not yet elected to join the common liver tests. <u>Hepatology</u> 2:512 (1983).

20. D. Festi, A.M. Morselli Labate, A. Roda, et al, Diagnostic effectiveness of serum bile acids in liver disease as evaluated by multivariated statistical methods. <u>Hepatology</u> 3:707 (1983).

21. A. Roda, L.J. Kricka, M. DeLuca, et al, Bioluminescent measurement of bile acids using immobilized 7 -hydroxysteroid dehydrogenase: application to serum bile acids. <u>J. Lipid Res.</u> 23:1354 (1982).

22. A. Roda, E. Roda, R. Fugazza, et al, Salivary bile acids: methodology and usefulness in the diagnosis of liver and intestinal function. <u>Hepatology</u> 3:821 (1983) abstr.

QUANTITATION AND METABOLISM OF BILE ACIDS IN HYPER-LIPOPROTEINEMIAS

Tatu A. Miettinen

Second Department of Medicine
University of Helsinki
00290 Helsinki 29, Finland

INTRODUCTION

Bile acids are formed from cholesterol in the liver via a sequence of reactions initiated by 7α-hydroxylase. Two primary bile acids, cholic acid and chenodeoxycholic acid, are formed and secreted as glycine or taurine conjugates into the bile and intestine. Most of them are reabsorbed, taken up by the liver and resecreted, completing enterohepatic circulation of bile salts. During each cycle a small amount of bile acids escape into the colon and feces and is regenerated by new hepatic synthesis. Thus, fecal bile acids equal with bile acid synthesis. Under normal conditions the serum bile acid levels are quite low even postprandially and only negligible amounts escape into the urine.

Bile acids form a pathway for cholesterol catabolism and accordingly they play an important role in the regulation of cholesterol metabolism and of serum cholesterol and lipoprotein levels. They also regulate bile production, keep biliary cholesterol in solution, and facilitate absorption of fats, fat soluble vitamins and cholesterol. Disturbancies in bile secretion can increase serum bile acids and their urinary excretion and reduce fat absorption. Bile acids strongly contribute to gallstone formation. Their malabsorption may result in diarrhea, steatorrhea, and urinary and gallstone formation. Quantitation of bile acids in different body fluids and excreta is necessary for understanding physiological and especially pathophysiological aspects of bile acids and cholesterol metabolism. The present paper will deal briefly with quantitation of bile acids in biological materials and metabolism of bile acids in different forms of hyperlipoproteinemias mainly in familial hypercholesterolemia and hypertriglyceridemia.

DETERMINATION OF BILE ACIDS

Enzymic methods. Three enzymes 3α-, 7α-, 12α-hydroxysteroid dehydrogenases (HSD) have been used for quantitation of bile acids especially in serum and bile or isolated bile acids from different sources.[1] Three α-HSD is most widely used and it measures total bile acids quite specifically and sensitively provided the enzyme preparation is pure. However, the presence of 3β-OH, $3 = 0$ or sulfation or glucuronidation at the 3 position results in underestimation. This may be the case in subjects with liver diseases and feces frequently contains 3β-OH bile acids even under normal conditions (see Fig. 1). Isolation of different bile acids or their conjugates by thinlayer chromatography (TLC) or high pressure liquid chromatography (HPLC) should preceed enzymic estimation of individual bile acids. Alternatively, the three major bile acids (cholic, cheno and deoxy) can be quantitated by a combined use of the three dehydrogenases.

Radioimmunoassay. Antibodies can be produced against bile acid-protein complexes - usually bile acid-bovine serum albumin complex - and used for radioimmunoassay of that bile acid in usual manner (cf. 1). Each bile acid should have its own antibody so that the method is suitable for the quantitation of individual bile acids provided the antibodies are specific enough. One of the major problems actually is the cross-reactivity of antibodies and difficulties in the determination of total bile acids in biological materials. Thus, for the fecal bile acids with mainly bacterial transformation products (see Fig. 1) and to some extent for the urinary bile acids, especially under diseased conditions,[2] this is quite impossible.

HPLC. Separation of complex bile acid mixtures with HPLC appears to be quite successfull from many biological materials (cf. 1). However, the simultaneous presence of free bile acids, perhaps with a wide variety of transformation products, and taurine- and glycineconjugated and sulphated bile acids forms such a mixture that is not separated totally but require preliminary group isolation, e.g. with TLC or ionexchange chromatography. Another problem of HPLC is the lack of specified detection of separated components. Ultraviolet spectrophotometry, directly or after derivatization, differential refractometry and 3α-HSD are most commonly used detection methods. Any masking of 3α-OH results in underestimation of effluent bile acids.

Gas-liquid chromatography (GLC). The use of capillary columns has markedly increased sensitivity and specificity of GLC in the determination of the bile acids (see Fig. 1). Owing to high resolution power great many individual bile acids can be separated and quantitated in each run yet the complex mixtures of fecal and urinary bile acids still show some overlapping and require preliminary group separation. Also, free and conjugated bile acids

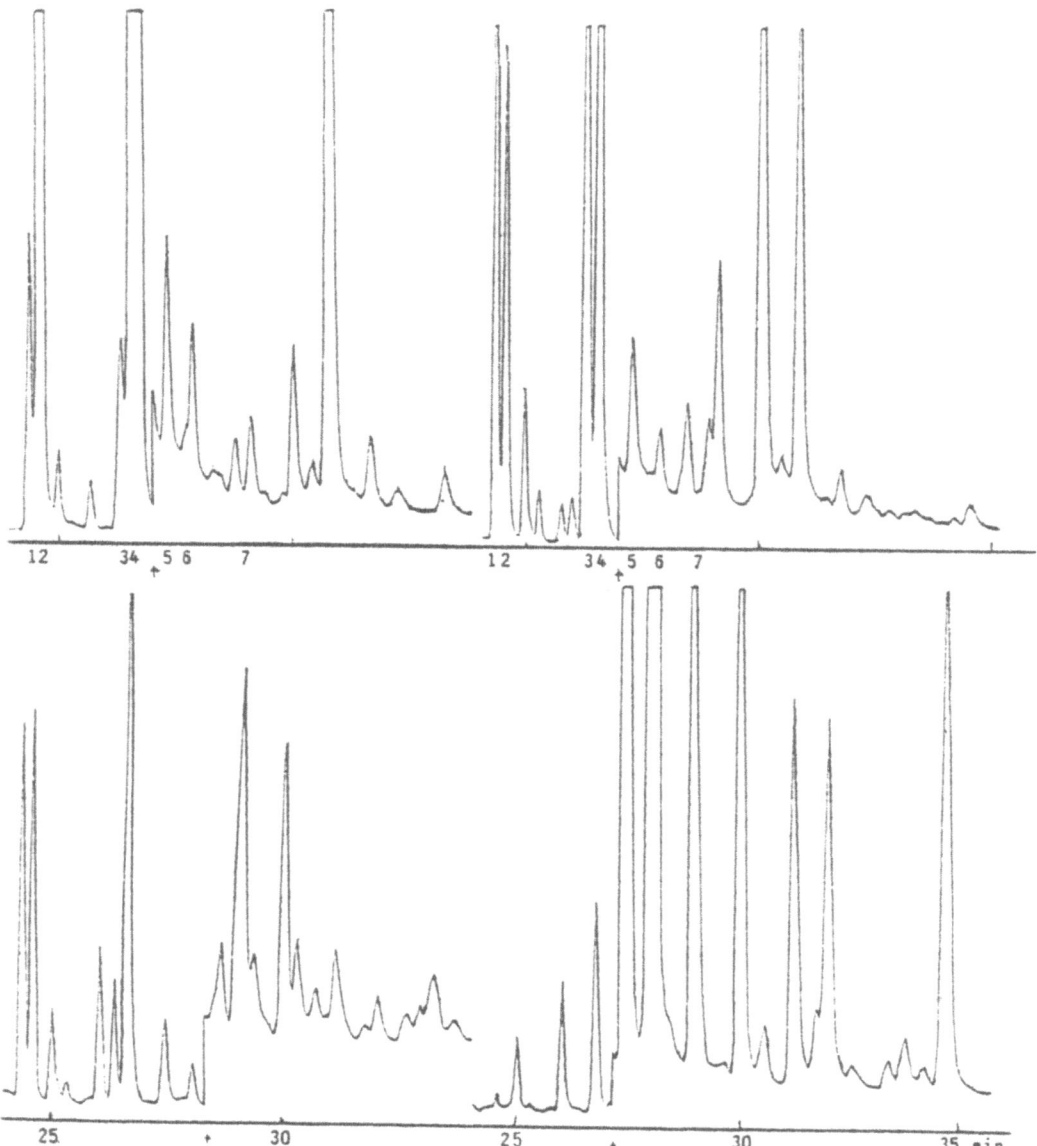

Fig. 1. Gas-liquid chromatographic runs of fecal bile acids on
OV-1 capillary column. Identifications according to retention times
of available standards: 1. isolithocholic acid, 2. cholic acid, 3.
isodeoxycholic acid, 4. deoxycholic acid, 5. chenodeoxycholic
acid, 6. cholic acid, 7. ursodeoxycholic acid. Run from a patient
with ileal dysfunction (lower panel on right hand side) shows
presence of mainly primary bile acids and derivatives without
7-dehydroxylation. Increase of sensitivity by a factor of four
indicated by small arrows.

have to be first group isolated. Preparation of samples for GLC is usually time-consuming and require extraction, purification, deconjugation of glycine-, taurine- and sulphate conjugates, methylation of the carboxyl group and derivatization of hydroxyl groups. Combination of GLC with mass spectrometry allows to identify and quantitate bile acids with a high accuracy.[2-4]

Quantitation of bile acid synthesis. Bulk measurement of fecal bile acids with GLC (cf. 5) is quite simple at the moment and has been widely used for quantitation of total bile acid synthesis. The use of nonpolar capillary column is preferable for routin work. The complexity of the fecal bile acid mixture requires extensive technique for quantitation of individual bile acids of cholic acid and chenodeoxycholic acid origin or their different conjugates.[4] According to our experience about 80% of the fecal bile acids in normal feces can be identified with a reasonable accuracy from the GLC run on capillary column to originate from either cholic or chenodeoxycholic acid. Usually litho and deoxycholic acids are major fractions but sometimes 3β-OH bile acids can predominate. In bile acid malabsorption 7-dehydroxylated derivatives are frequently lacking or small and the presence of 7β-OH and/or ketonic transformation products can be conspicious (see Fig. 1).

Bile acid synthesis can also be measured isotopically. Of these procedures Lindstedt's method[6] is widely used because it permits the measurement of the pool size, turnover and synthesis rates of the two primary bile acids separately provided that the two differently labeled bile acids are administered and that the ^{3}H-label is tightly bound and is not subjected to losses due to tritium exchange. The method may not be valid in gross bile acid malabsorption due to incomplete mixing of the labels within the bile acid pool. Comparison of the quantitative data obtained with this and GLC methods have given similar and even markedly different results (cf. 7). Usually the values of the isotopic procedure are somewhat higher than those of the GLC method, a discrepancy which has no explanation at the moment even when the nonspecific losses of tritium is taken into consideration. Hypertriglyceridemic subjects in particular produce much more bile acids on the basis of the isotopic than chemical balance.[7-9]

BILE ACID PRODUCTION IN HYPERLIPIDEMIA

Chylomicronemia with type I hyperlipoproteinemia (lipoprotein lipase deficiency) appears to have quite normal bile acid production.[10] Normalization of serum lipid levels with a low fat diet does not seem to change consistently bile acid synthesis. However, chylomicronemia with type V lipoprotein pattern has markedly high bile acid synthesis especially that of cholic acid when measured with the isotope dilution technique.[11] On the other hand, chemical balance data indicate that the production is within normal limits.[10] The discrepancy between the different results could be explainable partly by methodological problems and partly by patient selection.

Familial hypercholesterolemia (Type II) with tendon xanthomata is characterized by lacking LDL receptor activity in homozygous and by 50% reduced activity in heterozygous subjects.[12] LDL is catabolized slowly via non-receptor pathway only, resulting in a markedly high LDL cholesterol level. Cholesterol and bile acid synthesis appear to differ between homozygotes and heterozygotes. Earlier studies showed that in heterozygotes bile acid production was fairly low and was negatively correlated with the serum cholesterol level.[13] Subsequent studies on a larger number of subjects (Table 1) revealed that the mean bile acid synthesis was actually subnormal, the basal values being poorly correlated with age.[14-16] In heterozygous children the basal values appear to be within normal limits with no clear age-association.[17] Obesity[18] and hypertriglyceridemia[8-11,14-17] are frequently, though not invariably, associated with increased bile acid production. As shown in Table 1 these conditions when associated with familial hypercholesterolemia do not appear to increase fecal bile acids.

Table 1. Serum lipids and fecal bile acids in patients with familial hypercholesterolemia subgrouped according to obesity and hypertriglyceridemia. Mean$\pm$SE.

Group	No	Relative weight	Serum lipids, mmol/l		Fecal bile acids	
			Triglycer.	Cholesterol	µmol/day	µmol/kg /day
Controls	13	0.96$\pm$0.02	1.00$\pm$0.09	5.2$\pm$0.3	638$\pm$67	10.2$\pm$0.5
All subjects	69	1.22$\pm$0.02	1.49$\pm$0.07	11.9$\pm$0.4	472$\pm$24	7.2$\pm$0.3
Lean IIA	42	1.06$\pm$0.02	1.28$\pm$0.08	11.6$\pm$0.5	469$\pm$27	7.5$\pm$0.3
Lean IIB	12	1.06$\pm$0.03	2.27$\pm$0.10	13.3$\pm$0.8	381$\pm$56	6.4$\pm$0.8
Obese IIA	11	1.32$\pm$0.04	1.23$\pm$0.13	12.1$\pm$0.4	461$\pm$64	7.0$\pm$0.5
Obese IIB	4	1.39$\pm$0.10	2.47$\pm$0.12	11.3$\pm$1.1	751$\pm$46	7.8$\pm$0.3
Obese	15	1.34$\pm$0.04	1.56$\pm$0.19	11.9$\pm$0.3	539$\pm$59	7.2$\pm$0.5
IIB	16	1.14$\pm$0.05	2.32$\pm$0.10	12.8$\pm$0.7	472$\pm$59	6.7$\pm$0.5

Recent concept on hepatic cholesterol traffic[12] suggests that hepatic LDL receptors and hepatocyte cholesterol synthesis are interrelated. Low transport of LDL to hepatocyte by markedly reduced receptor activity should increase synthesis in heterozygous subjects. However, sterol balance data indicate that the whole body synthesis is within the low normal limits and hepatic synthesis could be even subnormal.[19] Low hepatic synthesis has

Table 2. Serum lipids, fecal bile acids and cholesterol synthesis before and after cholestyramine treatment in patients with different types of hyperlipoproteinemias. Mean$\pm$SE.

Type	No.	Serum lipids, mmol/l		Synthesis, µmol/kg/day		Cheno[a]
		Cholesterol	Triglyc.	Bile acids	Cholesterol	
Normal	6	5.2$\pm$0.4	0.86$\pm$0.09	11.0$\pm$1.3	37.8$\pm$6.2	39
		3.7$\pm$0.2	0.98$\pm$0.14	105.9$\pm$9.9	137.5$\pm$14.2	35
IIAX	12	11.2$\pm$0.5	1.20$\pm$0.11	7.2$\pm$0.8	30.3$\pm$3.2	49
		8.4$\pm$0.6	1.15$\pm$0.11	46.9$\pm$4.0	69.7$\pm$5.4	40
IIBX	6	12.1$\pm$1.4	3.04$\pm$0.67	7.8$\pm$0.8	32.7$\pm$4.8	46
		8.0$\pm$0.9	2.95$\pm$1.20	44.2$\pm$10.5	72.1$\pm$16.4	39
IIAXH	1	30.9	2.06	4.6	47.7	76
		31.1	2.00	95.2	144.0	37
IIAXM	1	9.9	0.80	5.1	24.9	44
		6.4	0.73	32.4	51.7	35
IIAXF	1	11.5	1.60	7.0	22.5	46
		8.9	2.14	48.0	66.2	55
IIAXH	1	26.7	1.00	19.0	67.8	43
		24.4	1.52	185.3	255.5	40
IIAXM	1	10.6	1.11	12.6	38.1	45
		5.9	1.19	100.8	142.9	39
IIAXF	1	8.7	0.92	9.9	35.7	44
		6.8	0.98	115.6	134.6	33
IIXH[b]	23	19.4$\pm$1.0	1.44$\pm$0.18	14.2$\pm$2.1	38.3$\pm$4.0	–
IIXH[c]	8	21.4$\pm$1.9	2.19$\pm$0.49	12.7$\pm$2.0	38.6$\pm$5.1	–
		21.7$\pm$1.7	2.33$\pm$0.36	124.0$\pm$17.3	166.6$\pm$20.6	
IIB[d]	7	7.9	3.47$\pm$0.48	10.2$\pm$1.3	36.2$\pm$4.3	42
		6.3	3.67$\pm$0.78	48.5$\pm$6.2	72.1$\pm$9.1	38
IV[e]	7	7.0	4.90$\pm$1.27	12.6$\pm$1.3	46.1$\pm$5.9	41
		6.0	6.54$\pm$1.67	57.9$\pm$4.0	85.5$\pm$8.0	42

X = tendon xanthomata, H = homozygous, M = mother, F = father; second values after cholestyramine treatment. [a]Cheno (% of total) include fecal bile acids of chenodeoxycholic acid origin. [b]Basal values collected from ref. 25-34; bile acids measured in 22 subjects. [c]Two present cases and patients from ref. 26,28,29. [d]Mainly from combined hyperlipoproteinemic families. [e]Mainly from hypertriglyceridemic families.

been found also in Watanabe rabbits with animal model of familial hypercholesterolemia.[20] In view of the markedly increased LDL level of heterozygous subjects it can be hypothesized that the absolute transfer of LDL via the receptor-mediated mechanism is almost within the normal limits and that via the non-receptor mechanisms is increased proportionately to LDL level. This would provide sufficiently cholesterol to hepatocyte to keep cholesterol synthesis within a relatively low level. Since newly synthesized cholesterol appears to be preferentially utilized for bile acid synthesis[21] low hepatic cholesterol production could be a reason for the low bile acid synthesis in heterozygous familial hypercholesterolemia. In fact, the base line bile acid values of Table 2 were significantly correlated with the basal cholesterol synthesis ($r = 0.746$) but the fraction of newly formed cholesterol converted to bile acids is not associated with cholesterol synthesis. This could indicate that impaired bile acid reabsorption hardly determines base line cholesterol synthesis. Fecal bile acid output can be limited by low biliary secretion. However, studies on direct measurement have revealed that biliary bile acid secretion is normal or may be even higher than in the controls.[22] Thus, in view of low fecal bile acids reabsorption should be effective contributing to low hepatic bile acid and cholesterol synthesis. The small bile acid pool size and low serum bile acid concentrations (cf. 23) should indicate rapid and numerous enterohepatic cycles in familial hypercholesterolemia.

Earlier studies suggested that the response of cholesterol and bile acid synthesis to cholestyramine is clearly subnormal in familial hypercholesterolemia (cf. 24). Subsequent investigations revealed, however, that two factors older age and low base line values could have been involved (Table 2, Fig. 2).[24] Subgrouping of 46 patients with familial hypercholesterolemia by ten-year age-periods showed that the youngest age group of 27 years was matched with controls, had about 3 µmol/kg/day lower basal bile acid synthesis than the controls but on cholestyramine increased bile acid production more than the older age-groups but clearly less than the age-matched normocholesterolemic controls. On the other hand, a hypercholesterolemic subgroup with a lowest basal bile acid synthesis responded to cholestyramine less than the other subgroups with the higher basal values. However, the few controls and patients with similar base-line bile acid synthesis appeared to respond fairly similarly to cholestyramine. Thus, Table 2 shows that the parents of the high-producing hypercholesterolemic family have quite similar pre- and postcholestyramine bile acid and cholesterol synthesis rates with the controls.

Homozygous patients usually children with familial hypercholesterolemia exhibit low to high bile acid (3-42 µmol/kg/day) and cholesterol (19-91 µmol/kg/day) synthesis rates under basal conditions[25-34] so that the effect of double dose of hypercholesterolemic gene cannot be easily visualized. However, the mean bile acid synthesis of 22 homozygotes[25,26,28-34] published so far (14$\pm$2 µmol/kg/day) appears to exeed that of heterozygous or even normal subjects (Table 2), some cases having exceptionally high levels. Despite markedly high serum cholesterol the absolute transport of LDL cholesterol to the liver, exclusively via the non-receptor pathway, may be subnormal. Thus, hepatic cholesterol synthesis actually tends to be high (38 ± 4 μmol/kg/day) in the 23 homozygotes of Table 2. The cholesterol and bile acid synthesis rates are not correlated with age (r = -0.151, and -0.137) or serum cholesterol (r = 0.232 and 0.022) but are interrelated (r = 0.731), the fraction of newly synthesized cholesterol eliminated as bile acids ($33 \pm 3\%$) being not associated with cholesterol synthesis (r = 0.032). The finding on two families in Table 2 indicate that in the homozygous children with double dose of the mutant familial hypercholesterolemia gene cholesterol and bile acid synthesis is about twice that of their heterozygous parents with only one dose of the mutant gene both under the base-line conditions and especially during the cholestyramine-induced increase in cholesterol synthesis. Cholesterol and bile acid productions appear to be genetically determined so that depending on the parents the synthesis rates can vary from low to high in different hypercholesterolemic families. The differences in cholesterol and bile acid metabolism between families and family members appear to be accentuated by cholestyramine and the pre- and posttreatment values are interrelated. Since the newly formed hepatic cholesterol may be preferentially utilized for bile acid synthesis[21] it can be hypothesized that the basal bile acid synthesis and the cholestyramine response is high in the subjects in whom the hepatocyte cholesterol requirement is predominantly covered by own synthesis and to a smaller extent by the uptake of plasma lipoproteins. Thus, the homozygous children with lacking or very low receptor-mediated uptake of LDL cholesterol actually had a very high response to cholestyramine.

A closer analysis of bile acid metabolism with the isotope dilution technique has shown that the low bile acid production in hypercholesterolemia is mainly due to low cholic acid synthesis.[8,9,11,23] This may be related to low hepatic cholesterol synthesis because the cholic acid and cholesterol synthesis rates appear to be interrelated.[21] Cholestyramine actually increases cholic acid synthesis especially in hypercholesterolemic subjects with a low basal cholic acid and cholesterol production. Table 2 shows that the relative amount of cheno is actually quite high in hypercholesterolemic subjects and is lowered by cholestyramine in most subgroups.

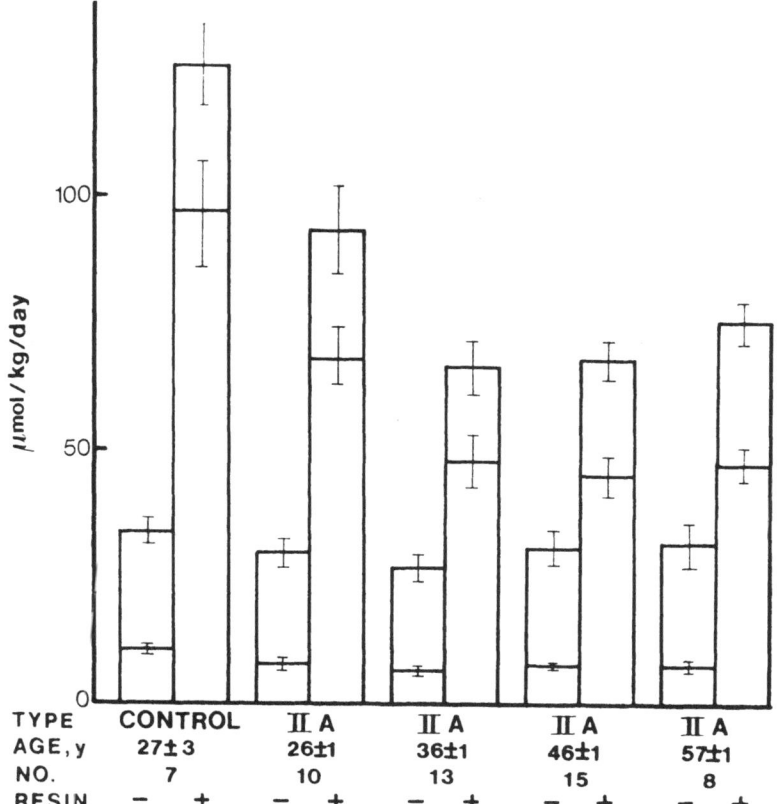

TYPE   **CONTROL**   **Ⅱ A**   **Ⅱ A**   **Ⅱ A**   **Ⅱ A**

AGE, y   27±3   26±1   36±1   46±1   57±1

NO.   7   10   13   15   8

RESIN   − +   − +   − +   − +   − +

Fig. 2. Effects of cholestyramine (resin 32 g/day) on cholesterol (whole bar) and bile acid (lower part of bar) synthesis in controls and patients with familial xanthomatotic type IIA subgrouped by age. Vertical lines indicate standard errors of means.

Familial combined hyperlipoproteinemia has been considered to exhibit enhanced apoB production,[35,36] resulting in expression of either type IIA, IIB or IV hyperlipoprotein pattern. The type IIA subjects apparently have no marked abnormality in their bile acid production because poorly defined mildly hypercholesterolemic subjects (may include polygenic forms) have fecal bile acid values which are not strikingly different from those in normal subjects or xanthomatotic hypercholesterolemic subjects but respond relatively poorly to cholestyramine.[14-16,24] The same appears to be true with sporadic or polygenic hypercholesterolemia, eventhough the two groups have not been studied carefully. Despite enhanced VLDL turnover subjects with type IIB abnormality have normal or relatively low bile acid production and as the subjects with xanthomatotic IIB hypercholesterolemia the response of bile acid and cholesterol synthesis to cholestyramine is quite limited (Table 2).[15,24] However, relatively high rates of bile acid synthesis has also been reported,[8,16] indicating that the entity might be heterogenous.

Type III hyperlipoproteinemia may be associated with increased VLDL production and abnormal elimination of VLDL remnants. Bile acid and cholesterol synthesis appear to be within normal limits.[10] However, the use of the isotopic technique has indicated that bile acid production is about twice that in hyperlipoproteinemia type II and is not different from that in type IV.[37] The net cholesterol synthesis may have been within the normal level on a fairly high dietary cholesterol intake.

Primary type IV hyperlipoproteinemia is associated with enhanced VLDL production and/or impaired VLDL removal and caused mostly by familial hypertriglyceridemia or combined hyperlipoproteinemia. There has been a lot of discussion on a causative association between enhanced VLDL production and bile acid and cholesterol synthesis.[8-11,16,23] Some evidence has also been presented that a primary change in bile acid and cholesterol synthesis would alter secondarily VLDL synthesis.

Earlier sterol balance studies showed that bile acid synthesis is frequently but not consistently increased in hypertriglyceridemic patients particularly when measured with the isotope dilution technique.[8,11,16,18,23] Furthermore, a negative correlation between serum cholesterol and fecal bile acids indicated that the lower the LDL level the higher the bile acid synthesis in hypertriglyceridemic patients.[15] In view of the current concept on VLDL metabolism in type IV,[35,36] the finding suggests that enhanced VLDL catabolism via a non-LDL pathway (low LDL) is associated with increased bile acid and also cholesterol synthesis. An increase of LDL i.e., development of type IIB pattern would then inhibit the production rates possibly via enhanced hepatic uptake of LDL cholesterol.

Despite quite high basal bile acid production the response of bile acid and cholesterol synthesis to cholestyramine is not excessively high in type IV (Table 2). Cholic acid which is predominantly increased in type IV appears to respond quite little to cholestyramine (cf. 8).

Table 3. Correlation of bile acid and cholesterol synthesis with serum lipids and triglyceride metabolism in two families (n = 17) with familial hypertriglyceridemia

Lipid	Bile acids		Cholesterol	
	mg/day	mg/kg/day	mg/day	mg/kg/day
Cholesterol				
VLDL, mmol/l	0.775*	0.525*	0.753*	0.544*
LDL, mmol/l	0.349	0.156	0.180	-0.034
HDL, mmol/l	-0.634	-0.374	-0.795*	-0.624*
Total, mmol/l	0.286	0.133	0.036	-0.171
Triglycerides				
VLDL, mmol/l	0.820*	0.576*	0.794*	0.595*
Total, mmol/l	0.815*	0.563*	0.774*	0.561*
†VLDL, FCR	-0.585*	-0.149	-0.696*	-0.461
†Total, FCR	-0.499*	-0.373	-0.507*	-0.382
†VLDL, mg/kg/h	0.451	0.041	0.677*	0.297
†Total, mg/kg/h	0.584*	0.225	0.702*	0.421
Fecal bile acids	1.000	1.000	0.801*	0.729*

VLDL-triglyceride range 0.18-2.91 mmol/l. None had increased LDL cholesterol. †Fractional catabolic rate (FCR) and turnover of triglyceride measured with ^{3}H-glycerol technique, *$p<0.05$ (Tilvis et al. Unpublished observations)

Type IV subjects in families with combined hyperlipoproteinemia have an elevated production of VLDL-triglycerides as the major cause of hypertriglyceridemia and this is frequently associated with increased bile acid and/or cholesterol synthesis.[38] On the other hand, type IV subjects with a poorly defined mostly familial hypertriglyceridemia and with a frequent overproduction and reduced clearance of VLDL-triglycerides appear to have only infrequently increased synthesis of bile acids and cholesterol.[38] However, in the two entities bile acid and/or cholesterol synthesis rates appear to correlate with the production rate of VLDL triglycerides. Our studies on familial hypertriglyceridemia (Table 3) with a predominant overproduction of VLDL-triglycerides of affected family members indicate that the high serum concentrations and increased production rates of VLDL and total triglycerides are frequently associated with enhanced bile acid and cholesterol synthesis. The latter appear to correlate negatively with the VLDL-triglyceride clearance and HDL cholesterol.

REFERENCES

1. J. M. Street, D. J. H. Trafford and H. L. J. Makin, The quantitative estimation of bile acids and their conjugates in human biological fluids. J Lipid Res 24:491 (1983).
2. A. Bremmelgaard and J. Sjövall, Bile acid profiles in urine of patients with liver diseases. Eur J Clin Invest 9:341 (1979).
3. B. Alme, A. Bremmelgaard, J. Sjövall and P. Thomassen, Analysis of metabolic profiles of bile acids in urine using lipophilic anion exchanger and computerized gas-liquid chromatography-mass spectrometry. J Lipid Res 18:339 (1977).
4. K. D. R. Setchell, A. M. Lawson, N. Tanida and J. Sjövall, General methods for the analysis of metabolic profiles of bile acids and related compounds in feces. J Lipid Res 24:1085 (1983).
5. S. M. Grundy, E. H. Ahrens, Jr. and T. A. Miettinen, Quantitative isolation and gas-liquid chromatographic analysis of total fecal bile acids. J Lipid Res 6:397(1965).
6. S. Lindstedt, The turnover of cholic acid in man. Acta Physiol Scand 40:1 (1957).
7. N. O. Davidsen, P. Samuel, S. Lieberman, S. P. Shane, J. R. Crouse and E. H. Ahrens, Jr. Measurement of bile acid production in hyperlipidemic man: does phonotype or methodology make the difference? J Lipid Res 22:620 (1981).
8. K. Hellström, Bile acid metabolism in hyperlipoproteinemia. in: "Bile Acids and Lipids," P. Paumgartner, A. Stiehl and W. Gerok, eds., MTP, Lancaster, 5 (1981).
9. B. Angelin, K. Einarsson and B. Leijd, Bile acids and triglyceride metabolism in man. in: "Bile Acids and Lipids," P. Paumgartner, A. Stiehl and W. Gerok, eds., MTP, Lancaster, 225 (1981).
10. S. M. Grundy, E. H. Ahrens, Jr., G. Salen, P.H. Schreibman and P. Nestel, Mechanism of action clofibrate on cholesterol metabolism in patients with hyperlipidemia. J Lipid Res 13:531 (1972).
11. K. Einarsson and K. Hellström, The formation of bile acids in patients with three types of hyperlipoproteinaemia. Eur J Clin Invest 2:225 (1972).
12. M. S. Brown and J. L. Goldstein, Lipoprotein receptors in the liver. Control signals for plasma cholesterol traffic. J Clin Invest 72:743 (1983).
13. T. A. Miettinen, R. Pelkonen, E. A. Nikkilä and O. Heinonen, Low excretion of fecal bile acids in a family with hypercholesterolemia. Acta Med Scand 182:645 (1967).
14. T. A. Miettinen, Clinical implications of bile acid metabolism in man. in: "The Bile Acids," P. P. Nair and D. Kritchevsky, eds., Plenum Press, New York, 2:191 (1973).

15. T. A. Miettinen, Bile acid metabolism. in: "Handbook of Experimental Pharmacology: Pharmacology of Hypolipidemic Agents," Springer-Verlag, Berlin-Heidelberg-New York 109 (1975).

16. H. S. Sodhi, B. Kudchodkar and D. T. Mason, Cholesterol metabolism in clinical hyperlipidemias. Adv Lipid Res 17:107 (1980).

17. J. H. Zavoral, D. C. Laine, L. K. Bale, D. L. Wellik, R. D. Ellefson, K. Kuba, W. Krivit and B. A. Kottke, Cholesterol excretion studies in familial hypercholesterolemic children and their normolipidemic siblings. Am J Clin Nutr 35:1360 (1982).

18. T. A. Miettinen, Cholesterol production in obesity. Circulation 44:842 (1971).

19. T. A. Miettinen, New insights into cholesterol dynamics. Arch Surg 113:45 (1978).

20. J. M. Dietschy, T. Kita, K. E. Suckling and J. L. Goldstein, Cholesterol synthesis in vivo and in vitro in the WHHL rabbit, an animal with defective low density lipo-protein receptors. J Lipid Res 24:469 (1983).

21. I. Björkhem and A. Lewenhaupt, Preferential utilization of newly synthesized cholesterol as substrate for bile acid bio-synthesis. J Biol Chem 254:5252 (1979).

22. T. A. Miettinen, Hyperlipidemia, bile acid metabolism and gallstones. Ital J Gastroenterol 10:Suppl 1:53 (1978).

23. B. Angelin, Cholesterol and bile acid metabolism in normo- and hyperlipoproteinaemia. Acta Med Scand Suppl:1 (1977).

24. T.A. Miettinen, Effects of hypolipidemic drugs on bile acid metabolism in man. Adv in Lipid Res 18:65 (1981).

25. B. Lewis and N. B. Myant, Studies in the metabolism of cholesterol in subjects with normal plasma cholesterol levels and in patients with essential hypercholesterolemia. Clin Sci (Oxf) 32:201 (1967).

26. C. D. Moutafis and N. B. Myant, The metabolism of choles-terol in two hypercholesterolaemic patients treated with cholestyramine. Clin Sci 37:443 (1969).

27. P. Samuel, W. Perl, C. M. Holtzman, N. D. Rochman and S. Lieberman, Long-term kinetics of serum and xanthoma cholesterol radioactivity in patients with hypercholes-terolemia. J Clin Invest 51: 266 (1972).

28. S. M. Grundy, E. H. Ahrens, Jr. and G. Salen, Inter-ruption of the enterohepatic circulation of bile acids in man: comparative effects of cholestyramine and ileal exclusion on cholesterol metabolism. J Lab Clin Med 78:94 (1971).

29. C. D. Moutafis, L. A. Simons, N.B. Myant, P. W. Adams and V. Wynn, The effect of cholesteryramine on the faecal excretion of bile acids and neutral steroids in familial hypercholesterolaemia. Atherosclerosis 26:329 (1977).

30. G. M. Martin and P. Nestel, Changes in cholesterol metabolism with dietary cholesterol in children with familial hypercholesterolaemia. Clin Sci 56:377 (1979).

31. K. B. Schwartz, J. Witztum, G. Schonfeld, S. M. Grundy and W. E. Connor, Elevated cholesterol and bile acid synthesis in a young patient with homozygous familial hypercholesterolemia. J Clin Invest 64:756 (1979).
32. G. A. Carter, W. E. Connor. A. K. Bhattacharyya and D. S. Lin, The cholesterol turnover synthesis and absorption in two sisters with familial hypercholesterolemia (type II a). J Lipid Res 20:66 (1979).
33. P. W. Stacpoole, S. M. Grundy, L. L. Swift, H. L. Greene, A. E. Slonim and I. M. Burr, Elevated cholesterol and bile acid synthesis in an adult patient with homozygous familial hypercholesterolemia. Reduction by a high glucose diet. J Clin Invest 68:1166 (1981).
34. D. J. McNamara, E. H. Ahrens, Jr., R. Kolb, C. D. Brown, T. S. Parker, N. O. Davidson, P. Samuel and R. M. McVie, Treatment of familial hypercholesterolemia by portacaval anastomosis: Effect on cholesterol metabolism and pool sizes. Proc Natl Acad Sci USA 80:564 (1983).
35. A. Chait, J. J. Albers and J. D. Brunzell, Very low density lipoprotein overproduction in genetic forms of hypertriglyceridaemia. Eur J Clin Invest 10:17 (1980).
36. A. H. Kissebah, S. Alfarsi and P. W. Adams, Integrated regulation of very low density lipoprotein triglyceride and apolipoprotein-B kinetics in man: normolipemic subjects, familial hypertriglyceridemia and familial combined hyperlipidemia. Metabolism 30:856 (1981).
37. E. Andersson, Metabolism of cholesterol and bile acids in normo and hyperlipidaemic subjects. Acta Med Scand Suppl 643 (1980)
38. U. Beil, S. M. Grundy, J. R. Crouse and L. Zech, Triglyceride and cholesterol metabolism in primary hypertriglyceridemia. Arteriosclerosis 2:44 (1982).

EFFECTS OF LIPID LOWERING DIETS AND OF BILE ACID SEQUESTRANTS ON PLASMA LIPOPROTEINS AND BILIARY METABOLISM

Cesare R. Sirtori

Director Center E. Grossi Paoletti, Institute of Pharmacology and Pharmacognosy
Professor of Chemotherapy, University of Milano
20129 Milano, Italy

INTRODUCTION

The effects of diets and/or of bile acid sequestrants on plasma lipid levels is well established (1,2). The role of changes in the biliary composition in eliciting the lipoprotein changes is, however, less clear. Object of this report will be to describe the pattern of abnormalities of bile acid (BA) composition in hyperlipoproteinemic patients; moreover, the effects of different diets (high polyunsaturates; high fiber; soy proteins) and of BA sequestrants will be evaluated.

Bile acid composition in hyperlipoproteinemia

Abnormalities in the excretion of BA were observed in the early studies on fecal fat and steroid excretion of hyper-lipoproteinemic patients. Miettinen and Aro (3) first noted that subjects with familial type II hypercholesterolemia have a subnormal fecal BA excretion, whereas this same tends to be elevated in type IV hypertriglyceridemics. Similar findings were later on reported by Nestel and Hunter (4), who, in particular, could find a highly significant increase of BA elimination in type IV patients.

The abnormally low BA levels in hypercholesterolemics could be linked to a reduced biosynthesis (5), based upon kinetic studies with ^{14}C-cholic and ^{3}H-chenodeoxycholic acids. On the average, cholic acid (CA) production represents less than 50% of total BA synthesis in both types IIA and IIB hyperlipoproteinemic patients (in controls it is 64+2%). In contrast, out of the 27 examined patients with a type IV hyperlipidemia pattern, 18 had a biosynthesis of CA and of CA+chenodeoxycholic acid (CDCA) exceeding the upper range of normals. In these same subjects, CA formation represented 73+3% of the total BA synthesis. A reduction of synthesis (for both CA and CDCA) was also noted in type IIB and IV patients following weight reduction (5).

A possible exception to this pattern may be that of patients with homozygous familiar type II hypercholesterolemia, where it appears that both cholesterol and BA biosynthesis is distinctly increased (approximately three times higher than normal) (6). In a recent study, administration of a high glucose diet (Vivonex) to one of such patients, resulted in a dramatic reduction of both neutral and acidic steroid elimination (7).

Studies on the composition of BA in the bile of hyperlipo-proteinemic patients have initially suggested that the duodenal bile is relatively enriched with primary BA (CA and CDCA) in type II individuals, whereas the percentage composition of the secondary BA deoxycholic acid (DCA) is higher in type IV (8). More recently, Ahlberg et al. (9) could describe a relative cholesterol supersaturation in type IIB and IV patients (to a lesser extent in type IIA) and, moreover, provided definitive evidence for an enrichment of secondary BA in both types IIB and IV individuals (Table 1). In type IIA, the percentage distri-bution of BA is essentially normal, whereas in the other hyperlipoproteinemia phenotypes reductions of, respectively, CA for type IIB and CDCA for type IV are detectable. In partial confirmation of these findings in the duodenal bile, a signifi-cant reduction of serum CA levels, was recently described in type IIB and IV individuals (10).

Table 1. Bile Acid Composition in Hyperlipoproteinemia

	CA	CDCA	DCA
N	39.1 + 2.9	37.7 + 3.0	3.2 + 3.9
IIA	44.2 + 1.9	35.0 + 1.0	20.8 + 2.4
IIB	29.4 + 3.6*°°	31.9 + 3.0	38.7 + 4.2*°°
IV	35.7 + 2.9	30.5 + 1.7*°	33.8 + 3.2*°°

$*$ $p < 0.05$ vs normal; $°$ $p < 0.05$; $°°$ $p < 0.01$ vs type IIA

Effects of different diets on bile acid composition

The effects of therapeutic diets for hyperlipidemias on BA composition may be widely different. We may consider here the case of diets enriched with polyunsaturated fatty acids (PUFA), undigestible fibers and vegetable vs animal proteins.

The effect of **PUFA rich diets** on plasma cholesterol is well established (1). The mechanism whereby this effect is elicited is, however, still far from clear. Early studies (11) compared the fecal steroid excretory pattern of normal individuals receiving, in sequence, a PUFA rich (corn oil) formula diet, and a similar diet enriched with cocoa butter. There was definite indication for an increased fecal excretion both of neutral steroids (NS) and BA during the formulated corn oil regimen (Table 2).

Although these findings may apply to normolipidemic individuals, there is no consensus that this may be a general mechanism of action of PUFA (12). In fact, Grundy and Ahrens (13) later on reported that a comparative evaluation of fecal steroid excretion in hypercholesterolemic patients, treated with a saturated and with a PUFA rich diet, failed to show significant changes in either the NS or BA elimination with the latter (Table 3). In a more recent report on the effects of saturated and PUFA diets in hypertriglyceridemic patients, Grundy (14), could however show that some significant changes do occur in the biliary BA distribution. In particular, the primary bile acid CA is significantly increased during PUFA, whereas DCA is reduced approximately 30% compared to a saturated diet (Table 4). Whether this last finding may be consequent to an accelerated BA turnover, is yet to be defined.

Table 2. Fecal Steroid Excretion During Diets Rich in Polyunsaturated Fatty Acids

| mg/24 h | Normals, n=10; x±SEM (Connor et al.,1969) | | |
	Cocoa Butter	Corn Oil	Cocoa Butter
Neutral Steroids	410±24	489±24**	385±43
Bile Acids	299±44	426±49**	244±36
Total	709±64	915±62**	629±70

** $p < 0.01$ vs Cocoa Butter.

103

Table 3. Fecal Steroid Excretion during Polyunsaturated Diets in Type II patients

Type II, n=9; x+SEM (Grundy and Ahrens, 1970)		
mg/24 h	First Period (saturated fat)	Second Period (polyunsaturated fat)
Neutral Steroids	486+38	470+46
Bile Acids	171+25	226+31
Total	658+41	687+52

Table 4. Biliary Lipid Composition during Polyunsaturated Diet

Type IV and V, n=10; x+SEM (Grundy, 1975)			
Mole %	Cholesterol	Bile Acids	Phospholipids
Saturated Diet	8.5+1.2	68.6+2.2	22.8+1.9
PUFA Diet	9.5+0.7	63.4+3.6	27.1+3.1
Bile Acid Distribution %	CA	CDCA	DCA
Saturated Diet	32.7+4.1	31.6+3.0	33.8+3.7
PUFA Diet	45.9+4.3**	29.8+3.0	23.4+4.5**

** $p < 0.01$ vs Saturated Diet.

Treatment with **undigestible fibers** may similarly lead to reduced plasma lipid levels (15). There may be, however, a significant difference between the effects of water insoluble (e.g. bran) and water soluble (e.g. pectin, guar gum) fibers. Careful evaluation of the former, in constipated patients due to diverticular disease, failed to show an increase in either BA or NS elimination (16). Indeed, BA excretion was reduced by bran (Table 5). Interestingly, and similarly to the effects of PUFA, the biliary content of CA was significantly raised by bran.

Among undigestible water soluble fibers, the effect of pectin on plasma cholesterol is well established. In a carefully controlled study of fecal steroids in mildly hypercholesterolemic patients treated with pectin (15 g/day), the plasma cholesterol reduction was accompanied by an increase of both NS and total BA elimination (Table 6)(17). It is noteworthy that fecal fat excretion was almost doubled in these patients during pectin administration.

Table 5. Effect of Bran on Fecal and Biliary Lipids in Diverticular Disease (Tarpila et al., 1978)

n=12, 85 g of wheat bran per day; x+SEM		
	Control	Fiber
Fecal		
Bile Acids	344+89	240+39*
Neutral Steroids	693+136	614+39
Balance	-637+170	-411+85**
Biliary		
CA %	38+5	48+3**
CDCA	40+4	42+3
DCA	22+7	10+3**

* $p < 0.05$ vs Control; ** $p < 0.01$ vs Control.

Table 6. Effects of Pectin on Fecal Steroid Excretion (Kay and Truswell, 1977)

n=9, 3 weeks of pectin (15 g/day) treatment; mean values			
	Control 1	Pectin	Control 2
Fat (g/day)	3.8	8.6**	4.0
Neutral Steroids (mg/day)	335	390**	331
LCA (mg/day)	96	130	92
DCA (mg/day)	160	233	191
Total Bile Acids (mg/day)	265	371**	294

** $p < 0.001$ vs Control.

Vegetable proteins, particularly from soy, exert a remarkable cholesterol lowering activity in type II individuals (18). Our experience, more than a decade long, is supported by a large number of experimental investigations (19,20), ranging from rodents to primates. Animal studies on steroid excretion with soy proteins are definitively suggestive of an enhanced elimination of both BA and NS, compared to a reference casein diet (20). Somewhat similar findings were reported in infants administered a soybean milk, vs children receiving bovine milk (21). On the other hand, cholesterol balance studies, carried out by our group, in type II patients receiving soy with no added cholesterol, could confirm the remarkable cholesterol lowering activity of the experimental diet, but no effect on either the fecal steroid excretion or on the slope of the plasma cholesterol specific activity decay curve (22) (Figure 1) could be demonstrated. It might be of interest to repeat such a study in patients receiving cholesterol together with soy proteins.

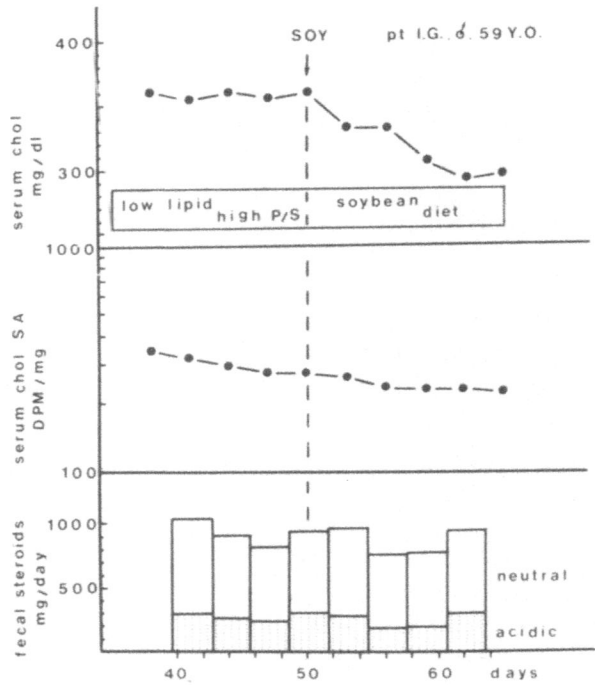

Fig.1 Cholesterol balance study in a type II patient treated with the soybean diet. Following the change from a low lipid diet with animal proteins to the soybean diet, there is a remarkable drop of plasma cholesterol levels, without, however, changes either in fecal steroid output or in the slope of the cholesterol specific activity decay curve (from Fumagalli, et al., 1982)

Effects of anion exchange resins on bile acid metabolism

Synthetic compounds, capable of binding BA in the duodenum (BA sequestrants) are an effective mode of treatment of hypercholesterolemia (2). The recently completed Lipid Research Clinic Study on cholestyramine, provided clearcut evidence for the beneficial activity of a marked plasma cholesterol reduction in preventing myocardial infarction (23).

The mechanism of action of anion exchange resins appears rather simple, at first consideration. BA, when bound, are not reabsorbed and are lost in the feces. In this way, after prolonged treatments (but a significant plasma cholesterol lowering may be noted already after one week) the circulating sterol pool is reduced, with consequent hypocholesterolemia. BA binding and consequent cholesterol drainage do not probably provide a full explanation for the mechanism of action of anion exchange resins. In the first place, they do not clarify the observed insensitivity of homozygous type IIA patients (24), in spite of the significant increase of fecal BA loss even in these. Secondly, in all cases, the intestinal binding of BA is followed by an immediate rise of liver cholesterol biosynthesis and of 7--α hydroxylase (see other presentations in this Symposium); these biochemical changes, although effectively antagonizing the primary drug effect, still fail to counteract the hypo-cholesterolemic activity. Recently, two further hypotheses have been presented. The first relates to an increase of liver high affinity receptors for lipoproteins following treatment, thus improving the physiological mechanism of cholesterol elimination from plasma (25). The second, based on animal findings, indicates that low density lipoproteins (LDL) derived from very low density lipoprotein (VLDL) breakdown are more rapidly and effectively cleared (26), and that a larger fraction of LDL is derived from VLDL catabolism following resin treatment (27).

Differences in the therapeutic response to BA sequestrants may also be dependent upon a variable binding of primary and secondary BA. Earlier studies had indicated that dihydroxy BA are more strongly bound by cholestyramine, compared to trihydroxy BA (28). Among conjugates, binding is higher with taurine- vs glycine-conjugates. The in vitro findings received clinical support by studies in normal men, also showing an elevation of glycine- to taurine-conjugated BA following treatment, as well as a predominance of biliary trihydroxy BA after cholestyramine (29)

More recently, Clain et al. (30), by detailed investigations on the BA binding properties of different antacids and of cholestyramine, could confirm that dihydroxy BA (CDCA and DCA) are far more strongly bound than CA (Table 7). Interestingly, it is apparent that BA binding by aluminum hydroxide shows a similar pattern to that of cholestyramine, thus possibly suggesting a role in BA regulation, and an eventual additivity to cholestyramine. Altogether, definitive support for the specificity of BA binding by cholestyramine, comes from a study in normal obese individuals, where Wood et al. (31) could show that after resin treatment the percentage of CA in bile is close to doubled, versus a consistent decrease of both CDCA and DCA (Table 8). The glycine/taurine (G/T) ratio is also markedly increased after drug treatment, thus supporting the specificity of cholestyramine binding for CDCA, DCA and taurine conjugates.

Table 7. Binding of Bile Acids by Antacids and Resin (Clain et al., 1977)

	% bound; 5 mM of each acid		
	CA	CDCA	DCA
Al (OH)$_3$	51.9	91.1	88.5
Mg (OH)$_2$	4.5	42.5	54.2
Al (OH)$_3$ + Mg (OH)$_2$	26.8	70.5	75.0
Cholestyramine	52.7	85.2	84.6

Table 8. Bile Acid Composition after Cholestyramine in Normal Obese Subjects (Wood et al., 1972)

	4 subjects; 20-26 obese, $x \pm$ SD	
	Off Resin	On Resin
% CA	38.0$\pm$8.4	67.3$\pm$6.2**
% CDCA	37.4$\pm$7.2	26.1$\pm$5.0**
% DCA	25.0$\pm$10.1	6.6$\pm$3.7**
Glycine/Taurine	2.7$\pm$1.0	7.3$\pm$2.6**

** $p < 0.01$ vs Off Resin.

In conclusion, all these studies support major effects of diets and drugs on BA composition. In general, it appears that BA turnover is accelerated both in hyperlipoproteinemias and after diet/drug treatments. The pattern of changes is variable: the percentage of CA in BA is raised during PUFA diets, but reduced after cholestyramine. It might be of interest to examine the sensitivity of patients with different BA patterns to the therapeutic regimens indicated in this report.

REFERENCES

1. J.T. Salonen, P. Puska, and H. Mustaniemi, Changes in morbidity and mortality during comprehensive community programme to control cardiovascular diseases during 1972-73 in North Karelia, Brit. Med. J. 2: 1178 (1979).

2. S.M. Grundy, E.H. Ahrens jr., and G. Salen, Interruption of the intrahepatic circulation of bile acids in man: Comparative effects of cholestyramine and ileal exclusion on cholesterol metabolism, J. Lab. Clin. Med. 78: 94 (1971).

3. T.A. Miettinen and A. Aro, Faecal fat, bile acid excretion, and body height in familial hypercholesterolaemia and hyperglyceridaemia, Scand. J. Clin. Lab. Invest. 30: 85 (1972).

4. P.J. Nestel and J.D. Hunter, Differences in bile acid excretion in subjects with hypercholesterolaemia, hypertriglyceridaemia and overweight, Aust. N.Z. J. Med. 4: 491 (1974).

5. K. Einarsson, K. Hellström, and M. Kallner, Bile acid kinetics in relation to sex, serum lipids, body weights, and gallbladder disease in patients with various types of hyperlipoproteinemia, J. Clin. Invest. 54: 1301 (1974).

6. K.B. Schwarz, J.G. Witztum, G. Schonfeld, S.M. Grundy, and W.E. Conner, Elevated cholesterol and bile acid synthesis in a young patient with homozygous familial hypercholesterolemia, J. Clin. Invest. 64: 756 (1979).

7. P.W. Stacpoole, S.M. Grundy, L.L. Swift, H.L. Greene, A.E. Slonin, and I.M. Burr, Elevated cholesterol and bile acid synthesis in an adult patient with homozygous familial hypercholesterolemia - Reduction by a high glucose diet, J. Clin. Invest. 68: 1166 (1981).

8. K. Einarsson, K. Hellström and M. Kallner, Effect of cholic

acid feeding on bile acid kinetics and neutral fecal steroid excretion in hyperlipoproteinemia (type II and IV). <u>Metabolism</u> 23: 863 (1974).

9. J. Ahlberg, B. Angelin, K. Einarsson, K. Hellström, and B. Leijd, Biliary lipid composition in normo- and hyperlipoproteinemia, <u>Gastroenterology</u> 79: 90 (1980).

10. M. Angelico, F. Angelico, P. Amodeo, A.A. Attili, C. Puoti, G. Ricci, and L. Capocaccia, Individual serum bile acids in patients with primary hyperlipoproteinemias, <u>Atherosclerosis</u> 37: 293 (1980).

11. W.E. Connor, D.T. Witiak, D.B. Stone, and M.L. Armstrong, Cholesterol balance and fecal neutral steroid and bile acid excretion in normal men fed dietary fats of different fatty acid composition, <u>J. Clin. Invest.</u> 48: 1363 (1969).

12. R.L. Jackson, O.D. Taunton, J.D. Morrissett, and A.M. Gotto jr., The role of dietary polyunsaturated fat in lowering blood cholesterol in man, <u>Circ. Res.</u> 42: 447 (1978).

13. S.M. Grundy and E.H. Ahrens jr., The effects of unsaturated dietary fats on absorption, excretion, synthesis, and distribution of cholesterol in man. <u>J. Clin. Invest.</u> 49: 1135 (1970).

14. S.M. Grundy, Effects of polyunsaturated fats on lipid metabolism in patients with hypertriglyceridemia, <u>J. Clin. Invest.</u> 55: 269 (1975).

15. R. Mc Pherson Kay, Dietary fiber, <u>J. Lipid Res.</u> 23: 221 (1982).

16. S. Tarpila, T.A. Miettinen, and L. Metsäranta, Effects of bran on serum cholesterol, faecal mass, fat, bile acid and neutral sterols, and biliary lipids in patients with diverticular disease of the colon, <u>Gut</u> 19: 137 (1978).

17. R.M. Kay and A.S. Truswell, Effects of citrus pectin on blood lipids and fecal steroid excretion in man, <u>Am. J. Clin. Nutr.</u> 30: 171 (1977).

18. C.R. Sirtori, E. Agradi, F. Conti, E. Gatti, and O. Mantero, Soybean protein diet in the treatment of type II hyperlipoproteinaemia, <u>Lancet</u> i: 275 (1977).

19. D.N. Kim, K.T. Lee, J.M. Reiner, and W.A. Thomas, Increased

steroid excretion in swine fed high-fat, high-cholesterol diet with soy protein, Exp. Mol. Pathol. 33: 25 (1980).

20. A.H.M. Terpstra, C.E. West, J.T.C.M. Fennis, J.A. Schouten, and E.A. Van der Veen, Hypercholesterolemic effect of dietary soy protein versus casein in rhesus monkeys (Macaca mulatta), Am. J. Clin. Nutr. 39: 1 (1984).

21. J.M. Potter and P.J. Nestel, Greater bile acid excretion with soybean than with cow milk in infants, Am. J. Clin. Nutr. 32: 1645 (1976).

22. R. Fumagalli, L. Soleri, R. Farina, R. Musanti, O. Mantero, G. Noseda, E. Gatti, and C.R. Sirtori, Fecal cholesterol excretion studies in type II hypercholesterolemic patients treated with the soybean protein diet, Atherosclerosis 43: 341 (1982)

23. The Lipid Research Clinics, Coronary Primary Prevention Trial - I and II, J. Am. Med. Ass. 251: 351 (1984).

24. C.D. Moutafis, N.B. Myant, M. Mancini, and P. Oriente, Cholestyramine and nicotinic acid in the treatment of familial hyperbetalipoproteinemia in the homozygous form, Atherosclerosis 20: 105 (1971).

25. I. Shepherd, C.J. Packard, S. Bicker, T.D.V. Lawrie, and H.G. Morgan, Cholestyramine promotes receptor-mediated low density lipoprotein metabolism, N. Engl. J. Med. 302: 1219 (1980).

26. G.C. Ghiselli, Evidence that two synthetic pathways contribute to the apolipoprotein B pool of the low density lipoprotein fraction of rabbit plasma, Biochim. Biophys. Acta 711: 311 (1982).

27. J.L. Witztum, G. Schonfeld, S.W. Weidman, W.E. Giese, and M.A. Dillingham, Bile sequestrant therapy alters the composition of low density and high density lipoproteins, Metabolism 28: 221 (1979).

28. L.M. Hagerman, D.A. Iulow, and D.L. Scheider, In vitro binding of mixed micellar solutions of fatty acids and bile salts by cholestyramine. Proc. Soc. Exp. Biol. Med. 143: 89 (1973).

29. J.T. Garbutt and T.J. Kenney, Effect of cholestyramine on

bile acid metabolism in normal man, J. Clin. Invest. 51: 2781 (1972).

30. J.E. Claim, J.-R. Malagelada, V.S. Chadwick, and A.F. Hofmann, Binding properties in vitro of antacids for conjugated bile acids, Gastroenterology 73: 556 (1977).

31. P.D. Wood, R. Shioda, D.L. Estrich, and S.D. Splitter, Effect of cholestyramine on composition of duodenal bile in obese individuals, Metabolism 21: 107 (1972).

FECAL BILE ACIDS IN HEALTH AND DISEASE

Michael H. Thompson

PHLS Centre for Applied Microbiology and Research
Bacterial Metabolism Research Laboratory
Porton Down, Salisbury, Wiltshire, UK

INTRODUCTION

Normal healthy adults consuming a mixed western diet excrete up
to 500 mg of bile acids in feces each day. These acids are derived
from the small proportion of micelles and bile acid conjugates that
are not reabsorbed in the terminal ileum and enter the colon. Prior
to excretion these substances and deconjugated and undergo a range of
transformations mediated by the intestinal bacteria[1]. In addition
to the secondary bile acids, lithocholic acid and deoxycholic acid
(Figure 1), which normally dominate the fecal bile acid profile, a
complex mixture of minor bile acids are excreted along with trace
amounts of cholic acid and chenodeoxycholic acid[2]. Although fecal
loss of bile acids is quite normal there is a growing body of evidence that abnormal fecal levels of the substrates may be associated
with the risk of developing colorectal cancer[3]. This chapter will
review some of the dietary and microbiological factors that influence
the excretion of bile acids.

DEVELOPMENT OF THE FECAL BILE ACID PROFILE

The newly born infant gut contents include a complex mixture of
neutral and acidic steroids generally present as glycine and taurine
conjugates or as sulphates[4]. The pattern of bile acids in meconium
probably represents the accumulation of maternal and foetal products
and is dominated by cholic acid, chenodeoxycholic acid, deoxycholic
acid, lithocholic acid and hyocholic acid[5]. Epimeric, unsaturated
or side-chain shortened bile acids have also been detected in
meconium[6]. This bile acid profile is rapidly lost in infants and,
at 18 months, the principle bile acids excreted are cholic acid and

113

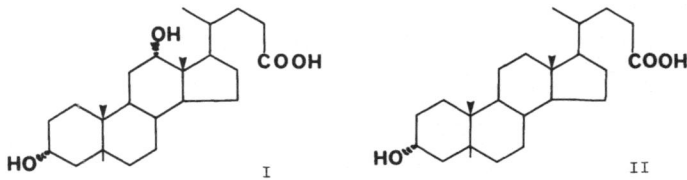

Fig. 1. Major fecal bile acids: Deoxycholic acid (I) and
Lithocholic acid (II).

chenodeoxycholic acid, along with a significant proportion of di-
hydroxy- and keto-bile acids[7]. At the age of four, secondary bile
acids compromise some 50% of the total bile acid excretion, rising to
more than 70% in adults.

In addition to these major bile acids Eneroth et al.[8], utilizing extraction and fractionation techniques incorporating saponification steps, identified a number of isomeric bile acids in feces
from adults (Table 1). Saponification eliminates the possibility of
quantifying individual fecal bile acid conjugates and sulphates, by
combining the released acids into the free bile acid fractions.
Vigorous saponification steps designed to hydrolyze bile acid derivatives are incorporated into other commonly used methods for quantifying bile acids[9,10]. More recently, by a modification of the method
of Alme et al.[11], the quantitative extraction and fractionation of
free fecal bile acids and their conjugates or sulphates has been
attained[2,12,13] (Table 1). Utilizing these techniques Tanida et
al.[2] identified some twenty six different bile acids, many of them
present as conjugates or sulphates, in fecal samples from eight
subjects. Glycine, taurine and sulphated derivatives accounted for a
maximum of 6, 3 and 10% respectively of the total fecal bile acid
output in those subjects. More than 80% of the substrates were
present in the unconjugated form in each case. Relatively low concentrations of allo-bile acids have been detected in human fecal
samples[14].

THE INTESTINAL FLORA

At birth the sterile infant bowel is rapidly colonized by predominantly anaerobic organisms, the composition of this flora being
determined by contamination from the immediate environment and
whether the baby is breast fed or bottle fed[15]. In healthy adults
the luminal flora is complex and stable, containing bacteria from
many different genera[16,17] and is often dominated by one particular
organism[18]. Bile acids may be degraded by intestinal organisms
both in vivo and in vitro. These activities are not confined to
specific bacteria but are more frequently expressed by sub populations of a number of organisms[1]. Therefore, while there may be

Table 1. Unconjugated Bile Acids Reported in Feces[2,13,18,68].

Monosubstituted 5β-cholanic acids (I)

3αOH-; 3βOH-; 12βOH-; 3oxo-;

Disubstituted 5β-cholanic acids (I)

3αOH, 12αOH-; 3αOH, 12βOH-; 3βOH, 12αOH-; 3βOH, 12βOH-; 3αOH, 7αOH-;
3βOH, 7αOH-; 3αOH, 7βOH-; 3αOH, 6αOH-; 3αOH, 7oxo-; 3αOH, 12oxo;
3βOH, 12oxo-; 3oxo 7αOH-; 3oxo, 12αOH-; 3oxo, 12oxo-;

Trisubstituted 5β-cholanic acids (I)

3αOH, 7αOH, 12αOH-; 3αOH, 7βOH, 12αOH-; 3βOH, 7αOH, 12αOH-;
3βOH, 7βOH, 12αOH-; 3αOH, 6αOH, 7αOH-; 3αOH, 7αOH, 12oxo-;
3αOH, 12αOH, 7oxo-;

5α-cholanic acids (II)

3αOH-; 3βOH-; 3αOH, 12αOH-; 3αOH, 12βOH-; 3βOH, 12αOH-; 3βOH, 12βOH-;
12oxo, 3αOH-; 3αOH, 7αOH, 12αOH-:

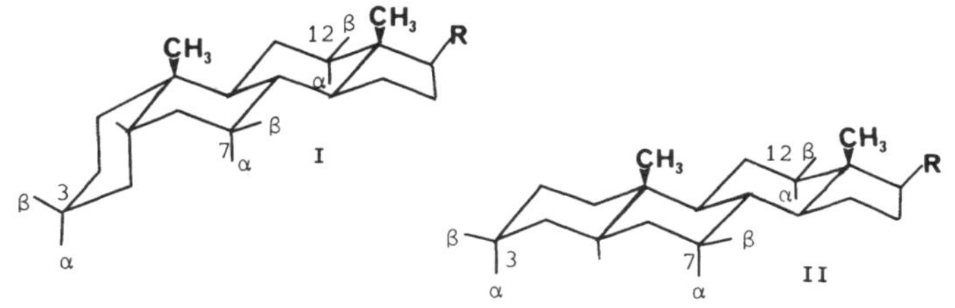

(R = CH(CH₃)CH₂CH₂COOH)

---

marginal differences in the general profiles of intestinal organisms
between populations[19] or between individuals consuming defined
diets[18], there may be considerable differences in the bile acid
degrading activity of the flora.

MICROBIAL DEGRADATION OF BILE ACIDS

Comparison of the fecal bile acid profiles of germ free and
conventional animals has confirmed that intestinal bacteria are
involved in the degradation of these substrates[20]. Thus germ free
rats secrete bile acids mainly in the conjugated form whereas in
conventional animals less than 5% are excreted in this form. Similarly β-muricholic acid is a major fecal component in germ free
animals whereas the dehydroxylation product hyodeoxycholic acid is
the major fecal bile acid in conventional animals.

Bile acids may be degraded _in vitro_ by intestinal bacteria via a
number of pathways including deconjugation, desulphation, dehydroxylation, oxidoreduction, epimerization and dehydrogenation of the
steroid nuclus (Figure 2).

Desulphation

Bile acid sulphates are degraded in mixed fecal cultures of
organisms derived from man, rats or mice[21]. Under these conditions
3α-monosulphates of cholic acid, chenodeoxycholic acid and allocheno-
deoxycholic acid are readily degraded although 7α- and 12α-mono-
sulphate esters of cholic and chenodeoxycholic acids are not. The
latter observation indicates that this activity is not present in the
normal colonic flora. Identification of the organisms associated
with the degradation of 3α-sulphates of bile acids has yet to be
resolved although it has been demonstrated that some Clostridia can
degrade lithocholic acid-3α-sulphate[22] (Figure 2).

Deconjugation

In contrast to desulphation, deconjugation activity is widely
distributed throughout the intestinal flora being expressed both in
mixed fecal culture and by individual organisms, including bacteroides, bifidobacteria, clostridia, enterococci, eubacteria,
lactobacilli and streptococci[1]. Some organisms are capable of
hydrolyzing a range of conjugates whereas others exhibit a specificity for either taurine or glycine conjugates and, under some
circumstances, a specificity for particular bile acids. In general
glycine and taurine conjugates are rapidly degraded at physiological
pH's[23] accounting for the very low levels of these substrates
normally detected in feces (Figure 2).

Dehydroxylation

7α-hydroxy bile acids are readily dehydroxylated by organisms
isolated from feces[24,25]. The bacteria capable of expressing this
activity represent only a small proportion of the colonic flora[26]
but carry out the reaction with a high degree of efficiency and are
responsible for the conversion of primary bile acids in the colon
(Figure 2). 3α- and 12α- bile acids do not appear to be dehydroxylated by intestinal organisms and there is some confusion as to
whether conjugated bile acids can be dehydroxylated[26]. More
recently dehydroxylation of ursodeoxycholic acid by a strain of
Eubacteria has been demonstrated, this 7β-dehydroxylation occurring
at a slightly lower rate than 7α-dehydroxylation in the same
organism[27].

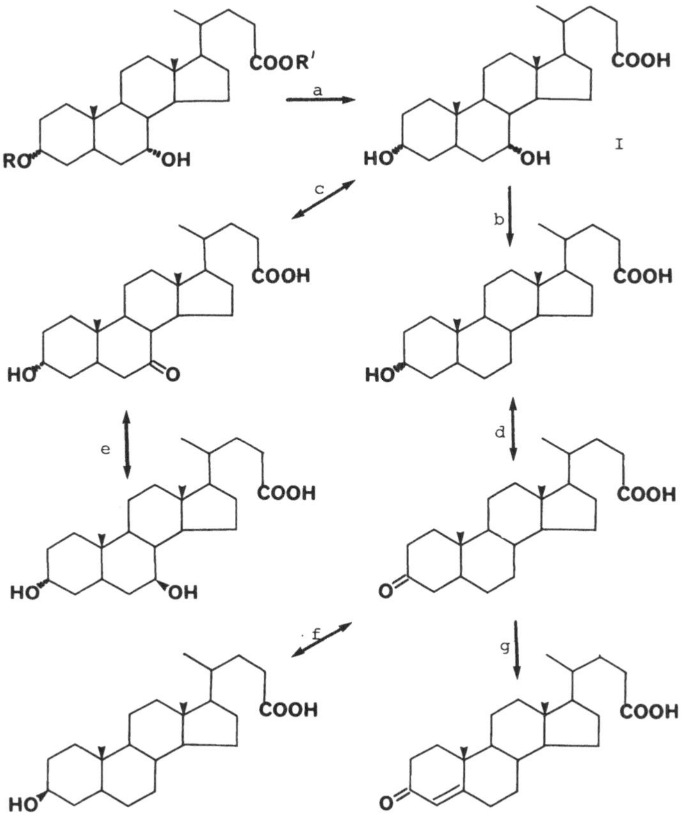

Fig. 2. <u>In vitro</u> degradation of bile acids by intestinal bacteria:
Deoxycholic acid (I). (a) Desulphation (R = SO₄) and
deconjugation (R¹ = Taurine or Glycine); (b) 7α-dehydroxy-
lation; (c) 7α-hydroxysteroid dehydrogenation; (d) 3α-
hydroxysteroid dehydrogenation; (e) 7-keto reduction and
epimerization; (f) 3-keto reduction and epimerization; and
(g) nuclear steroid dehydrogenation.

Oxidoreduction

Oxidoreduction of hydroxyl groups by intestinal organisms is
associated with the formation of epimerized bile acids via ketonic
intermediates (Figure 1). 3α-, 6β-, 7α-, 7β- and 12α-hydroxysteroid
dehydrogenases have all been identified in intestinal organisms[26].
In vitro studies have demonstrated that the oxidation pathway is
favored at non physiological alkaline pH whereas reduction of the
keto compounds is preferred under neutral or acidic conditions. This
activity is responsible for the low concentrations of keto bile acids
detected in feces, substrates that are readily reduced to epimeric
compounds at physiological pH levels (Figure 2). 7β-hydroxysteroid

117

dehydrogenase has only recently been characterized in intestinal organisms[28] whereas 6β-hydroxysteroid dehydrogenase is well characterized. The latter activity is responsible for the epimerization of β-muricholic acid to ω-muricholic acid in rats and pigs.

Nuclear Dehydrogenation

The steroid nucleus of bile acids can also be modified by intestinal organisms, the reaction generally requiring a 3-keto substituted bile acid as substrate (Figure 2). Under strictly anaerobic conditions some Clostridia can convert 3-oxo-cholanic acid to 3-oxo-4-cholanic acid, 3-oxo-1-cholanic acid or 3-oxo-1, 4-choladienic acid and 3-oxo-7α-hydroxy-choladienic acid to 3-oxo-4, 6-cholanic acid. Although this reaction proceeds readily _in vitro_ unsaturated substrates have yet to be reliably identified in feces.

DIET AND FECAL BILE ACIDS

Population Studies

Interpopulation studies have demonstrated considerable differences in the fecal concentrations of bile acids. Our own studies in nineteen populations[30] have revealed that subjects consuming a diet typical of a rural third world population excreted relatively low concentrations of bile acids when compared to subjects consuming a western style diet (Table 2). Bile acid degradation to secondary substrates is also apparently reduced in these third world groups consuming a low animal fat and protein diet which is also high in fiber.

In a more detailed study of four Scandinavian populations, in which the environmental and cultural variations are considerably reduced, the concentration of fecal bile acids was inversely correlated with fiber consumption but not with animal fat which was uniformly high[32]. Reddy et al. have similarly compared fecal bile acid excretion in populations consuming different diets[33]. Due principally to a higher intake of cereal products rural Finns excrete lower concentrations of bile acids when compared to New York subjects consuming a mixed western diet. Comparison of five North American groups with defined dietary practices demonstrated that Seventh Day Adventists, vegetarians, Japanese or Chinese subjects all excreted less bile acid than controls on a typical mixed diet[33]. However, only in the vegetarian group was the degree of conversion to secondary bile acids reduced.

More specific information on the relationship between fecal bile acid excretion and the consumption of specific dietary items, such as animal fat, protein and fiber, has been derived from dietary manipulation studies.

Table 2. Bile Acid Concentrations in Fecal Samples from Populations
at Different Risk of Developing Colon Cancer[30].

Population	Fecal bile acid (total)*	Deoxycholic acid*	Incidence of colon cancer**
Uganda	0.5	0.1	0.6
Japan	1.4	0.5	4.7
India	0.5	0.3	5.7
South Africa (black)	2.6	1.0	8.6
Hong Kong (Group C)***	2.2	0.9	7.2
Hong Kong (Group B)	3.1	1.2	11.2
Hong Kong (Group A)	4.7	1.7	13.3
England	6.2	1.5	18.2
South Africa (white)	5.9	1.6	19.4
United States (black)	6.3	–	28.0
United States (white)	6.0	2.2	28.1
Scotland	6.2	2.5	31.2

Determined by a modification of the method of Grundy, Ahrens and
Miettenen[9].

Kuopio (rural Finland)	7.8	–	5.5
Parrikala (rural Finland)	6.3	–	6.7
Them (rural Denmark)	8.0	–	12.9
Helsinki (urban Finland)	7.8	–	17.0
Copenhagen (urban Denmark)	8.4	6.0	20.7
Copenhagen (urban Denmark)	9.5	–	22.8
Greenland (Eskimos)	7.7	5.5	19.0

Determined by a modification of the method of Evrard and
Jannssen[10].

* mg.g^{-1} dry feces; ** cases per 100,000 population;
*** Hong Kong population sub-groups divided by income.

Fat and Fecal Bile Acids

Altering the consumption of fat is generally associated with a
variation in fecal bile acid excretion although the extent of the
effect may depend upon the composition of the fat eaten. Reducing
general fat intake is associated with reduced fecal bile acid concentration[34] whereas raising dietary fat intake leads to an increase
in bile acid loss[35]. In more detailed studies varying the fat
intake from the mainly saturated (cocoa butter) form to the polyunsaturated (corn oil) form was associated with an increased loss of
bile acids[36]. This increase is reflected by a disproportionate
increase in deoxycholic acid loss. More recently Brussard et al.[37]
reported that in groups of volunteers consuming standard diets in
which the fat content was defined as low or high and in which the

relative proportions of saturated and unsaturated fat were altered there was no significant variation in bile acid excretion.

These conflicting observations indicate that fat related influence on fecal bile acid levels may be dependent upon the availability and composition of the dietary fat. Furthermore, varying the intake of cholesterol, normally comprising only a small proportion of the total fat intake, may exert a disproportionate effect on bile acid loss.

Protein and Fecal Bile Acids

Reddy et al.[38] demonstrated that in subjects transferring from a mixed western diet to a meat free diet the overall excretion of bile acids is unaltered, although the degradation of cholic acid is reduced. Conversely transferring from a normal western diet to a meat supplemented diet is associated with an overall increase in fecal bile acid loss, primarily as enhanced loss of secondary bile acids[39]. However, modifying meat intake is inevitably associated with changes in intrinsic fat consumption which may also influence bile acid excretion. In order to overcome this unavoidable variation in both animal protein and fat consumption associated with variation in dietary meat, Cummings et al.[40] varied protein intake in a small group of volunteers consuming a fat and fiber controlled diet. Doubling the protein intake was associated with only a marginal increase in bile acid concentration indicating that increased animal protein consumption does not in itself influence bile acid loss.

Fiber and Fecal Bile Acids

Considerably more data is available with respect to the relationship between dietary fiber intake and fecal bile acid excretion. The basic hypothesis of the role of dietary fiber in ameliorating gastrointestinal disease[41] suggests that increased fiber intake bulks the stool and dilutes the concentration of luminal contents, including bile acids. In practice depending upon the fiber supplement a range of effects on stool bulk and fecal bile acid concentrations are observed.

Wheat bran is widely associated with enhanced total loss of bile acids although the stool bulking effect of this fiber effects a considerable reduction of fecal bile acid concentrations[42,43]. Oat bran supplementation, in contrast, whilst raising the total daily loss of bile acids is associated with a significant increase in fecal bile acid concentration due to the marginal stool bulking effect of this fiber[44]. Bagasse[45] (sugar cane fiber) and pectin supplementation, whilst increasing total daily bile acid loss by approximately one third, are not associated with an increase in fecal bile acid concentration. Guar gum supplementation, like oat bran, is associated with an increase in total loss and, due to its limited stool

bulking effect, an increase in fecal bile acid concentrations[47].
All other fiber supplements studied caused increased bile acid loss,
probably by binding the bile acids and reducing ileal reabsorption.
The more soluble and digestable fibers do not significantly increase
stool bulk and therefore are associated with an increase in fecal
bile acid concentration.

DIET AND FECAL FLORA

Whilst the fecal flora appears to be stable in individuals the
metabolic potential of the organisms may be affected by dietary
change. Thus in some subjects reduction of the meat content of their
diet[38] is associated with the excretion of a higher proportion of
primary bile acids when compared to controls, indicating reduced
microbial dehydroxylation. Bacterial degradation of bile acids is
also reduced in subjects with diarrhoea[13]. Interpopulation studies
have demonstrated that the profile of fecal organisms in samples from
populations consuming radically different diets may exhibit significant differences. Thus individuals consuming an animal fat and
protein enriched diet appear to carry, on average, more bacteroides
and fewer enterococci or similar anaerobes when compared to Africans
or Indians consuming an essentially vegetarian diet[48]. Subjects
living under essentially the same environmental conditions but consuming different diets, such as Seventh Day Adventists in North
America, have similar profiles of fecal organisms[18,32]. Microbial
bile acid deconjugation and oxidoreduction activity is generally
distributed in these populations but those subjects consuming a mixed
western diet carry a higher concentration of organisms able to 7α-
dehydroxylate and dehydrogenate bile acids[49,50]. The effect of
varying specific dietary items on the relative proportions or carriage of bacteria has also been studied. Dietary supplements of
wheat bran[42,43], bagasse[45] or fat[35] or changing from a mixed
western diet to a meat free diet are not associated with any significant changes in the profile of fecal organisms[38], the interindividual variations being greater than any apparent diet related
effect. Only extreme dietary modification causes variation in the
fecal flora as observed in a small group of subjects consuming a
chemically defined soluble diet. Over the ten days of the study
fecal enterococci and lactobacilli decreased whereas carriage of
enterobacteria increased [51]. In a similar study of extreme dietary
modification in which subjects consumed boiled rice, vegetable or
lean beef diets for three day periods only marginal changes in the
carriage of organisms is noted[52].

It may therefore be concluded from these observations that the
profile of fecal bile acids in adults is influenced by the consumption of specific dietary items, particularly animal fat and protein.
The development of the profile reflects the changing pattern of bile
acid excretion into the colon and the development of a metabolically

active flora. Bile acid conjugates and sulphates entering the colon are comprehensively degraded by luminal organisms to dehydroxylated, oxidized or epimerized free bile acids. Although the relative proportions of the organisms responsible for these activities are not significantly influenced by dietary variation, fecal pH, Eh, water content and transit time are. Thus dietary variation influences the conditions in the bowel and may therefore alter the underlying microbial degradation of bile acids.

FECAL BILE ACIDS AND COLON CANCER

Cholesterol cancer is more prevalent in the urbanized societies of North America and Western Europe when compared to the rural populations of the developing world. Studies of incidence rates in migrant groups or defined sub-populations such as Seventh Day Adventists in North America, indicate that environmental factors, especially diet, are most closely associated with risk. In particular consumption of a diet high in animal, fat or protein and depleted in fiber is associated with the greatest risk. There is no correlation of risk with the consumption of known carcinoogens or their precursors and it has therefore been hypothesized that the biologically active substrates responsible for tumor development may be generated in situ. However, as no known carcinogens, with the possible exception of N-nitrosamines[53], have been isolated from feces only indirect evidence is available to suggest the presence of biologically active species in the colon. In this context there is a growing body of evidence to suggest that bile acids may be associated with the initiation and development of colorectal tumors or their precursor lesions[54]. In animal model studies for large bowel cancer whilst no genotoxic activity has been attributed to bile acid derivatives these substrates do exert a tumor promoting activity[55]. In particular rectal instillation of secondary bile acids is associated with promotion of tumor growth as is the consumption of a diet that enhances overall bile acid excretion into the bowel.

As already noted high risk populations excrete elevated concentrations of more degraded bile acids, especially secondary bile acids with known tumor promoting activities, and also carry more organisms capable of bile acid dehydroxylation and dehydrogenation. Similar studies have indicated that fecal bile acid concentrations are higher in colorectal cancer patients and those subjects at high risk of developing this condition.

Fecal Bile Acids and Adenomas

Colorectal cancer is associated with the presence and growth of adenomatous polyps in the bowel, the greatest malignant potential being associated with the larger adenomas. The adenomacarcinoma (or dysplasia-carcinoma) sequence[56] stages the development of colon

tumors from the appearance of small polyps in the bowel. A proportion of healthy individuals, increasing with age, carry small
polyps a limited number of which increase in size to eventually
become tumors. A range of factors may influence the stages in this
sequence, including bile acids which may influence the growth of
adenomas and the development of the tumors[56]. In one study adenoma
subjects appear to excrete higher concentrations of bile acids than
controls[57] although there is some evidence that only those subjects
with large adenomas have elevated bile acid levels[58] (Table 3).
There are also indications that the relative proportions of lithocholic acid to deoxycholic acid are different in subjects with large
adenomas when compared to controls[59].

Fecal Bile Acids and Ulcerative Colitis

Patients with ulcerative colitis, particularly those of long
duration, are also at high risk of developing colon cancer. In
general these subjects do not excrete significantly higher concentrations of bile acids although there is some evidence that long term
colitics, with more dysplastic colon tissue, do excrete higher levels
of bile acids[58] (Table 3). In this group, therefore, higher concentrations of known tumor promoters are observed in subjects with
the highest risk of developing colon cancer.

Fecal Bile Acids and Familial Polyposis

Subjects with familial polyposis, an hereditary condition in
which a large number of polyps develop in the bowel relatively early
in life, form a group at high risk of developing bowel cancer. This
group of patients with a high risk pre-cancerous lesion appears to be
atypical. Fecal bile acid concentrations in these subjects are not
significantly higher than controls (Table 3) and there is some evidence that the degree of degradation is reduced[60]. However, these
subjects may be unusually sensitive to low levels of biologically
active agents, the hereditary expression of the premalignant lesion
being the most important risk factor in this group. Certainly the
degree of degradation of fecal cholesterol is suppressed in these
subjects[61] suggesting that compared to non-hereditary colon cancer
this predisposing condition has a separate etiology.

Fecal Bile Acids and Colorectal Cancer

Colorectal cancer subjects excrete higher concentrations of
fecal bile acids[19,57] and carry more organisms able to dehydrogenate these substrates[59]. Although the correlation has not been
confirmed in all studies[62,63] this may be due to some patient
groups containing a disproportionate number of advanced and metasta-
sized tumors. These conditions may be associated with impaired liver
function and bile acid secretion, and is supported by the observation
that subjects with Dukes C cancer excrete significantly lower concen-

Table 3. Fecal Bile Acid Concentration in Subjects with Colorectal
Cancer, Colorectal Adenomas, Familial Polyposis and
Ulcerative Colitis[30,58].

Patient Groups	Number of Subjects	Average fecal bile acid concentration $(mg.g^{-1}$ dry feces)
Colorectal Polyps	98*	8.1
Non-adenomatous polyps	9	6.8
Adenomas only	79*	8.4
<5mm diameter	20	6.6
6-20mm diameter	37	8.5
>20mm diameter	22	10.1
Adenoma type		
Tubular adenoma	36	8.4
Tubulovillous adenoma	11	8.4
Villous adenoma	17	9.4
Long-term ulcerative colitis	79*	7.7
With severe dysplasia/carcinoma	9	10.0
Familial Polyposis	6	5.0
Colorectal Cancer	84*	10.1
Colon Cancer	30	10.6
Rectal Cancer	38	10.3
Healthy Controls	-	7.0/8.0

* Detailed pathological specification not available for all subjects.

trations of bile acids when compared to those with Dukes A tumors
[58]. More detailed studies have revealed that the profile of fecal
bile acids and bacteria does not vary significantly between subjects
with colorectal cancer or adenomas and controls although there is
some evidence that the relative proportions of lithocholic acid to
deoxycholic acid is higher in cancer subjects[59]. The latter observation is unlikely to be due to the presence of the cancer influencing bile acid secretion as it is also observed in subjects with
the precursor lesion.

CONCLUSION

Whilst interindividual variations in the profiles of fecal
bacteria are considerable there are no major differences in the
average profiles of different populations, in patients with
colorectal cancer, adenomas or ulcerative colitis or in subjects
consuming specifically modified diets. In contrast the profile of
fecal bile acids varies considerably between populations, is influ-

enced by the consumption of fat and fiber and, in case control studies, correlates with the risk of developing colorectal cancer. The profile of fecal bile acids naturally reflects the relative proportions of bile acids excreted into the colon and the ability of the fecal organisms to degrade those substrates. The correlation between the risk of developing colon cancer and the consumption of a high risk - high fat - low fiber diet is associated with the enhanced excretion of secondary bile acids. The latter are known tumor promoters in animal models of large bowel cancer[55]. They have also been shown to possess comutagenic[65,66] or promotional[67] activity in short term assays for these properties. In case control studies, with the exception of familial polyposis, risk of developing colorectal is also associated with elevated concentrations of fecal bile acids.

Acknowledgements

The work of the Bacterial Metabolism Research Laboratory referred to in this chapter is supported by the Cancer Research Campaign (UK).

REFERENCES

1. I. A. Macdonald, V. D. Bokkenheuser, J. Winter, A. M. McLernon, and E. H. Mosbach, Degradation of steroids in the human gut, J.Lipid Res., 24:675 (1983).
2. N. Tanida, Y. Hikasa, M. Hosomi, M. Satomi, I. Oohama, and S. Shimoyama, Fecal bile acid analysis in healthy Japanese subjects using lipophilic anion exchanger, capillary column gas chromatography and mass spectrometry, Gastroenterologia Japonica, 16:363 (1983).
3. B. S. Reddy, "Oncology Overview: The Role of Bile Acids in the Promotion of Gastrointestinal Carcinogenesis," International Cancer Research Data Bank, Bethesda (1983).
4. P. Back and K. Walter, Developmental pattern of bile acid metabolism as revealed by bile acid analysis of meconium, Gastroenterology, 78:671 (1980).
5. R. Lester, J. Pyrek, J. M. Little, and E. W. Adcock, Diversity of bile acids in the fetus and newborn infant, J.Pediatric Gastro.Nutr., 2:355 (1983).
6. J. Pyrek, R. Lester, E. W. Adcock, and A. T. Sanghvi, Constituents of human meconium - I. Identification of 3-hydroxy-etianic acids, J.Steroid Biochem., 8:341 (1983).
7. C. T. L. Huang, J. T. Rodriguez, W. E. Woodward, and B. L. Nichols, Comparison of patterns of fecal bile acid and neutral sterol between children and adults, Am.J.Clin.Nutr., 29:1196 (1976).
8. P. Eneroth, B. Gordon, R. Ryhage, and J. Sjövall, Identification of mono- and dihydroxy bile acids in human feces by gas-

liquid chromatography and mass spectrometry, J.Lipid Res., 7:511 (1966) et seq.

9. S. M. Grundy, E. H. Ahrens, and T. A. Miettenen, Quantitative isolation and gas liquid chromatographic analysis of total fecal bile acids, J.Lipid Res., 6:397 (1965).

10. E. Evrard and S. Janssen, Gas liquid chromatographic determination of human fecal bile acids, J.Lipid Res., 9:226 (1968).

11. B. Almé, A. Bremmelgaard, J. Sjövall, and P. Thomassen, Analysis of metabolic profiles of bile acids in urine using lipophilic anion exchanger and computerized gas-liquid chromatography-mass spectrometry, J.Lipid Res., 18:339 (1977).

12. R. W. Owen, M. H. Thompson, and M. J. Hill, Analysis of metabolic profiles of steroids in feces of healthy subjects undergoing chenodeoxycholic acid treatment by liquid-gel chromatography and gas-liquid chromatography-mass spectrometry, J.Steroid Biochem., 21: (1984) in press.

13. K. D. R. Ketchell, A. M. Lawson, N. Tanida, and J. Sjövall, General methods for the analysis of metabolic profiles of bile acids and related compounds in feces, J.Lipid Res., 24:1085 (1983).

14. R. Wait, M. J. Hill, and M. H. Thompson, The role of minor bile acids in the etiology of colon cancer, Europ.J.Cancer Clin. Oncol., 19:1323 (1983).

15. P. L. Stark and A. Lee, The microbial ecology of the large bowel of breast-fed and formula fed infants during the first year of life, J.Med.Microbiol., 15:189 (1982).

16. W. E. C. Moore, E. P. Kato, and L. V. Holdeman, Anaerobic bacteria of the gastrointestinal flora and their occurrence in clinical infections, J.Inf.Dis., 119:641 (1969).

17. T. Mitsuoka, Recent trends in research on intestinal flora, Bifidobacteria Microflora, 1:3 (1982).

18. M. J. Goldberg, J. W. Smith, and R. L. Nichols, Comparison of the fecal microflora of Seventh-Day Adventists with individuals consuming a general diet, Annals of Surgery, 186:97 (1977).

19. A. Schwan, A. Rydén, and G. Laurell, Fecal bacterial flora of four Nordic population groups with diverse incidence of large bowel cancer, Nutr.Cancer, 4:74 (1982).

20. H. Eyssen and J. V. Eldere, Metabolism of bile acids, in: "The Germ Free Animal in Biomedical Research," M.E. Coates and B.E. Gustaffson, eds., Laboratory Animals Ltd., London (1984).

21. S. Huijghebaert, G. Parmentier, and H. Eyssen, Specificity of bile salt sulfatase activity in man, mouse and rat intestinal microflora, J.Steroid Biochem., 40:907 (1984).

22. S. P. Borriello and R. W. Owen, The metabolism of lithocholic acid and lithocholic acid-3-αsulphate by human fecal bacteria, Lipids, 17:477 (1982).

23. V. Aries and M. J. Hill, Degradation of steroids by intestinal bacteria 1: Deconjugation of bile salts, Biochim.Biophys. Acta, 202:526 (1970).

24. I. A. Macdonald, G. Singh, D. E. Mahony, and C. E. Meier, Effect of pH on bile salt degradation by mixed fecal cultures, Steroids, 32:245 (1978).

25. M. Morotomi, Y. Kawai, and M. Masahiko, Intestinal microflora and bile acids: in vitro cholic acid transformation by mixed fecal culture of rats, Microbiol.Immunol., 23:839 (1979).

26. P. B. Hylemon and T. L. Glass, Biotransformation of bile acids and cholesterol by the intestinal microflora, in: "Human Intestinal Microflora in Health and Disease," D.J. Hentges, ed., Academic Press, New York (1983).

27. B. A. White, R. J. Fricke, and P. B. Hylemon, 7β-dehydroxylation of ursodeoxycholic acid by whole cells and cell extracts of the intestinal anaerobic bacterium, Eubacterium species VPI 12708, J.Lipid Res., 23:145 (1982).

28. I. A. Macdonald, Y. P. Rochon, D. M. Hutchison, and L. V. Holdeman, Formation of ursodeoxycholic acid from chenodeoxycholic acid by a 7β-hydroxy-steroid dehydrogenase-elaborating Eubacterium aerofaciens strain co-cultured with 7α-hydroxy-steroid dehydrogenase-elaborating organisms, Appl.Environ. Microbiol., 44:1187 (1982).

29. V. C. Aries, P. Goddard, and M. J. Hill, Degradation of steroids by intestinal bacteria. III. 3-oxo-5β-steroid Δ^1-dehydrogenase and 3-oxo-5β-steroid Δ^4-dehydrogenase, Biochim. Biophys.Acta., 248:482 (1971).

30. M. H. Thompson, Bacteria and carcinogenesis, in: "Advances in Gastroenterology: Gastrointestinal and Hepatobiliary Cancer," H.J.F. Hodgson and S.R. Bloom, eds., Chapman and Hall, London (1983).

31. M. J. Hill, J. S. Crowther, B. S. Drasar, G. Hawksworth, V. Aries, and R. E. O. Williams, Bacteria and etiology of cancer of large bowel, Lancet, 1:95 (1971).

32. M. J. Hill, A. J. Taylor, M. H. Thompson, and R. Wait, Fecal steroids and urinary volatile phenols in four Scandinavian populations, Nutr.Cancer, 4:67 (1982).

33. B. S. Reddy, L. A. Cohen, D. McCoy, P. Hill, J. H. Weisburger, and E. L. Wynder, Nutrition and its relationship to cancer, Adv.Cancer Res., 32:237 (1980).

34. M. J. Hill, The effect of some factors on the fecal concentration of acid steroids, neutral steroids and urobilins, J.Pathol., 104:239 (1971).

35. J. H. Cummings, H. S. Wiggins, D. J. A. Jenkins, H. Houston, T. Jivraj, B. S. Drasar, and M. J. Hill, Influence of diets high and low in animal fat on bowel habit, gastrointestinal transit time, fecal microflora, bile acid and fat excretion, J.Clin.Invest., 61:953 (1978).

36. W. E. Connor, D. T. Witiak, D. B. Stone, and M. L. Armstrong, Cholesterol balance and fecal neutral steroid and bile acid excretion in normal men fed dietary fats of different fatty acid composition, J.Clin.Invest., 48:1363 (1969).

37. J. H. Brussard, M. B. Katan, and J. G. A. J. Hautvast, Fecal excretion of bile acids and neutral steroids on diets differ-

ing in type and amount of dietary fat in young healthy persons, Europ.J.Clin.Invest., 13:115 (1983).

38. B. S. Reddy, J. H. Weisburger, and E. L. Wynder, Effects of high risk and low risk diets for colon carcinogenesis on fecal microflora and steroids in man, J.Nutr., 105:878 (1975).

39. B. S. Reddy, Diet and excretion of bile acids, Cancer Research, 41:3766 (1981).

40. J. H. Cummings, M. J. Hill, T. Jivraj, H. Houston, W. J. Branch, and D. J. A. Jenkins, The effect of meat protein and dietary fiber on colonic function and metabolism. I. Change in bowel habit, bile acid excretion, and calcium absorption, Am.J. Clin.Nutr., 32:2086 (1979).

41. D. P. Burkitt, A. R. P. Walker, and N. S. Painter, Effect of dietary fiber on stools and transit time and its role in the causation of disease, Lancet, ii:1408 (1972).

42. J. H. Cummings, M. J. Hill, D. J. A. Jenkins, J. R. Pearson, and H. S. Wiggins, Changes in fecal composition and colonic function due to cereal fiber, Am.J.Clin.Nutr., 29:1468 (1976).

43. R. M. Kay, Dietary fiber, J.Lipid Res., 23:221 (1982).

44. R. W. Kirby, J. W. Anderson, B. Sieling, E. D. Rees, W.-J. L. Chen, R. E. Miller, and R. M. Kay, Oat-bran intake select- ively lowers serum low-density lipoprotein cholesterol con- centrations of hypocholesterolemic men, Am.J.Clin.Nutr., 34:824 (1981).

45. I. McLean Baird, R. L. Walters, P. S. Davies, M. J. Hill, B. S. Drasar, and D. A. T. Southgate, The effects of two dietary fiber supplements on gastrointestinal transit, stool weight and frequency, and bacterial flora, and fecal bile acids in normal subjects, Metabolism, 26:117 (1977).

46. J. H. Cummings, D. A. T. Southgate, W. J. Branch, H. S. Wiggins, H. Houston, D. J. A. Jenkins, T. Jivraj, and M. J. Hill, The digestion of pectin in the human gut and its effect on calcium absorption and large bowel function, Br.J.Nutr., 41:477 (1979).

47. M. H. Thompson, R. W. Owen, M. J. Hill, and J. C. Cummings, Factors affecting fecal bile acid concentrations: Effects of fat and fiber, Biochem.Soc.Trans., 13: (1985) in press.

48. B. S. Drasar and M. J. Hill, "Human Intestinal Flora," Academic Press, London (1974).

49. M. J. Hill, The role of colon anaerobes in the metabolism of bile acids and steroids, and its relation to colon cancer, Cancer, 36:2387 (1975).

50. P. Goddard, F. Fernandez, B. West, M. J. Hill, and P. Barnes, The nuclear dehydrogenation of steroids by intestinal bacteria, J.Med.Micro., 8:429 (1975).

51. J. S. Crowther, B. S. Drasar, P. Goddard, M. J. Hill, and K. Johnson, The effect of a chemically defined diet on the fecal flora and fecal steroid concentration, Gut, 14:790 (1973).

52. W. E. C. Moore and L. V. Holdeman, Discussion of current bac- teriological investigations of the relationships between

intestinal flora, diet and colon cancer, Cancer Res., 35:3418 (1975).

53. K. Suzuki and T. Mitsuoka, Increase in fecal nitrosamines in Japanese individuals given a Western diet, Nature, 294:453 (1981).

54. N. D. Nigro, Animal studies implicating fat and fecal steroids in intestinal cancer, Cancer Res., 41:3769 (1981).

55. B. S. Reddy, J. H. Weisburger, and E. L. Wynder, Colon cancer: Bile salts as tumor promotors, in: "Carcinogenesis, Vol 2. Mechanisms of Tumor Promotion and Co-carcinogenesis," T.J. Slaga, S. Sivak, and R. K. Boutwell, eds., Raven Press, New York (1978).

56. M. J. Hill, B. C. Morson, and H. J. R. Bussey, Etiology of adenoma-carcinoma sequence in large bowel, Lancet, i:245 (1978).

57. B. S. Reddy and E. L. Wynder, Metabolic epidemiology of colon cancer: Fecal bile acids and neutral sterols in colon cancer patients and patients with adenomatous polyps, Cancer, 39:2533 (1977).

58. M. J. Hill, B. C. Morson, and M. H. Thompson, The role of fecal bile acids (FBA) in large bowel carcinogenesis, Br.J.Cancer, 48:143 (1983).

59. R. W. Owen, M. Dodo, M. H. Thompson, and M. J. Hill, The fecal ratio of lithocholic acid to deoxycholic acid may be an important etiological factor in colorectal cancer, Europ.J. Cancer Clin.Oncol., 19:1307 (1983).

60. E. Bone, B. S. Drasar, and M. J. Hill, Gut bacteria and their metabolic activities in familial polyposis, Lancet, i:1117 (1975).

61. B. S. Reddy, A. Mastromarino, C. Gustafson, M. Lipkin, and E. L. Wynder, Fecal bile acids and neutral sterols in patients with familial polyposis, Cancer, 38:1694 (1976).

62. M. Moskovitz, C. White, R. N. Barnett, S. Stevens, E. Russell, D. Vargo, and M. H. Floch, Diet, fecal bile acids, and neutral sterols in carcinoma of the colon, Dig.Dis.Sci., 24:746 (1979).

63. D. G. Mudd, S. T. D. McKelvey, W. Norwood, D. T. Elmore, and A. D. Roy, Fecal bile acid concentrations of patients with carcinoma or increased risk of carcinoma in the large bowel, Gut, 21:587 (1980).

64. A. J. Mastromarino, B. S. Reddy, and E. L. Wynder, Fecal profiles of anaerobic microflora of large bowel cancer patients and patients with nonheriditary large bowel polyps, Cancer Res., 38:4458 (1978).

65. S. J. Silverman and A. W. Andrews, Bile acids: Co-mutagenic activity in the Salmonella-mammalian-microsome mutagenicity test, J.Nat.Cancer Inst., 59:1557 (1977).

66. M. Wilpart, P. Mainguet, A. Maskens, and M. Roberfroid, Structure-activity relationship amongst biliary acids showing

co-mutagenic activity towards 1,2-dimethylhydrazine, Carcinogenesis, 4:1239 (1983).

67. L. R. Ferguson and M. J. Parry, Mitotic aneuploidy as a possible mechanism for tumor promoting activity in bile acids, Carcinogenesis, 5:447 (1984).

68. K. D. R. Setchell, J. M. Gilbart, and A. M. Lawson, Fat and cancer, Brit.Med.J., 286:1750 (1983).

BILE ACIDS AND INTESTINAL PATHOPHYSIOLOGY

George V. Vahouny and Marie M. Cassidy

Departments of Biochemistry and Physiology
The George Washington University
School of Medicine and Health Sciences
Washington DC, 20037, USA

Despite our increased knowledge of the synthesis, secretion and enterohepatic circulation of bile salts, several aspects of the effects of these sterol metabolites on the physiology of the intestine itself have not been emphasized and are poorly understood. This becomes of greater significance when we consider that bile acids, particularly chenodeoxycholic acid and ursodeoxycholic acids, are employed for gallstone therapy; there are several dietary influences on the enterohepatic circulation of bile acids and on bile acid excretion (e.g. fats and dietary fibers); increased colonic bile acid concentrations have been implicated in the promotion of colorectal cancer; and there appears to be an inverse relationship between cholesterolemia and colon cancer.

The purported role of bile acids in the promotion of colon cancer, in particular, has generated renewed interest in the pathophysiology of these steroids in the intestinal tract. The purpose of this paper is the review of our knowledge in this important area of bile acid pathophysiology.

BILE ACIDS AND SMALL INTESTINAL STRUCTURE AND FUNCTION

The small intestinal mucosa tends to maintain a constant morphological appearance, despite the fact that there is a rapid renewal of cells in intestinal crypts and rapid transit of cells up the intestinal villi. Among those factors which are reported to influence morphological structure and the rates of enterocyte proliferation, differentiation and extrusion, are physical trauma[1]; changes in gut flora[2]; hormones[3]; the state of nutrition and feeding patterns [4]; and bile acid concentration[5].

131

Generally, conjugated bile acids predominate in the small intestine under physiological conditions, although unconjugates can also be found normally (e.g. [6]). However, unconjugated bile acid concentrations increase when abnormal bacteria flora exist[6-8].

It has been extensively documented[9-15] that bile acids, and particularly the unconjugated forms, can cause histological damage to the small intestinal mucosa, both in vivo and in vitro, and can inhibit transport of several nutrients. This damage generally involves the villus tip cells of both jejunum and ileum[9] and includes cell necrosis, denudation, desquamation, and reduced numbers of goblet cells[10-15]. Although most investigators have suggested that these effects are observed only with unconjugated deoxycholate or cholate, similar effects on jejunal structure in vivo have been observed with glycine or taurine conjugates of deoxycholate[15]. As might be expected, these morphological effects have been associated with certain alterations in transport functions of the small intestine. These include interference with glucose and amino acid transport and metabolism[9,11,12], and with water and electrolyte transport[13,15-17].

There is also evidence that bile acids influence the proliferative enterocyte pool in the small intestine. Feeding cholic acid to germ-free mice resulted in increased turnover of ileal mucosal cells [18]. This was apparently due to increased excretion of the bile acid and higher concentration of steroids in the lower intestine. Similarly, transposition of the bile duct from the duodenum into the ileum[5] resulted in mucosal hyperplasia in the lower small intestine in response to mucosal damage. Conversely, bile diversion caused a decreased proliferative cell pool in both jejunum and ileum, and a 50% decrease in the labelling index, using tritrated thymidine incorporation measurements[19]. In these bile-diverted animals, re-infusion of 30 μM taurocholate, at a rate approximating bile flow, resulted in a marked increase in labelling in the jejunal crypts and an increased crypt to villus cell migration in both jejunal and ileal segments (Table 1).

These evidences collectively suggest that normal enterohepatic circulation of bile acids plays an important role in intestinal morphology and cytokinetics, and that modification of bile acid content and/or composition may have unexpected effects on structure function characteristics of the small intestine.

BILE ACIDS AND COLONIC STRUCTURE AND FUNCTION

The observations on small intestinal responses to bile acid cited above have been extended to include responses of the large bowel to altered bile acid concentrations and compositions. Increased concentrations of bile acids in the colon cause abnor-

132

Table 1. Cell Migration in Bile-diverted Rats Infused Without and
With Sodium Taurocholate (30 μM).

	Time after [^{3}H] Thymidine (hours)	Position of uppermost cells on villus column	
		Bile salt	+ Bile salt
Jejunum	12	12.5	29.2
	24	46.5	63.9
Ileum	12	8.7	24.0
	24	27.9	49.0

Bile salt was infused duodenally for 60–72 h prior to autoradiographic studies (data derived from Roy et al.[19]).

malities in the colonic epithelium[20,21]. Furthermore, as shown in
Figure 1, this topographical damage can be induced by direct colonic
infusions of a solution of mixed bile acids or by bile acids bound to
the anion-exchange resin, cholestyramine[21]. In addition to these
morphological deviations, both conjugated and unconjugated bile acids
can inhibit water absorption in the canine colon[22], and induce
secretion of water and electrolytes in the human colon[23].

Normally, bile salts are absorbed slowly and passively in the
duodenum or jejunum, and are absorbed more rapidly and actively in
the lower small intestine, particularly the terminal ileum (see
[24]). It has been estimated[25] that 120 mg of bile salts are
absorbed from the rat small intestine daily, and that only 12 mg
reach the large bowel. On this, two-thirds is passively absorbed in
the colon and the remainder is excreted[25]. Thus, only about 2–4%
of the bile salts of the total enterohepatic pool are excreted daily.

These kinetics can be altered, in some cases quite dramatically
with a variety of nutritional, pharmacological and pathological
conditions. Increases in fecal bile acid output are proportional to
dietary fat levels[26], and to increased intake of certain types of
dietary fiber derivatives, such as pectin[27]. Fecal bile acids are
also increased in ileal disease and malfunction[28], following
iliectomy[29], and during therapy for hypercholesterolemia with
bile-acid sequestering resins, such as cholestyramine[30]. Although
the effects of each of these conditions on the morphology and function of the large bowel have not been extensively investigated, it
has been reported that free bile acids per se[20,21], and increased
colonic bile acid concentrations induced by bile acid-sequestering
dietary fiber[31] or anion-exchange resins[32], will cause extensive
morphological damage to the colonic epithelium in experimental
animals.

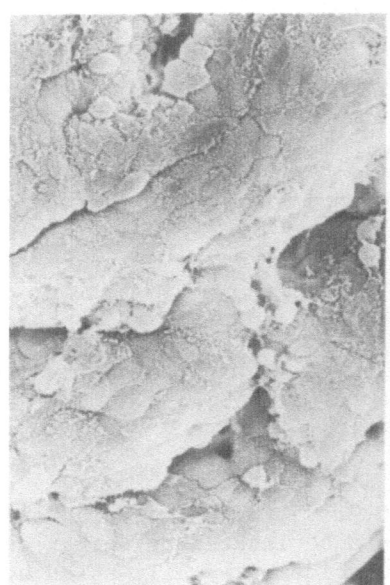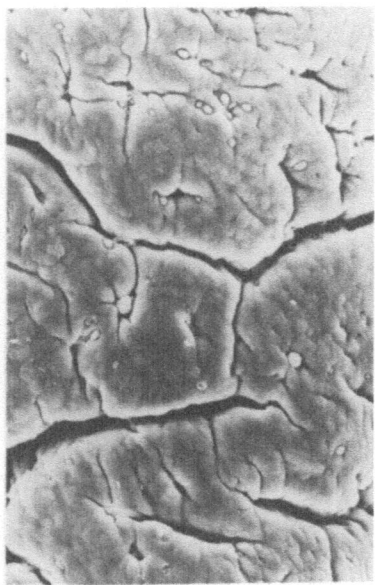

Fig. 1. Topography of rat colon by scanning microscopy. The section
on the left is from a rat with an indwelling cecal catheter
and infused with saline twice each day for five days. The
section on the right is from a rat infused with 154 μmol of
an equimolar bile salt mixture containing cholate, chenodeoxycholate and deoxycholate, twice daily for five days.

It is well recognized that various types of mucosal irritants,
including bile acids, which are known to evoke necrosis of villus
cells, can result in feedback stimulation of crypt cell turnovers,
cell migration and villus repair rates[33]. These increased cell
proliferative rates in the colon are also compatable with mechanisms
of tumor promotion in tissues previously exposed to carcinogens[34].
Sprintz[33] has suggested that any damage to the colonic mucosa, even
if non-specific, may represent a co-carcinogenic factor in colon
carcinoma. Thus, it is not surprising that there has been a great
deal of attention given to the possible role of colonic bile acid
concentrations in the promotion of colon carcinogenesis, possibly via
their hyperplastic effects on the colonic epithelium.

BILE ACIDS AND COLON CANCER

An important advance in the search for causative agents in human
colon cancer were the reports of Hill and colleagues[35,36], who

suggested that a correlation between diet and colon carcinoma might be explained by an involvement of bile steroids. These reports have been confirmed by others (e.g. [37,38]), and although the relation-ship between bile acids and human colorectal cancer may be more complex [39] than originally proposed, there is a considerable literature on experimental large bowel carcinogenesis, which suggest a promoting role for increased colonic bile acid concentrations.

Experimental Models for Colonic Neoplasia

Chemical induction of intestinal neoplasia in experimental animals, usually rodents, can be accomplished by administration of any of several carcinogenic agents (see [40]). These agents appear to provide a high degree of specifity and tumor yield, and produce a pathology which is largely compatible with the human disease[40]. The most commonly used agents are 1,2-dimethyl-hydrazine (DMH), azoxymethane (AOM) and methylazoxymethanol (MAM) which are chemically related, and can be administered orally and/or subcutaneously. N-methyl-N'-nitrosoguanidine (MNNG) and N-Methylinitrosourea are effective by rectal instillation, suggesting a direct action on the colonic mucosa.

Although extrapolation of studies using these carcinogens to the human disease state should be interpreted with reservation, these models have provided important information on dietary factors influ-encing experimental colon cancer, and on the role of bile fiber supplements which dilute colonic contents and increase fecal volume, such as bran and cellulose, appear to protect against colonic neo-plasia (e.g. [50-52]), particularly when dietary fat levels are not high[53]. These fibers, coincidentally perhaps, are also not hypo-lipidemic (e.g. [54]). In contrast, fiber supplements which have bile acid-binding properties in vitro, or increase bile output (concentration) in vivo, are either without effect, or in several cases have been reported to enhance the effect of the chemical carcinogen. These include agar[55], alfalfa[56], pectin[57,58], Guar gum[58] and metamucil[58]. These general relationships between fecal bile acid concentrations and chemically-induced neoplasia have been summarized by Hill[39] and are shown in Table 2.

These relationships between colonic bile acid concentrations and colonic neoplasia may well be related to hyperplastic to responses in the colon to these surgical and dietary manipulations. Our studies [21,31,32] have demonstrated morphological and topographical devi-ations in the colon following: fecal infusion of free bile acids or bile acids bound to cholestyramine; inclusion of 2% levels of choles-tyramine, colestipol or DEAE-sephadex in rat diet; inclusion of alfalfa, pectin or metamucil, but not wheat bran or cellulose, in rat diets. The direct relationship between acids as promoters of colonic neoplasia.

Table 2. Relationship Between Fecal Bile Acid Concentrations and
          Experimental Colonic Neoplasias (Modified form [39]).

Experimental manipulation	Effect on fecal bile acid concentration	Effect on colonic neoplasia (Reference)
Rectal instillation of bile acids	increase	increase [41,42]
Bile diversion to caecum	increase	increase [43]
Diversion of fecal stream (colostomy)	decrease	decrease [44]
Administration of cholestyramine	increase	increase [46,47]
Dietary manipulations		
Increased fat	increase	increase [48]
Wheat bran	decrease	decrease [50,51]
Cellulose	decrease	decrease [52]
Pectin	increase	increase [57,58]
Guar gum	increase	increase [58]
Alfalfa	increase	increase [56]
Metamucil	increase	increase [58]

Bile Acids as Promoters of Experimental Colonic Neoplasia

The involvement of bile acids in the promotion of chemically-induced colon cancer has been demonstrated by several approaches. These include: direct rectal instillation of bile acids; surgical displacement of the bile duct; modification of the fecal stream; effect of bile acid sequestering agents; and dietary-induced increases in colonic and fecal bile acids.

In the first approach[41], it has been reported that multiple rectal instillations of lithocholic or taurodeoxycholic acids were themselves not carcinogenic. However, both bile acids doubled the frequency of MNNG-induced neoplasms, suggesting that these agents were acting as promoters of carcinoma. Similar results were obtained in germ-free rats with deoxycholate instillations[42], implying that further bacterial modification of the bile acid was not a requisite for the promoting action of the bile acid.

Surgical displacement of the bile duct to the mid-small intestine results in an increased fecal output of bile acids[43]. Administration of AOM to these animals markedly increased tumor formation largely in the distal colon[43]. Conversely, diversion of the fecal stream by colostomy in rats decreased by half, the numbers of colonic tumors induced by the carcinogen[44].

As mentioned earlier, cholestyramine sequesters bile acids and other micellar constituents[45], and increases fecal output of these acidic steroids[30]. Inclusion of this agent as 2% of the diet in rats produced a striking increase in malignant intestinal tumors, induced by either DMH, AOM or MAM[45]. Furthermore, this effect was also observed in germ-free rats administered DMH[47], suggesting that colonic microorganisms are not required for the promotion, and that the bile acid can act to promote colonic tumors, even when remaining bound to the resin[47].

With respect to nutritional effects, it has been reported[48], that an increase in dietary fat in rat diets increases the levels of fecal bile acids (primarily deoxycholate and β-muricholate). These animals also develop more colonic tumors than animals on the low or "normal" fat diets[48].

The results of various studies on dietary fibers and experimental carcinogenesis have been extensively reviewed[40,49] and have not been entirely consistent. In general, however, dietary these morphological phenomena, hyperplasia and increased colonic neoplasia, however, remains to be demonstrated.

SUMMARY

This treatise has summarized available evidence relating modified bile acid metabolism with the structural and functional alterations in small and large bowel physiology. Based on experimental models, these evidences suggest that nutritional, surgical or pharmacological modifications in normal bile acid metabolism, such as might be emphasized to decrease various hyperlipoproteinemias, may not be of overall benefit with respect to large bowel pathophysiology. Whether these relationships apply directly to human health and disease remains conjectural.

Acknowledgements

The author wishes to express his appreciation to his colleagues Drs. D. Kritchevsky and J. Story, and to F. Lightfoot, L. Grau, S. Haus-Smith and S. Satchithanandam with whom portions of our studies were accomplished. Supported in part by U.S.D.A. grant 82-CRCR-1001.

REFERENCES

1. B. Creamer, The turnover of the epithelium of the small intestine, Brit.Med.Bull., 23:266 (1967).
2. S. Lesher, H. E. Walburg, and G. A. Sacher, Generation cycle in the duodenal crypt cells of germ-free and conventional mice, Nature, 202:884 (1964).

3. C. P. Leblond and R. Carriere, The effect of growth hormone and thyroxine on the mitotic rate of the intestinal mucosa of the rat, Endocrinology, 56:261 (1955).

4. J. P. A. McManus and K. J. Isselbacher, Effect of fasting versus feeding on the rat small intestine, Gastroenterology, 59:214 (1970).

5. G. G. Altmann, Influence of bile and pancreatic secretions on the size of intestinal villi in the rat, Am.J.Anat., 132:167 (1971).

6. Y. S. Kim, N. Spritz, M. Blum, J. Terz, and P. Sherlock, The role of altered bile acid metabolism in the steatorhea of experimental blind loops, J.Clin.Invest., 45:956 (1966).

7. L. H. Rosenberg, W. G. Hardison, D. M. Bull, Abnormal bile salt patterns and intestinal bacterial overgrowth associated with malabsorption, New Eng.J.Med., 276:1391 (1967).

8. S. Tabaqhali and C. C. Booth, Jejunal bacteriology and bile salt metabolism in patients with intestinal malabsorption, Lancet, 2:12 (1966).

9. A. M. Dawson and K. J. Isselbacher, Studies on lipid metabolism in the small intestine with observations on the role of bile salts, J.Clin.Invest., 30:730 (1960).

10. R. J. Fry and E. Staffeldt, Effect of a diet containing sodium deoxycholate on the intestinal mucosa of the mouse, Nature, 202:1369 (1964).

11. A. S. Nunn, R. D. Baker, and G. W. Searle, Inhibition of intestinal glucose absorption by bile salt, Life Sci., 1:646 (1963).

12. J. L. Pope, T. M. Parkinson, and S. A. Olson, Action of bile salt on the metabolism and transport of water-soluble nutrients by perfused rat jejunum in vitro, Biochim.Biophys. Acta, 130:218 (1966).

13. G. E. Sladen and J. T. Harries, Studies on the effects of unconjugated dihydroxy bile salts on rat small intestinal function in vivo, Biochim.Biophys.Acta, 288:443 (1972).

14. T. Low-Beer, R. E. Schneider, and W. O. Dobbins, Morphological changes of the small-intestine mucosa of guinea pig and hamster following incubation in vitro perfusion in vivo with unconjugated bile salts, Gut, 11:486 (1970).

15. M. W. Teem and S. F. Phillips, Perfusion of hamster jejunum with conjugated and unconjugated bile acids: Inhibition of water absorption and effects on morphology, Gastroenterology, 62:261 (1972).

16. R. I. Russel, J. G. Allan, V. P. Gerskowitch, and K. M. Cochran, The effect of conjugated and unconjugated bile acids on water and electrolyte absorption in human jejunum, Clin.Sci.Molec. Med., 45:301 (1973).

17. S. Feldman and M. Gibaldi, Bile salt-induced permeability changes in isolated rat intestine, Proc.Soc.Exp.Biol.Med., 132:1031 (1969).

18. R. Rankin, R. Wilson, and P. M. Bealmear, Increased turnover of intestinal mucosal cells of germ-free mice induced by cholic acid, Proc.Exp.Biol.Med., 138:270 (1971).

19. C. C. Roy, G. Laurendau, G. Doyon, L. Chartrand, and M. R. Rivest, The effect of bile and of sodium taurocholate on the epithelial cell dynamics of the rat small intestine, Proc.Soc.Exp.Med., 149:1000 (1975).

20. D. R. Saunders, J. R. Hedges, J. Sillery, L. Esther, K. Matsumura, and L. E. Ruben, Morphological and functional effects of bile salt on rat colon, Gastroenterology, 68:1236 (1975).

21. G. V. Vahouny, S. Satchithanandam, F. Lightfoot, L. Grau, S. Haas-Smith, D. Kritchevsky, and M. M. Cassidy, Morphological disruption of colonic mucosa by free or cholestyramine-bound bile acids, Dig.Dis.Sci., (1984) in press.

22. H. S. Mekhjian and S. F. Phillips, Perfusion of the canine colon with unconjugated bile acids: Effect on water and electrolyte transport, morphology and bile acid absorption, Gastroenterology, 59:120 (1970).

23. H. S. Mekhjian, S. F. Phillips, and A. F. Hofmann, Colonic secretion of water and electrolytes induced by bile acids: Perfusion studies in man, J.Clin.Invest., 50:1569 (1971).

24. W. T. Beher, "Bile Acids. Chemistry and Physiology of Bile Acids and Their Influence on Atherosclerosis II," D. Kritchevsky, O.J. Pollak, and H.S. Simms, eds., S. Karger, Basel (1976).

25. S. Linstedt and B. Samuelsson, Bile acids and steroids LXXXIII. On the interconversion of cholic and deoxycholic acid in the rat, J.Biol.Chem., 234:2026 (1959).

26. B. S. Reddy, J. H. Weisburger, and E. L. Wynder, Colon cancer: Bile salts as tumor promoters, in: "Mechanisms of Tumor Promotion and Cocarcinogenesis," T.J. Slaga, A. Sivak, and R.K. Boutwell, eds., Raven Press, New York, pp.453 (1978).

27. G. A. Leveille and H. E. Sauberlich, Mechanism of the cholesterol-depressing effect of pectin in the cholesterol-fed rat, J.Nutr., 88:209 (1966).

28. A. F. Hofmann, The syndrome of ileal disease and the broken enterohepatic circulation: Cholerheic enteropathy, Gastroenterology, 52:752 (1967).

29. M. R. Playoust, L. Lack, and I. M. Weiner, Effect of ileal resection on bile salt absorption in dogs, Am.J.Physiol., 208:363 (1965).

30. W. G. Thompson, Cholestyramine, Can.Med.Assn.J., 104:305 (1971).

31. M. M. Cassidy, F. G. Lightfoot, L. Grau, J. Story, D. Kritchevsky, and G. V. Vahouny, Effect of chronic intake of dietary fibers on the ultrastructural topography of rat jejunum and colon, Am.J.Clin.Nutr., 34:218 (1981).

32. M. M. Cassidy, F. G. Lightfoot, L. E. Grau, T. Roy, D. Kritchevsky, and G. V. Vahouny, Effect of bile-salt binding resins on the morphology of rat jejunum and colon, Dig.Dis.Sci., 25:504 (1980).

33. H. Sprinz, Factors influencing intestinal wall renewal, Cancer, 28:71 (1971).

34. T. J. Slaga, A. Sivak, and R. K. Boutwell, eds., "Carinogenesis: Mechanisms of Tumor Promotion and Carcinogenesis," Raven Press, New York (1978).

35. M. J. Hill and V. C. Aries, Fecal steroid composition and its relationship to cancer of the large bowel, J.Pathol., 104:129 (1971).

36. M. G. Hill, The effect of some factors on the fecal concentration of acid sterols, neutral sterols and urobilins, J.Pathol., 104:239 (1971).

37. B. S. Reddy and E. L. Wynder, Large Bowel carcinogenesis: fecal constituents of populations with diverse incidence rates of colon cancer, J.Natl.Cancer Inst., 50:1437 (1973).

38. B. S. Reddy and E. L. Wynder, Metabolic epidemiology of colon cancer: fecal bile acids and neutral sterols in colon cancer patients with adenomatous polyps, Cancer, 39:2533 (1977).

39. M. J. Hill, Bile acids and human colorectal cancer, in: "Dietary Fiber in Health and Disease," G.V. Vahouny and D. Kritchevsky, eds., Plenum Press, New York, pp.299 (1982).

40. H. J. Freeman, Studies on the effects of single fiber sources in the dimethylhydrazine rodent model of human bowel neoplasia, in: "Dietary Fiber in Health and Disease," G.V. Vahouny and D. Kritchevsky, eds., Plenum Press, New York, pp.287 (1982).

41. T. Narisawa, N. E. Magadia, J. J. Weisburger, and E. L. Wynder, Promoting effect of bile acid on colon carcinogenesis after intrarectal instillation of N-methyl-N'-nitrosoguanidine in rats, J.Nat.Cancer Inst., 53:1093.

42. B. S. Reddy, T. Narisawa, J. H. Weisburger, and E. L. Wynder, Promoting effects of sodium deoxycholate on colon adeno-carcinoma in germ free rats, J.Nat.Cancer Inst., 56:441 (1976).

43. C. Chomcai, N. Bhadrachari, and N. D. Nigro, Effect on bile on the induction of experimental intestinal tumors in rats, Dis.Colon Rectum, 17:310 (1974).

44. R. L. Campbell, D. V. Singh, and N. D. Nigro, Importance of fecal stream in the induction of colon tumors by azoxymethane in rats, Cancer Res., 35:1369 (1975).

45. J. W. Huff, J. L. Gilfillin, and V. M. Hunt, Effect of choles-tyramine, a bile acid binding polymer on plasma cholesterol and fecal bile acid excretion in the rat, Proc.Soc.Exp.Med., 114:352 (1963).

46. N. D. Nigro, N. Bhadrachari, and C. Chomcai, A rat model for studying colonic cancer: Effect of cholestyramine on induced tumors, Dis.Colon Rectum, 16:438 (1973).

47. T. Asano, M. Pollard, and D. C. Madsen, Effects of choles-tyramine on 1,2-dimethylhydrazine-induced enteric carcinoma in germ-free rats, Proc.Soc.Exp.Biol.Med., 150:780 (1975).

48. B. S. Reddy, J. J. Weisburger, and E. L. Wynder, Effect of dietary fat level and dimethylhydrazine on coloncarcino-

genesis and fecal acid and neutral steroid excretion in rats, J.Natl.Cancer Inst., 52:507 (1974).

49. B. S. Reddy, Dietary fiber and colon carcinogenesis: A critical review, in: "Dietary Fiber in Health and Disease," G.V. Vahouny and D. Kritchevsky, eds., Plenum Press, New York, pp.265 (1982).

50. T. A. Barbolt and R. Abraham, The effect of bran on dimethyl-hydrazine-induced colon carcinogenesis in the rat, Proc.Soc. Exp.Biol.Med., 157:656 (1978).

51. D. Fleiszer, J. Macfarlane, D. Murray, and R. A. Brown, Protective effect of dietary fiber against chemically induced bowel tumors in rats, Lancet, 2:552 (1978).

52. H. J. Freeman, G. A. Spiller, and Y. S. Kim, A double-blind study on the effect of purified cellulose dietary fiber on 1,2-dimethylhydrazine-induced rat colonic neoplasia, Cancer Res., 38:2912 (1978).

53. N. D. Nigro, Animal studies implicating fat and fecal steroids in intestinal cancer, Cancer Res., 38:2912 (1978).

54. R. M. Kay and A. S. Truswell, Dietary fiber: Effects on plasma and biliary lipids in man, in: "Medical Aspects of Dietary Fiber," G.A. Spiller and R.M. Kay, eds., Plenum Press, New York, pp.153 (1981).

55. H. P. Glauert, M. R. Bennick, and C. H. Sander, Enhancement of 1,2-dimethylhydrazine-induced colon carcinogenesis in mice by dietary agar, Food Cosmet.Toxicol., 19:281 (1981).

56. K. Watanabe, B. S. Reddy, J. H. Weisburger, and D. Kritchevsky, Effect of dietary alfalfa, pectin, and wheat bran on azoxy-methane- or methylnitrosourea-induced colon carcinogenesis in F 344 rats, J.Natl.Cancer Inst., 63:141 (1979).

57. H. G. Nauer, N. G. Asp, A. Dahlqvist, P. E. Fredlund, M. Nyman, and R. Oste, Effect of two kinds of pectin and guar gum on 1,2-dimethylhydrazine initiation of colon tumors and on fecal B-glucuronidase activity in the rat, Cancer Res., 41:2518 (1981).

58. W. M. Castledon, Prolonged survival and decrease in intestinal tumors in dimethylhydrazine-treated rats fed a chemically defined diet, Br.J.Cancer, 35:491 (1977).

THE THERAPY OF CHOLESTEROL GALLSTONES WITH BILE ACIDS

E. Roda in collaboration with

F. Bazzoli, G. Mazzella, M. Malavolti, and F. Luzza

Clinica Medica 3, University of Bologna

The only definitive treatment of gallstones was, up to few years ago, the surgical procedure of chlecystectomy.

The application of the fundamental knowledge, gained during the last decade, of the pathogenesis of cholesterol gallstones, allowed the actual placing of medical cholelitholysis with chronic administration of bile acids.

The first medical cholelitholysis in man was obtained in 1972 by Danzinger and Hofmann with chenodeoxycholic acid (cheno) (1). Trhee years later, in Japan, Makino showed that also urso-deoxycholic acid (urso), the 7 epimer of cheno, could dissolve cholesterol gallstones in vivo, in man (2).

How cheno and urso dissolve cholesterol gallstones, is not fully established. Repletion of bile acid pool and suppression of cholesterol synthesis (by reducing the activity of HMG-CoA) have firstly been hypothesized as possible mechanisms of action. More recently a reduced bile acid/colesterol secretory coupling, and therefore a reduced transmembrane cholesterol transport, seems to follow the administration of the two cholelitholytic bile acids (3). Whether or not cheno and urso act by reducing the amount of cholesterol transported per mole of bile acid into the bile canalicolus, the net effect of treatment is bile with less cholesterol relative to bile acid and phospholipidis, i.e. the reversion of the physicochemical conditions which produced cholesterol gallstones.

Thus only radiolucent cholesterol-rich gallstones may be treated medically, while radioopaque pigment stones are insoluble even in unsaturated bile. Radiolucent gallstone, however, does not mean always cholesterol-rich gallstone, but it has been shown that up to 20% of such stones are not cholesterol in type.

Furthermore, oral bile acid therapy is not efficacious in dissolving those stones with calcification either at the periphery or in the centre. To dissolve stones in the gallbladder it must be assumed that bile, unsaturated in cholesterol by the administration of cheno or urso, can easily enter the gallbladder lumen. A functioning gallbladder (i.e. opacified during oral cholecystography) is, therefore, together with gallstone radiolucency, an irrecusable prerequisite of oral bile acid therapy.

Stone size is another important factor to be considered for the prognosis of a successful cholelitholytic treatment.

Both cheno and urso are poorly and slowly effective on large stones (15-20 mm and more). Large stones, in fact, because of the low surface/volume ratio and probably because of densely packed, laminated outer layers, are more resistent to the effects of unsaturated bile.

The results of the National Cooperative Gallstone Study (4) showed that dissolution is significantly more frequent in cheno-treated patients with small stones and particularly in those with floating stones.

Also urso-treated patients seem to respond to treatment in a manner which is inversely related to stone size. In a recent review Bachrach and Hofmann (5) analyzed the results of several studies with ursodeoxycholic acid and observed that patients with stones less than 5 mm in diameter have a 30% chance of their gallstones disappearing within one year or even 6 months; patients with stones 5-10 mm in diameter have a dissolution rate of about 18% in a period of time not shorter than a year and in patients with stones more than 10 mm in diameter any dissolution which might occur will require more than a year and the expected success rate is probably 10%.

The results we have obtained in a comparative study on cheno and urso-therapy (6) are in concordance with those of the literature as far as chenodeoxycholic acid is concerned, while revalue the efficacy of urso on large stones.

We showed, in fact, that cheno produced complete dissolution mostly in patients with small stones, while the effectiveness of urso was not statistically different in patients with small stones (<10 mm) and in patients with large stones (>10 mm), although large stones require a longer time for complete dissolution. In addition to stone type and size, also the dose is an important factor influencing dissolution.

In the National Cooperative Gallstone Study (4) the doses of chenodeoxycholic acid were suboptimal (the highest dose was 750 mg/day) and the frequence of cholelitholysis was definitely lower than those obtained in other studies (6, 7), in which a weight-related dosage of 15 mg/kg/day was adopted.

A further evidence that a fixed dose of 750 mg/day chenodeoxycholic acid is inadequate results from the observation that higher dissolution rates were obtained in those patients with less than ideal body weight and consequently receiving and higher dosage per kg/body weight (4).

Presently it is accepted that the optimal dosage of chenodeoxycholic acid is 15 mg/kg/day.

As far as ursodeoxycholic acid is concerned, the dosage should not be higher than 8-10 mg/kg/day, since it has been shown that increasing the dose up to 15 mg/kg/day does not produce significant increases of dissolution rates (6, 8). The above dosage, however, must be increased in obese gallstone patients up to 20 mg/kg/day chenodeoxycholic acid and probably 15 mg/kg/day ursodeoxycholic acid. If the optimal dose is adopted and if patient selection (radiolucency, stone size and gallbladder function) is rigorous, it is than reasonable to expect a total dissolution rate of about 30-40% and even higher in those patients with "floating stones".

This success rate is achieved with both bile acids, however urso treated patients showed an earlier response to treatment.

In our comparative study, in fact, of the 42 total dissolutions obtained with urso treatment, 31 (73%) were achieved during the first six months period, while of the 33 total dissolutions obtained with cheno treatment, only 14 (42%) were achieved during the same period.

In addition to the lower dose and to the earlier response, urso therapy has the advantage not to induce those side effects frequently observed in patients treated with cheno: diarrhea and hypertransaminasemia.

A clinically important diarrhea has been reported in about 40% of the patients treated with cheno (4) and in several studies cases of patients who refused to continue the treatment because of these annoying side effects have been reported.

Diarrhea caused by cheno administration, however, is a dose related phenomenon and in most cases settle spontaneously after few weeks of treatment.

The mechanism by which cheno (a di- -hydroxy-bile acid) induces diarrhea are probably related to the inhibition of water and electrolyte transport and to the activation of the adenylate cyclase cyclic AMP and guanylate cyclase cyclic GMP systems which would promote secretion of water and electrolytes.

These effects are not induced by di- -hydroxy bile acids and diarrhea is almost unknown in patients given urso. As mentioned, hypertransaminasemia is the second most common side effect during cheno administration. It has been observed in about one third of cheno-treated patients but, as shown in the NCGS, only in 2.6% of the cases abnormalities of liver morphology were observed. However since in other studies (9, 10) severe or moderate lightmicroscopic changes have been reported in 3 and 12%, respectively, of gallstone patients evaluated before treatment, it remains to be demonstrated that hypertransaminasemia during cheno administration correlates with liver damage.

An accumulation of lithocholic acid, the bacterial biotransformation product of chenodeoxycholic acid, has been suspected to cause hypertransaminasemia during treatment.

Lithocholic acid, however, although hepatotoxic in the experimental animal, should not produce liver damage in man. The human liver, in fact, sulphates efficiently lithocholic acid and since sulphated bile acids are malabsorbed, man should be protected from potential hepatotoxicity of this secondary bile acid.

A lack of the cytosolic enzyme into the circulation as a consequence of altered hepatocyte membrane permeability due to a direct effect of cheno has been also proposed as a possible mechanism of hypertransaminasemia.

This hypothesis is supported by some in vitro studies in which cultured hepatocytes incubated with cheno have been shown to release lactic dehydrogenase and transaminases into the culture medium (11). The "direct" toxicity against liver membrane was not observed when urso was tested using the same experimental design. This experimental evidence is of particular interest since it reflects the clinical observation that cheno in some cases produces hypertransaminasemia, but urso does not.

As far as the effect on serum lipids is concerned, the majority of the studies have shown a scarce effect of both cheno and urso on serum cholesterol.

The results of the NCGS, however, have raised some doubts about the safety of chenodeoxycholic acid because of significant increase of LDL cholesterol observed in the treated patients. This increase in LDL cholestero, however, is small (10 mg/dl) compared with the placebo patients and the potential atherogenic effect of cheno is far from being proved.

Urso, on the other side, does not seem to influence serum cholesterol, with the exception of a small and potentially beneficial increase of HDL cholesterol (12).

It is almost unanimously accepted that both cheno and urso lower serum tryglicerides (4, 6) and a statistically significant decrease has been observed after administration to hypertrygliceridemic patients (6).

Also acquired gallstone calcification should be regarded as a possible side effect during bile acid treatment since this phenomenon implies the failure of medical treatment.

The reported values of acquired calcifications vary in the different studies up to 10% of the treated patients.

In the NCGS the side effect was similarly observed both in the placebo and in the treated patients. This result suggest that acquired calcifications could be considered as part of the natural history of gallstone disease and not a side effect of treatment.

This problem, however, is far from being fully defined and we still need to know much more about the effect of bile acids on biliary calcium secretion and about the solubility of calcium salts in bile during cholelitholytic treatment.

Ten years after the availability of the medical treatment for cholesterol gallstones, an overcoming problem in the evaluation of its usefulness is the possibility of gallstone recurrence after dissolution.

In 1-14 weeks after withdrawing treatment bile reverts to its supersaturated state (13). Since other factors (obesity, pregnancy, diurnal variation of biliary cholesterol saturation, presence of nucleating factors, etc.) are required for gallstone recurrence, a supersaturated bile does not necessarily mean gallstone recurrence, but does represent a high risk factor.

Few studies are presently available on the frequency of this phenomenon. Ruppin and Dowling (14) have observed recurring gallstones in about 50% of their succesfully treated patients.

In our experience, however, recurrence frequency is not greater than 20% (unpulished observation). Both these values are obtained from retrospective study and it is likely that more definitive data will be provided by presently undergoing long term prospective studies.

In conclusion oral bile acid therapy, is effective in dissolving cholesterol gallstones and, in selected patients, its efficacy is at least of 30%. Although its safety is accepted, patients, particularly if treated with cheno, should be checked regularly during treatment for serum transaminases and serum lipids.

Postdissolution recurrence is an overcoming problem, and the possibility of a long term maintenance therapy is still to be evaluated.

REFERENCES

1. R.G. Danzinger, A.F. Hofmann, et al, Dissolution of cholesterol gallstones by chenodeoxycholic acid. N. Engl. J. Med. 286:1 (1972).
2. I. Makino, K. Shinozaki, et al, Dissolution of cholesterol gallstones by ursodeoxycholic acid. Jap. J. Gastroenterol. 72:690 (1975)
3. C. Sama, N.F. LaRusso, Y. Lopez, et al, The effect of acute bile acid administration on biliary lipid secretion in healthy volounteers. Gastroenterology 82:515 (1982).
4. National Cooperative Gallstone Study, Chenodiol (chenodeoxycholic acid) for dissolution of gallstone. Ann. Intern. Med. 95:257 (1981).
5. W.H. Bachrach, A.F. Hofmann, Ursodeoxycholic acid in the treatment of cholesterol cholelithiasis. Part. II. Dig. Dis. Sci. 27:833 (1982).
6. E. Roda, F. Bazzoli, A.M. Morselli Labate, et al, Ursodeoxycholic acid vs. chenodeoxycholic acid as cholesterol dissolving agents: a comparative randomized study. Hepatology 2:804 (1982).
7. J.H. Iser, R.H. Dowling, H.Y.J. Mok, et al, Chenodeoxycholic acid treatment of gallstones: a follow-up report and analysis of factors influencing response to therapy. N. Engl. J. Med. 293:378 (1975).
8. P.H. Maton, G.M. Murphy, R.H. Dowling, Ursodeoxycholic acid treatment of gallstones. Dose response study and possible mechanism of action. Lancet 2:1297 (197..).
9. S. Hadziyannis, T. Feize, P.J. Scheur, et al, Immunoglobulin-containing cells in the liver. Clin. Exp. Immunol. 5:499 (1969).

10. J. Reichman, B. Wahlgenmuth, Ch.F. Schwokowski, Leberschaden beim Gallensteinladen. Zeitschrift für die Gesamte Inner Medezin 28:327 (1973).

11. F. Nakayama, K. Myazaki, A. Koga, Effect of chenodeoxycholic and ursodeoxycholic acids on isolated human hepatocytes. Gastroenterology 78:1228 (1980) abstr.

12. O. Leiss, T. Bosch, K. von Bergman (1981), Effects of bile acids feeding on lipoprotein concentration, changes in cholesterol synthesis and biliary lipid secretion in patients with radiolucent gallstones. In: "Bile Acids and Lipids", G. Paumgartner, A. Stiehl, W. Gerok, Eds, MTP Press, Lancaster, pp. 247.

13. J.M. Iser, G.M. Murphy, R.H. Dowling, The speed of change in biliary lipids and bile acids with chenodeoxycholic acid-is intermittent tratment feasible? Gut 18:7 (1977).

14. D.C. Ruppin, R.H. Dowling, Is recurrence inevitable after gallstone dissolution by bile acid treatment? Lancet, i: 181 (1982).

DISSOLUTION OF CHOLESTEROL GALLSTONES IN BILE

Gianfranco Salvioli

Insegnamento di Semeiotica Medica
Università di Modena, Ospedale Estense
Viale V. Veneto, 9, 41100 Modena, Italy

Cholesterol monohydrate (CHM) is present in human gallstones[1] and in arterial wall[2]. Bile salt-induced cholesterol gallstone dissolution is a recent advance in clinical medicine: chenodeoxy-cholic acid (CDCA)[3] and its epimer, ursodeoxycholic acid (UDCA)[4] reduce the relative amount of cholesterol in human bile and when administered for sufficiently long periods of time can induce dis-solution of Ch gallstones. Equilibrium is approached very slowly in a detergent system, and thus the most important behavior in a model bile system dissolving solid ChM crystals is the dynamics of the solubilization process and in particular the dissolution rate. The presence of an interfacial barrier on the surface of Ch gallstones is an important discovery for the understanding of factors regulating dissolution rates[5,6,7].

CHOLESTEROL, BILE SALTS, AND LECITHIN

Bile contains three amphiphiles (cholesterol, lecithin and bile salts) assembled in mixed micelles. These greatly increase water-solubility of cholesterol (usually very low about 70-80 nM). If excess cholesterol is present, the solubilizing capacity of the micelles is exceeded and supersaturation reached: nucleation of cholesterol molecules can occur with formation of cholesterol mono-hydrate crystals and stones[8]. Only ChM is found in gallstones and its dissolution rate is slower than anhydrous cholesterol[9].

Lecithin (Lec) is a swelling insoluble amphiphile having truncated-cone shape complementary to Ch; in water it forms liquid crystals which can dissolve high proportions of cholesterol. A bilayer of lecithin is destroyed by bile salt (BS) simple micelles,

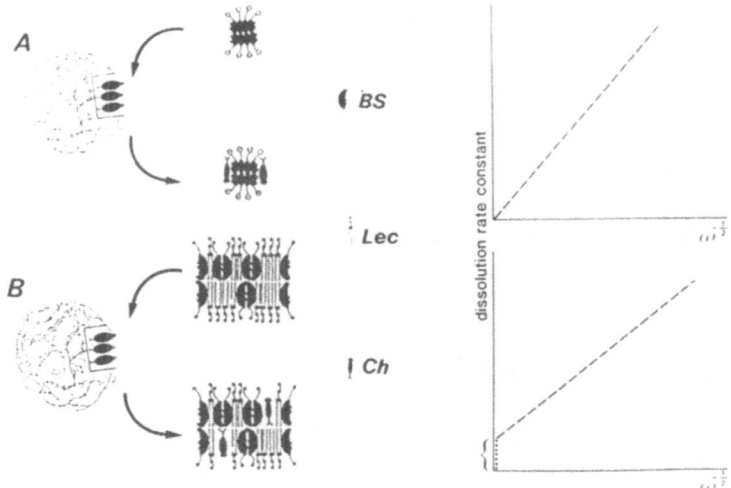

Fig. 1. Dissolution of cholesterol stones by bile salt micelles. In
A the cholesterol of stones is dissolved by simple micelles
(BS plus Lec). In both cases unsaturated micelles diffuse
to the surface of the stones where interfacial resistance
regulates the detachment of Ch molecules; these saturate the
micelles and in this form diffuse into the bulk solution.
Plotting the dissolution rate constant against $\omega^{\frac{1}{2}}$, a linear
correlation is obtained with k=0 at zero angular velocity.
In this case the dissolution process is only diffusion
regulated. In the case of BS micelles, instead, the process
of Ch dissolution is largely regulated by interfacial
resistance: the positive intercept on the vertical axis (D)
of the correlation between k and $\omega^{\frac{1}{2}}$ indicates interfacial
resistance.

only when a BS/Lec ratio greater than 0.3 is reached[10]. Therefore
at low concentrations BS can be accommodated into the bilayer without
dissolution.

Liposomes made of cholesterol and egg lecithin (molar ratio 0.3)
are solubilized by BS at different speeds and in the order TDC>TCDC>
TC>TUCD[11]. At equilibrium the dissolution capacity of the different BS is about the same[11].

Bile salts are soluble amphiphiles forming simple micelles in
water; the capacity to solubilize CH is increased (about 4 times) in
the presence of lecithin (mixed micelles)[8]. The solubilization
capacity of mixed micelles for cholesterol increases with increasing
total lipid concentration, temperature, and Lec/BS molar ratio[12].

The influence of bile acid composition has not been studied extensively; in the absence of lecithin the maximum Ch solubility and speed of solubilization is greatest for deoxycholic acid[13] and lowest for ursodeoxycholic acid[8,14].

When mixed micelles are enriched in lecithin, the particles become bigger and the solutions manifest the Tyndall phenomena[8]; mixed micelles are transformed into vesicles so that the solution shows a new phase (liquid crystals). In this manner a solution resembling bile can present different phases in relation to the molar percentage composition of the three components (Ch, Lec, and BS) and in particular solid (Ch crystals), liquid (micelles), and liquid crystalline phases may be present[12]. Cholesterol is solubilized in micellar and liquid-crystalline phases and this possibility has been demonstrated for some hydrophilic bile acids such as ursodeoxycholic acid[11].

HOW ARE CHOLESTEROL CRYSTALS DISSOLVED BY MICELLES?

A detailed understanding of the dissolution kinetics of ChM is important. Some dissolution rate experiments follow a diffusion-convection model[5]. However, interfacial phenomena are important when the dissolution of Ch by bile salt solutions is involved (Figure 1)[5,6,7].

Evolution of Ch dissolution kinetics requires an apparatus consisting of a) a static disk of Ch having a known surface for evaluation of the initial dissolution rate, b) powdered cholesterol monohydrate to evaluate equilibrium Ch solubility (Cs) and c) a rotating disk of Ch to evaluate the relative contribution of the resistances (interfacial or diffusion) during the dissolution process (Figure 2).

The dissolution rate (dC/dt) may be calculated using the formula:

$$\frac{dC}{dt} = k \frac{S}{V} (Cs-C) \tag{1}$$

where Cs is the equilibrium Ch solubility, C is the Ch concentration at the first hour; k is the dissolution rate constant which evaluates the general speed of dissolution (its value is greatly influenced by the amount of Ch solubilized at equilibrium).

The constant k can be evaluated from formula (1). Evaluation of k at different angular velocities allows interpretation of the mechanisms promoting transfer of cholesterol from the surface of the Ch disk to the micellar solution.

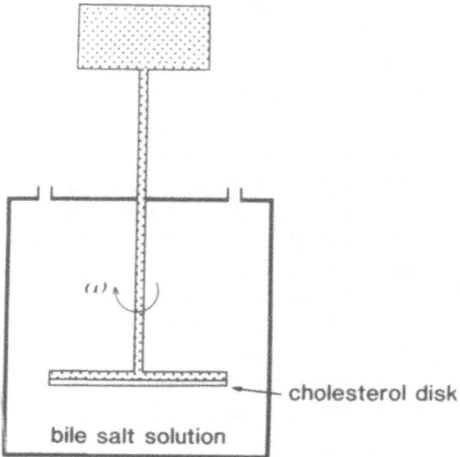

cholesterol disk

bile salt solution

Fig. 2. A ChM disk rotating in a chamber containing BS solution is used to evaluate the different components (diffusion, convection, interfacial resistance) involved in the dissolution process. We can evaluate k at different angular velocities (see Figure 1):

$$k = 0.625 \times D^{\frac{2}{3}} \times \omega^{\frac{1}{2}} \times \nu^{-\frac{1}{6}}$$

ω = angular velocity at the disk-solution interface
D = diffusion coefficient; ν = viscosity.

When dissolution rate constant is plotted against angular velocity, a linear correlation is obtained with k=0 at zero angular velocity. This is similar to the diffusion controlled process in which stagnant conditions greatly reduce dissolution. Phase 2 of Figure 1 is very fast in respect to diffusion to and from the solid surface: this modality occurs only when Ch is dissolved by solvents such as glyceril monoctanoate or ethanol-water[16]. However, cholesterol dissolution in BS solutions is about 3.5 times slower than predicted by diffusion-controlled processes. Thus, a non-diffusion mediated mechanism seems more probable, as suggested by the potentiating effects of electrolytes and counterions[17].

In this dissolution model, resistance occurs at the crystal-solution interface. When dissolution rate constant is plotted against angular velocity the positive intercept on the vertical axis indicates interfacial resistance (Figure 1)[9]. Detachment of Ch molecules from the surface of the cholesterol disk (or Ch stone) is a slow process and can be influenced by the presence of lecithin in BS micelles. Higuchi et al. have shown that dissolution of ChM crystals by cholate-lecithin solutions is unaffected by variations of angular velocity of the disk[17]. The speed of dissolution is fifteen times slower when Lec is added to BS due to the appearance of greater interfacial resistance[7].

DISSOLVING CAPACITIES OF CHENODEOXYCHOLIC AND URSODEOXYCHOLIC ACID: DIFFERENT MECHANISMS

Igimi and Carey[9] obtained the results reported in Table 1 using 100 mM solutions of bile acids and BS to dissolve cholesterol monohydrate crystals. Chenodeoxycholic acid and salts have a dissolution rate constant two to three fold faster than of UDCA[9]. When powdered ChM is dissolved by solution of TUDC/Lec or TCDC/Lec, the solubilizing capacity of TCDC/Lec is initially higher than that of TUDC-Lec. However in time the latter solution becomes turbid (due to the formation of liquid crystals)[18] and solubilizes more Ch, in this case not in micellar form but in liquid-crystalline phase[11].

The mixture UDC-Lec solubilizes increasing amounts of Ch in time and equilibrium is reached after a long period[18]. The liquid-crystalline phase (mesophase) can be separated by ultracentrifugation: it contains high concentrations of Ch (with a Lec/Ch ratio of about 1) and is probably metastable. The mesophase also appears when about 80% of total biliary BA are represented by UDC.

With added lecithin the initial dissolution rates of ChM disk are slower in GUDC-Lec systems than in GCDC-Lec. Dissolution rate is accelerated by the presence of Lec, especially in the case of GUDC[11]. On the contrary dissolution rate constants are decreased by the presence of Lec. The dissolution of ChM crystals can be followed by polarized light microscopy (Figure 3): solutions of

Table 1. Dissolution of Cholesterol Monohydrate Crystals.

	CDC	GCDC	TCDC	UDC	GUDC	GCDC
Cmax (a)	6.1	2.2	1.5	0.33	0.19	0.13
BS/Ch mole ratio	16:1	45:1	68:1	303:1	526:1	770:1
Dissolution rate (b)	11.2	2.5	1.8	0.39	0.09	0.07
Dissolution rate constant [k] (c)	2.03	1.25	1.29	1.27	0.46	0.58

(a) equilibrium solubility of cholesterol (mmoles)
(b) (mmoles cm^{-2} x sec^{-1}) x 10^7
(c) (cm x sec^{-1}) x 10^4
CDC = chenodeoxycholic acid
UDC = ursodeoxycholic acid
G and T indicate glyco- and tauro- conjugates (from [9]).

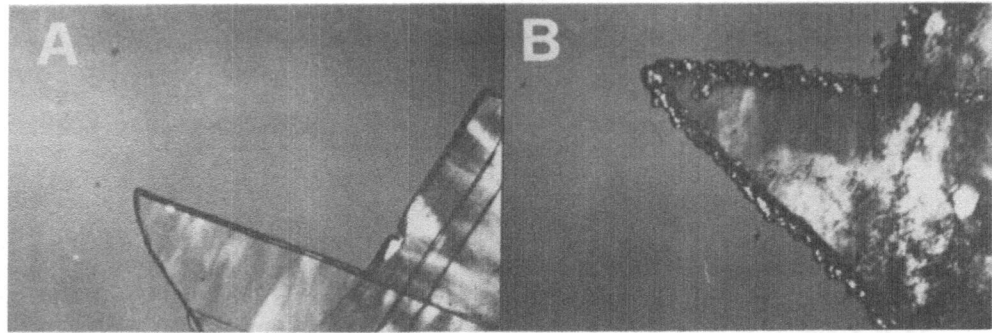

Fig. 3. Cholesterol monohydrates crystal dissolution in a mixture of
tauroursodeoxycholate: Lecithin (80:20) at 37°C, observed by
polarized light microscope. After 3 hours (B) the edges of
the crystal are covered by birefringent liquid crystals made
of cholesterol-lecithin in molar proportion of about
one[11].

TUDC-Lec induce the formation of liquid-crystals around the contours
of the ChM crystals. The same finding is present in ursodeoxycholic-
rich bile only at high, non-physiological concentrations of Lec but
liquid crystals disappear after a short period of observation[11].
Therefore in the presence of Lec, UDCA and CDCA solubilize Ch crystals via different mechanism. Preincubation of ChM with a TUDC-Lec
system (but not with TCDC-Lec) accelerates subsequent Ch dissolution
by BS solutions. Moreover the total amount of Lec adsorbed to ChM
interfaces by preincubation of cholesterol crystals with different
BS-Lec solutions is 5 fold greater after preincubation with TUDC-Lec
and interfacially absorbed lecithin is solubilized faster by TCDC
than by TUDC[11].

Thus TUDC-Lec mixtures modify the ChM surface owing to surface
variations by deposition of liquid crystals. Liquid crystals contain
lecithin and cholesterol and are rapidly destroyed by other BS
present in bile. In fact, Multilamellar liposomes made of lecithin
are dissolved by tauroconjugates at different speeds: the clearing-
time is faster the most hydrophobic BS (TDC and TCDC) and slower when
hydrophilic bile salts are employed (TUDC)[11].

DISSOLUTION OF ChM BY SOLUTIONS RESEMBLING BILE

We used the following three mixtures containing BS with glyco/
tauro ratio of 3.5: normal bile (31% DCA, 35% CDCA, 34% CA), urso-
rich bile (11% DCA, 21% CDCA, 15% CA, 50% UDCA) and cheno-rich bile
(9% DCA, 80% CDCA, 2% UDC, 9% CA).

In absence of Lec the initial dissolution rates follow this order: normal>cheno-rich/urso-rich. With added Lec, initial dissolution rate is faster in cheno-rich bile[11]. Evaluation of the dissolution rate constant shows that urso-rich bile dissolves more rapidly when Lec content is 10%. At 20-25 Lec, a thin liquid-crystalline film was observed microscopically on the surface of the compressed disk of ChM[11].

For a given bile salt: lecithin ratio the interfacial resistance decreases with increasing BS concentration and in the experience of Kwan and coworkers cheno-rich bile dissolves Ch three times as fast as bile with normal biliary bile acid composition.

THE CONTRIBUTION OF SIMPLE AND MIXED MICELLES TO CHOLESTEROL CRYSTAL DISSOLUTION

In normal bile, simple and mixed micelles coexist and both can dissolve cholesterol. When mixed micelles containing Lec and Ch collide with Ch gallstones, Lec is deposited on the stone surface: Lec incorporates cholesterol with formation of liquid crystals, which are dissolved by simple micelles. The prevalence of BS with poor detergency in bile allows for long residence times of liquid crystals on the Ch crystal surface so that more Ch can be incorporated[11]. Dissolution rate depends on the sum of interfacial resistance from BS monomers, presence of simple and mixed micelles, and on their relative concentrations in the dissolving solution[20]. Simple micelles are the principal species responsible for interfacial transport of Ch in a TC/Lec system as reported in Figure 4[20] so that k of simple micelles (ks) is higher than k of mixed micelles (km).

IS IT POSSIBLE TO ACCELERATE CH GALLSTONE DISSOLUTION?

Factors influencing interface resistance can induce variations of dissolution rates. Electrical repulsion between negative charges of the cholesterol crystal surface and micelles reduce dissolution rate[21]. Micelles and ChM crystals interact more readily in the presence of counterions (Na^+) or when cationic amphiphiles are added. In particular benzalkonium chloride reduces interfacial resistance: in this case dissolution becomes largely diffusion controlled[21] owing to the barrier-breaking effects caused by reduction of the negative charge of micelles[21].

DISSOLUTION OF TRUE CHOLESTEROL GALLSTONES

In vitro Toully et al.[22] found that deoxycholic acid is more effective than chenodeoxycholic and cholic acids; contrasting results reported in the literature[23] are probably due to different exper-

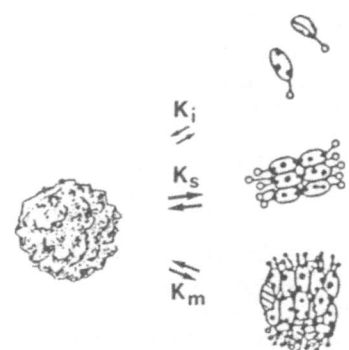

Fig. 4. "i", "s", and "m" indicate monomers of bile salt simple
micelles, and mixed micelles, respectively. Dissolution
rate depends on the sum of the interfacial resistance (k)
of "i", "s" and "m", and on the relative concentrations.
In a taurocholate-lecithin system, simple micelles are
responsible for interfacial transport of cholesterol.

imental conditions (composition and structure of the stones) and
methods used to evaluate stone dissolution (changes of stone weight
or diameter amounts of solubilized Ch). However the most critical
parameter is the surface area of the stones, which varies with the
radius squared and volume cubed. A problem in measurement of the
stone surface area lives in that often they are facetted. Park et
al.[23] have proposed a silvering method to determine the surface
area.

The mass of Ch removed per unit time per unit area is irrespective of stone size. The mass of cholesterol dissolved from a stone
by BS solution increases with stone size and is linearly related to
its surface area[23].

Dissolution rate is also influenced by other not yet fully
understood parameters such as surface components (glycoproteins,
crystals containing calcium) and stone compactness-similar to the
compression pressure used in preparation of Ch disks; hydrodynamic
conditions in the gallbladder are also relevant. In the gallbladder,
stones are probably surrounded by a thick unstirred layer which
greatly reduces diffusion of molecules.

REFERENCES

1. D. M. Small, The formation of gallstones, Adv.Inter Med., 16:243
    (1970).
2. D. M. Small and G. G. Shipley, Physical-chemical basis of lipid
    deposition in atherosclerosis, Science, 185:222 (1974).

3. R. G. Danziger, A. F. Hofmann, L. J. Schoenfield, and J. L. Thistle, Dissolution of cholesterol gallstones by chenodeoxycholic acid, N.Engl.J.Med., 286:1 (1972).

4. I. Makino, K. Shinozaki, J. Yoshino, and S. Nakagawa, Dissolution of cholesterol gallstones by ursodeoxycholic acid, Jap.J.Gastroent., 72:690 (1975).

5. W. I. Higuchi, F. Sjuib, D. Mufson, A. P. Simonelli, and A. F. Hofmann, Dissolution kinetics of gallstones: Physical model approach, J.Pharm.Sci., 62:942 (1973).

6. W. I. Higuchi, S. Prakongpan, and F. Young, Mechanism of dissolution of human cholesterol gallstones, J.Pharm.Sci., 62:945 (1973).

7. S. Prakongpan, W. I. Higuchi, K. H. Kwan, and A. M. Molokhia, Dissolution rate studies of cholesterol monohydrate in bile acid-lecithin solutions using the rotating-disk method, J.Pharm.Sci., 65:685 (1976).

8. M. C. Carey, Measurement of the physical-chemical properties of bile salt solutions, in: "Bile Acids in Gastroenterology," L. Barbara, R.H. Dowling, A.F. Hofmann, and E. Roda, eds., MTP Press Ltd., Lancaster (1983).

9. H. Igimi and M. C. Carey, Cholesterol gallstone dissolution in bile: Dissolution kinetics of crystalline (anhydrate and monohydrate) cholesterol with chenodeoxycholate, ursodeoxycholate, and their glycine and taurine conjugates, J.Lipid Res., 22:254 (1981).

10. D. M. Small, M. Bourges, and D. G. Dervichian, Ternary and quaternary aqueous system containing bile salt, lecithin, and cholesterol, Nature, 211:816 (1966).

11. G. Salvioli, H. Igimi, and M. C. Carey, Cholesterol gallstone dissolution in bile: Dissolution kinetics of crystalline cholesterol monohydrate by conjugated chenodeoxycholate-lecithin and conjugated ursodeoxycholate-lecithin mixtures: Dissimilar phase equilibria and dissolution mechanisms, J.Lipid Res., 24:701 (1983).

12. M. C. Carey and D. M. Small, The physical chemistry of cholesterol solubility in bile: Relationship to gallstone formation and dissolution in man, J.Clin Invest., 61:998 (1978).

13. M. J. Armstrong and M. C. Carey, The hydrophobic-hydrophylic balance of bile salts: Inverse correlations between reverse-phase high performance liquid chromatographic mobilities and micellar cholesterol solubilizing capacities, J.Lipid Res., 23:70 (1982).

14. M. C. Carey, Critical tables for calculating the cholesterol saturation of native bile, J.Lipid Res., 19:945 (1978).

15. V. G. Levich, "Physicochemical Hydrodynamics," Prentice-Hall, Englewood Cliffs, NJ (1962).

16. G. L. Flynn, Y. Shah, S. Prakongpan, K. Kwan, W. I. Higuchi, and A. F. Hofmann, Cholesterol solubility in organic solvents, J.Pharm.Sci., 68:1090 (1979).

17. A. F. Hofmann. W. I. Higuchi, K. H. Kwan, S. Prakongpan, J. L. Thistle, and A. Molokhia, Factors influencing the dissolution

rate of model gallstones in bile acid solutions: A critical
assessment, in: "Biological Effects of Bile Acids," G.
Paumgartner, A. Stiehl, and W. Gerok, eds., MTP Press Ltd.,
Lancaster (1979).

18. O. I. Corrigan, C. C. Su, W. I. Higuchi, and A. F. Hofmann,
     Mesophase formation during cholesterol dissolution in urso-
     deoxycholic-lecithin solution: New mechanism for gallstone
     dissolution in humans, J.Pharm.Sci., 69:869 (1981).

19. K. H. Kwan, W. I. Higuchi, A. M. Molokhia, and A. F. Hofmann,
     Dissolution kinetics of cholesterol monohydrate in simulated
     bile. I. Influence of bile acid type and concentration, bile
     acid-lecithin ratio and added electrolyte, J.Pharm.Sci.,
     66:1094 (1977).

20. W. I. Higuchi, C. C. Su, J. K. Park, M. H. Alkan, and E. Gulari,
     Mechanism of cholesterol gallstone dissolution: Analysis of
     the kinetics of cholesterol monohydrate dissolution in tauro-
     cholate/lecithin solutions by the Mazer, Bendek and Carey
     model, J.Phys.Chem., 85:127 (1981).

21. D. C. Patel and W. I. Higuchi, Mechanism of cholesterol gall-
     stone dissolution II. Correlation between the effect of alkyl
     amines as cholesterol gallstone dissolution rate accelerators
     and the degree of binding of the alkyl amines to the bile
     acid micelles, J.Coll.Interf.Sci., 74:211 (1980).

22. J. Toulli, P. Jablonski, and J. M. Watts, Dissolution of human
     gallstones: The efficacy of bile salt, bile plus lecithin and
     heparin solutions, J.Surg.Res., 19:47 (1975).

23. Y. H. Park, H. Igimi, and M. C. Carey, The "mirroring" of gall-
     stones: Description of a novel silvering method to determine
     the surface area of an irregular object, Gastroenterology,
     83:1071 (1982).

BILE ACIDS, FIBER AND CANCER

David Kritchevsky

The Wistar Institute of Anatomy and Biology
36th Street at Spruce
Philadelphia, Pennsylvania 19104

Dietary fiber is a term coined by Hipsley[1] to describe
material supposedly undegraded by our enzymes or digestive juices.
Trowell[2] later expanded this definition to add the source of the
material, namely plant cell walls. The designation "dietary fiber"
has also been broadened to include other cellular materials. A
precise definition that will satisfy everyone is still lacking, but
it is safe to assert that the term "dietary fiber" has entered our
scientific vocabulary and will not be dislodged easily. The principal dietary fibers are lignin, cellulose, hemicellulose and pectin;
all but lignin are carbohydrate in nature. The designation of fiber
now also includes polysaccharide food additives such as gums,
mucilages and algal polysaccharides. Each has a definite chemical
structure, specific chemical and physical properties and unique
physiological effects. With the exception of lignin, all dietary
fibers are degraded to some extent by the intestinal flora. Pectin
and plant gums are almost completely degraded, whereas cellulose is
degraded to a small extent[3]. It should also be noted that the
Fiber Hypothesis relating to its effects on health and disease as
propounded by Cleave[4] and Burkitt and Trowell[5] is based on a
dietary life style, not on additions of specific substances to the
diet. Furthermore, dietary patterns are often related to affluence,
and diets high in fiber are usually low in fats and other macro-
nutrients.

Portman[6] observed that the rate of bile acid excretion in rats
could be affected by dietary factors. He found[6,7] that when rats
were fed commercial diets they excreted greater quantities of cholic
acid and digitonin precipitable steroids than when fed semipurified
rations. The results of one of his experiments are summarized in
Table 1. In rats fed a semipurified diet, cholic acid half life was

doubled, its pool size reduced by 40% and excretion of this bile acid fell by 71%. Eastwood and Boyd[8] found addition of 25% cellulose to a stock diet composed of wholemeal flour, skim milk powder and brewers yeast increased fecal excretion of trihydroxy cholanic acids by 37% but decreased excretion of dihydroxy acids by 40%. To investigate the possibility suggested by Portman[6] that some dietary factor altered bile salt reabsorption and excretion, Eastwood and Hamilton[9] designed a system for measuring the absorption of bile salts to plant substances in vitro. They tested the binding of cholic and taurocholic acids to a number of substances at pH 3.9 and pH 8.0. There were differences among the substances used and for the same substances at the two pH's (Table 2). They concluded that binding was a hydrophobic phenomenon most probably due to the lignin content of the material used. Story and Kritchevsky[10] tested the binding of cholic, chenodeoxycholic and deoxycholic acids and their glycine and taurine conjugates to alfalfa, bran, cellulose and lignin. Cellulose bound very little of the substrates and bran bound appreciable quantities (greater than 10%) of only cholic acid, chenodeoxycholic acid and glycochenodeoxycholic acid. Alfalfa bound more than 10% of all but taurocholic acid. Lignin bound considerable (17-53%) of all the substrates, the most vigorously bound ones being glycodeoxycholic and cholic acids. Birkner and Kern[11] and Balmer and Zilversmit[12] found that many foodstuffs were capable of binding bile acids and salts. Story and Kritchevsky[13] found that materials such as curry powder, dried parsley and oregano bound appreciable quantities of taurocholic acid.

Human studies show that populations ingesting high fiber diets excrete greater volume of feces and more bile acids than those on low fiber diets[14]. Antonis and Bersohn[15] studied the effects of both fat and fiber on bile acid excretion in man. On a high fat - high fiber diet, neutral steroid excretion was increased by 50% but bile acid excretion was unaffected. When the diet was low in fat but high in fiber, neutral steroid excretion was increased by 90% and acidic steroid excretion by 36%. In men fed bran for 4-10 weeks, the deoxy-

Table 1. Diet and Cholic Acid Metabolism in Rats[a].

Diet	$t^{\frac{1}{2}}$ (days)	Pool (mg/kg)	Excretion (mg/kg/day)
Commercial pellets (CP)	2.0	100	35
Ethanol extracted CP	2.2	97	31
Semipurified[b] (SP)	4.2	62	31
SP plus CP lipids	2.8	50	12
SP plus CP non-saponifiables	3.7	64	12

[a] After Portman [7]
[b] Sucrose (67.6); casein (20); corn oil (8); salts (4).

Table 2. Adsorption of Bile Acids to Fiber[a].

| | Binding at pH 3.9[b] | | Binding at pH 8.0 | |
	C	TC	C	TC
Barley husk	0.97	1.05	1.05	0.75
Oat husk	0.77	0.38	0.51	0.40
Corn meal	1.10	0.74	1.28	1.25
Apple	1.00	1.14	0.59	0.53
Brussels sprout	1.09	1.33	1.03	1.18
Carrot	0.92	0.81	0.51	0.00
Pear	1.00	0.90	0.59	0.58
Turnip	0.91	0.67	0.31	0.30

[a] After Eastwood and Hamilton[4]
[b] C - Cholic acid; TC - Taurocholic acid.

cholic acid pool is decreased, the chenodeoxycholic acid pool increased and the cholic acid pool unchanged[16,17]. Men fed wheat bran exhibit increased excretion of acidic steroids[16,18,19]. Dietary pectin leads to large increases in fecal bile acid excretion[20,21].

Pectin also increase bile acid excretion in rats[22]. Kelley et al.[23] observed that rats fed 15% cellulose as part of a semi-purified diet excreted 2.52 mg of bile acids per gm of faces and the ratio of fecal cholic-chenodeoxycholic acid (C/CD) was 1.04. When cellulose was replaced by alfalfa the fecal bile acid concentration rose to 3.75 mg/gm and the C/CD ratio became 0.64. Substitution of whole ground oats for cellulose increased fecal bile acid concentration to 6.16 mg/gm and the C/CD ratio was 0.67. A similar effect of fiber on bile acid spectrum was seen in studies in which baboons were fed commercial or semipurified rations[24]. The effect of fiber on bile acid metabolism is a function of the type of fiber used. Binding may be one mechanism by which fiber increases bile acid excretion.

The link of bile acids to cancer begins with the demonstrations 50 years ago that deoxycholic[25,26] and cholic acid[27] could be converted by drastic chemical manipulation to the carcinogen methylcholanthrene. Thus, it could be hypothesized that bile acids could also be converted to carcinogen in vivo[28]. Narisawa et al.[29] demonstrated that when the carcinogen N-methyl-N'-nitro-N-nitrosoguanidine (MNNG) was instilled into rats intrarectally, together with lithocholic or taurodeoxycholic acids, the tumor incidence was doubled. These studies suggested a promotional, if not initiating, role for bile acids. Since some dietary fibers can bind bile acids, it is interesting to examine the epidemiological data relating to fiber in the diet and the incidence of colon cancer. These data have been revised recently[30]. The earliest study, done in 1933[31], found negative correlations with the ingestion of milk, whole-meal bread and vegetables. A similar negative correlation with milk and fiber was reported 44 years later[32]. Most, but not all studies found some relation between fiber intake and incidence of colon cancer. Two are notable-Howell[33] suggested a standard of living effect; Bingham et al.[34] found no significant association with dietary fiber intake in general but did observe a negative correlation between colon cancer and those foods containing pentose-rich fibers. The latter observation suggests a specific metabolic effect. Many studies in which fecal bile acids of colon cancer prone populations have been compared with controls. Comparison of bile acid distribution or of total bile acid excretion have yielded no clues. However, it has been observed that the concentration of bile acids in the feces is high in population exhibiting high incidence of colon cancer. Crowther et al.[35] studied large bowel cancer and fecal steroid excretion in three socioeconomic groups in Hong Kong. The concentration of fecal bile acids was positively correlated with income and incidence of colon cancer. Reddy et al.[36] compared fecal steroids of 15 subjects from New York City (high incidence of colon cancer) with those of 15 subjects from Kuopio, Finland (low incidence of colon cancer). Fecal volume (g/day dry feces) was 60.3 in the Finnish group and 22.3 in the Americans. The two groups excreted the same amount of bile acid daily (276 ± 1 mg) but the concentration of fecal bile acids was 4.59 mg/g in the Finns and 11.67 mg/g in the New Yorkers. The Finnish subjects excreted more than twice as much neutral steroid as the New York subjects (1103 vs. 477 mg/day) but the concentrations were similar, 18.3 vs. 21.4 mg/g. Thus, bile acid concentration rather than amount may offer the relevant correlation.

Collation of animal data on the effects of fiber on colon cancer offers little that is substantive[30]. Dietary fiber-colon cancer studies in rats have involved six rat strains, rats of both sexes, semipurified or commercial diets, different fibers fed in varying quantities, and carcinogens of various types administered orally, subcutaneously or intrarectally. However, some useful data have emerged.

Barbolt and Abraham[37] fed rats a diet containing 20% bran and administered 1,2-dimethylhydrazine (DMH) orally as well. There was 100% incidence of colon tumors in the control rats and 67% incidence in the bran-fed rats. The number of tumors per rat was 6.4 ± 0.9 in the controls and 1.2 ± 0.6 in the bran-fed group (p<0.001). There were no differences between the two groups in incidence of duodenal or cecal tumors. Thus, the effect of dietary bran was localized to the colon. Freeman et al.[38] obtained similar when they fed cellulose as the dietary fiber. Neither substance binds bile acids to any appreciable extent[10].

If bile acids are promoters of colon cancer, one would think that binding and possibly immobilizing them, would reduce their co-carcinogenic potential. To test this hypothesis, Nigro et al.[39] administered three different carcinogens – DMH, azoxymethane (AOM), and methylazoxymethanol (MAM) – to rats who were maintained on a normal diet or one containing 2% cholestyramine. The results (Table 3) show that the number of proximal bowel tumors enhanced between 74 and 350% in rats fed cholestyramine. The enhancement of occurrence of distal bowel tumors in cholestyramine-fed rats was even greater.

Watanabe et al.[40] tested the influences of fiber type and mode of carcinogen administration. They fed 15% alfalfa, pectin or bran rats treated with AOM (administered subcutaneously) and methyl-nitrosourea (MNU) administered intrarectally. Both bran and pectin significantly inhibited carcinogenesis in the AOM treated rats. Alfalfa significantly enhanced carcinogenesis in the MNU-treated rats (Table 4). These results, taken with those of Nigro et al.[34] suggest that substances which vigorously bind bile are more carcino-genic than ones which merely effect fecal bulk. The explanation may be found in the work of Cassidy et al.[41,42] who fed rats alfalfa, bran, cellulose, pectin and several bile acid binding resins and then examined their gut morphology by scanning electron microscopy. The number of structural deviations observed was inversely correlated with efficacy of bile acid binding (Table 5). The increased concen-tration of bile acids could possible exert a detergent-like effect and disrupt the structure of the mucosa.

The epidemiological data available suggest some protection from colon cancer in populations subsisting on diets high in fiber, but other confounding variables such as affluence and life style must be considered. The concentration, rather than the amount of bile acids

Table 3. Incidence of Chemically-induced Large Bowel Tumors in Rats as Affected by Cholestyramine (CH)[a].

| Carcinogen[b] | Regimen[c] | Number of tumors | |
		Proximal	Distal
DMH	ND	15	1
	ND + 2% CH	31	29
AOM	ND	19	8
	ND + 2% CH	33	36
MAM	ND	4	2
	ND + 2% CH	18	15

[a] After Nigro et al.[39]
[b] DMH - 1,2-dimethylhydrazine; AOM - azoxymethanol; MAM - methlazoxymethanol
[c] ND - normal diet.

Table 4. Effect of Fiber (15%) on Colon Cancer Induced by AOM and MNU[a],[b] (30 rats/group).

Fiber	AOM		MNU	
	Incidence (%)	Tumors/ rat	Incidence (%)	Tumors/ rat
Control[c]	57	0.8	69	1.0
Bran	33[d]	0.4	60	0.8
Pectin	10[e]	0.1	59	1.0
Alfalfa	53	0.7	83[e]	2.8

[a] After Watanabe et al.[40]
[b] AOM - Azoxymethane given subcutaneously
MNU - Methylnitrosourea given intrarectally
[c] Contains 5% cellulose
[d] Significantly different from control or alfalfa (p<0.05)
[e] Significantly different from all other groups (p<0.05)

Table 5. Influence of Dietary Fiber on Bile Acid Binding and Intestine Morphology[a].

Regimen	Average bile acid binding capacity (0-100%)	Percent of intestinal villi or colonic ridges with structural deviations[b]	
		Jejunum	Colon
Commercial	0	7.1±2.3	5.0±0.8
Bran	5	5.0±1.1	15.0±4.9
Cellulose	0	7.5±2.1	22.1±4.1
Pectin	-	30.7±4.7	29.4±8.0
Alfalfa	15	32.8±7.2	58.6±4.3
DEAE-Sephadex	30-40	13.0±3.6	40.6±9.1
Colestipol	50-60	35.9±12.6	55.0±10.1
Cholestyramine	80-100	64.2±4.7	39.5±10.5

[a] After Cassidy et al.
[b] Means ± SE for minimum of 250 villi or colonic folds

in the feces may be the best link between bile acid metabolism and susceptibility to colon cancer. Animal experiments suggest that not all fiber is equivalent and that both fiber type and mode of carcinogen administration influence the incidence of colon cancer. Animal experiments suggest that not all fiber is equivalent and that both fiber type and mode of carcinogen administration influence the incidence of colon cancer. Animal studies are not standardized which makes comparison difficult. At the very least, dietary studies should be carried out using defined rather than commercial diets. The current data suggest that we may eventually develop a structure-function relationship between fiber and its effects on bile acid metabolism and on colon cancer.

Acknowledgement

Supported, in part, by a Research Career Award (HL-0074) from the National Institutes of Health and by a grant-in-aid from the Commonwealth of Pennsylvania.

REFERENCES

1. E. H. Hipsley, Dietary "fiber" and pregnancy toxaemia, Br.Med. J., 2:420 (1953).
2. H. Trowell, Definition of dietary fiber and hypotheses that it is a protective factor in certain diseases, Am.J.Clin.Nutr., 29:417 (1976).
3. J. H. Cummings, Consequences of the metabolism of fiber in the human large intestine, in: "Dietary Fiber in Health and Disease," G.V. Vahouny and D. Kritchevsky, eds., Plenum Press, NY, pp.9-22 (1982).
4. T. L. Cleave, The neglect of natural principles in current methodical practice, J.Royal Naval Med.Service, 42:55 (1956).
5. D. P. Burkitt and H. C. Trowell, eds., "Redefined Carbohydrate Foods and Disease: Some Implications of Dietary Fiber," Academic Press, Inc., London, pp.356 (1975).
6. O. W. Portman and P. Murphy, Excretion of bile acids and hy-droxysterols by rats, Arch.Biochem.Biophys., 76:367 (1958).
7. O. W. Portman, Nutritional influences on the metabolism of bile acids, Am.J.Clin.Nutr., 8:462 (1960).
8. M. A. Eastwood and G. S. Boyd, The distribution of bile salts along the small intestine of rats, Biochim.Biophys.Acta, 137:393 (1967).
9. M. A. Eastwood and D. Hamilton, Studies on the adsorption of bile salts to nonabsorbed components of diet, Biochim. Biophys.Acta, 152:165 (1968).
10. J. A. Story and D. Kritchevsky, Comparison of binding of various bile acids and bile salts in vitro by several types of fiber, J.Nutr., 106:1292 (1976).
11. H. J. Birkner and F. Kern, jr., In vitro absorption of bile salts to food residues, salicylazosulfapyridine and hemo-cellulose, Gastroenterology, 67:237 (1984).
12. J. Balmer and D. B. Zilversmit, Effects of dietary roughage on cholesterol absorption, cholesterol turnover, and steroid excretion in the rat, J.Nutr., 104:1319 (1974).
13. J. A. Story and D. Kritchevsky, Binding of sodium taurocholate to various foodstuffs, Nutr.Rep.Int., 11:161 (1975).

14. W. D. Mitchell and M. A. Eastwood, Dietary fiber and colon function, in: "Fiber in Human Nutrition," ed., G. A. Spiller and R. J. Amen, Plenum Press, New York, pp.185-206 (1976).

15. A. Antonis and I. Bersohn, The influence of diet on fecal lipids in South African white and Bantu prisoners, Am.J.Clin.Nutr., 11:142 (1962).

16. E. W. Pomare and K. W. Heaton, Alteration of bile salt metabolism by dietary fiber (bran), Br.Med.J., 4:262 (1973).

17. E. W. Pomare, K. W. Heaton, T. S. Low-Beer, and H. J. Espiner, The effect of wheat bran upon bile salt metabolism and upon the lipid composition of bile in gallstone patients, Am.J. Dig.Dis., 21:521 (1976).

18. M. M. Stanley, D. Paul, D. Gacke, and J. Murphy, Effects of cholestyramine, metamucil and cellulose on fecal bile salt excretion in man, Gastroenterology, 65:889 (1973).

19. D. T. Forman, J. E. Garvin, J. E. Forestner, and C. B. Taylor, Increased excretion of fecal bile acids by an oral hydrophilic colloid, Proc.Soc.Exp.Biol.Med., 127:1060 (1968).

20. R. M. Kay and A. S. Truswell, Effect of citrus pectin on blood lipids and fecal steroid excretion in man, Am.J.Clin.Nutr., 30:171 (1977).

21. T. A. Miettinen and S. Tarpila, Effect of pectin on serum cholesterol, fecal bile acids and biliary lipids in normolipidemic and hyperlipidemic individuals, Clin.Chem.Acta., 79:471 (1977).

22. G. A. Leveille and H. E. Sauberlich, Mechanism of the cholesterol-depressing effect of pectin in the cholesterol-fed rat, J.Nutr., 88:209 (1966).

23. M. J. Kelley, J. N. Thomas, and J. A. Story, Modification of spectrum of fecal bile acids in rats by dietary fiber, Fed.Proc., 40:845 (1981).

24. D. Kritchevsky, L. M. Davidson, I. L. Shapiro, H. K. Kim, M. Kitagawa, S. Malhotra, P. P. Nair, T. B. Clarkson, I. Bersohn, and P. A. D. Winter, Lipid metabolism and experimental atherosclerosis in baboons: Influence of cholesterol-free, semi-synthetic diets, Am.J.Clin.Nutr., 27:29 (1974).

25. J. W. Cook and G. A. D. Haslewood, Conversion of bile acid into hydrocarbon derived from 1,2-benzanthracene, Chem.Ind., 758: (1933).

26. H. Wieland and E. Dane, Untersuchungen uber die Konstitution der Gallensauren, Z.Physiol.Chem., 219:240 (1933).

27. L. F. Fieser and M. S. Newman, Methylcholanthrene from cholic acid, J.Am.Chem.Soc., 57:961 (1935).

28. M. J. Hill, Metabolic epidemiology of dietary factors in large bowel cancer, Cancer Res., 35:3398 (1975).

29. T. Narisawa, N. E. Magadia, J. H. Weisburger, and E. L. Wynder, Promoting effect of bile acids on colon carcinogenesis after intrarectal instillation of MNNG in rats, J.Natl.Cancer Inst., 55:1093 (1974).

30. D. Kritchevsky, Fiber, steroids and cancer, <u>Cancer Res.</u>, 43:2491S (1983).

31. P. Stocks and M. K. Karns, A cooperative study of the habits, homelife, dietary and family histories of 450 cancer patients and of an equal number of control patients, <u>Ann.Eugen.</u>, 5:237 (1933).

32. International Agency for Research on Cancer, Dietary fiber, transit time, fecal bacteria, steroids and colon cancer in two Scandinavian populations, <u>Lancet</u>, 2:207 (1977).

33. M. A. Howell, Diet as an etiological factor in the development of cancers of the colon and rectum, <u>J.Chronic Dis.</u>, 28:67.

34. S. Bingham, D. R. R. Williams, T. J. Cole, and W. P. T. James, Dietary fiber and regional large bowel cancer mortality in Britain, <u>Br.J.Cancer</u>, 40:456 (1979).

35. J. S. Crowther, B. S. Drasar, M. J. Hill, R. Maclennan, D. Magnin, S. Peach, and C. H. Teah-Chan, Fecal steroids and bacteria and large bowel cancer in Hong Kong by socioeconomic groups, <u>Br.J.Cancer</u>, 34:191 (1976).

36. B. S. Reddy, A. R. Hedges, K. Laakso, and E. L. Wynder, Metabolic epidemiology of large bowel cancer, <u>Cancer</u>, 42:2832 (1978).

37. T. A. Barbolt and R. Abraham, The effect of bran in dimethyl-hydrazine-induced colon carcinogenesis in the rat, <u>Proc.Soc. Exp.Biol.Med.</u>, 157:656 (1978).

38. H. J. Freeman, G. A. Spiller and Y. S. Kim, A double-blind study on the effect of purified cellulose dietary fiber on 1,2-dimethylhydrazine-induced rat colonic neoplasia, <u>Cancer Res.</u>, 38:2912 (1978).

39. N. D. Nigro, N. Bhadrachari, and C. Chomachai, A rat model for studying colonic cancer: Effect of cholestyramine on induced tumors, <u>Dis.Colon Rectum</u>, 16:438 (1973).

40. K. Watanabe, B. S. Reddy, J. H. Weisburger, and D. Kritchevsky, Effect of dietary alfalfa, pectin and wheat bran on azoxy-methane or methylnitrosourea-induced colon carcinogenesis in F344 rats, <u>J.Natl.Cancer Inst.</u>, 63:141 (1979).

41. M. M. Cassidy, F. G. Lightfoot, L. E. Grau, T. Roy, D. Kritchevsky, and G. V. Vahouny, Effect of bile salt-binding resins on the morphology of the rat jejunum and colon: A scanning electron microscope study, <u>Dig.Dis.Sci.</u>, 25:509 (1980).

42. M. M. Cassidy, F. G. Lightfoot, L. E. Grau, J. A. Story, D. Kritchevsky, and G. V. Vahouny, Effect of chronic intake of dietary fiber on the ultrastructural topography of rat jejunum and colon: A scanning micro study, <u>Am.J.Clin.Nutr.</u>, 34:218 (1981).

INTESTINAL OPERATIONS AND BILE ACIDS: THEIR EFFECTS

ON ADAPTATION AND CARCINOGENESIS IN THE GUT

J. B. Bristol, J. B. Rainey and R. C. N. Williamson

University Department of Surgery
Bristol Royal Infirmary, Bristol BS2 8HN, UK

INTRODUCTION

The epithelial lining of the small and large bowel is renewed completely every 2-8 days in rodents and man[1]. Despite this considerable feat of replication the overall mass of intestinal mucosa remains remarkably constant in healthy adult animals and presumably also in humans. Since the gut environment is constantly changing, with variations in diet and the pattern of eating, alterations of blood flow, and a varying hormonal milieu, the mechanisms regulating mucosal maintenance and renewal must be sensitive and efficient. When they break down there are serious consequences such as ulceration and neoplasia. In this review, the role of intestinal operations as initiators of adaptive mucosal change will be emphasized and discussed in relation to their promotional effect on experimental intestinal (mainly colorectal) carcinogenesis. Finally, the role of bile salts in both these processes will be examined, and recent work from this department presented.

NORMAL INTESTINAL CELL RENEWAL

The basic architecture of the gut mucosa is very simple. In the small intestine, epithelial-lined crypts containing the four cell types – columnar, mucous, entero-endocrine and Paneth – surround the base of the villus, representing the functional unit. Within large bowel, the situation is simpler, with only three cell types (no Paneth cells) lining crypts which open directly onto the luminal surface and not onto villi. Using stathmokinetic and autoradiographic techniques, the lower half to two-thirds of the crypt has been recognized as the proliferative compartment, i.e. the portion where replication normally occurs. Above this are the maturation and functional zones. At the very base of each crypt is a small, slowly-cycling pool of cells acting as a functional stem for the rest of the crypt[2]. Mucous and entero-endocrine cells also replicate within the crypts whilst still immature[3-5] but replication ceases as they differentiate into the typical mature forms. The overall pattern of organization is similar in small and large bowel[1,6,7]; details of the events of the proliferative cell cycle can be found else-where[6,7]

Following disease or injury an adaptive response rapidly ensues within the epithelium of both small and large bowel in an attempt to restore the status quo ante. The principal stimuli are listed in Table 1. Of these, operative shortening is by far the greatest.

INTESTINAL OPERATIONS

The strongest stimulus to adaptive growth in the small bowel is loss of functioning intestine; in the large bowel compensatory changes are less easy to detect, although it is a relatively under-studied area when compared to its enteric counterpart.

Partial Enterectomy

Small intestine remaining after partial resection soon becomes hyperplastic increased mucosal mass being detectable within 8 hours [8-10]. It persists for at least 3-6 months, and probably indefi-nitely[11,12]. Adaptation develops on either side of a resected segment, is always maximal downstream, and the degree of hyperplasia reflects the length of the bowel excised[13-15]. It also diminishes with increasing distance from the anastomosis[1]. Thus, in the large bowel, maximal adaptation might be expected in the caecum and proximal colon after ileectomy. Increases of 22-51 per cent in surface area and segmental weight were indeed seen in rat caecum 30 weeks after 60 per cent distal small bowel resection, but no such changes were observed in the colon[16]. Likewise, increased mucosal

Table 1. Agents Initiating Adaptive Intestinal Change.

Agent	Examples
Intestinal operations	Resection, bypass, transposition
Food intake	Fasting, refeeding, hyperphagia, parenteral nutrition
Mucosal damage	Irradiation, cytotoxics, chemical carcinogens
Miscellaneous	Hormones, lactation, hypothermia

172

thickness was confined to the caecum 8 weeks after resection of the terminal 50 cm of ileum, although colonic hyperplasia did ensue after additional resection of the caecum[17]. These two are the only studies indicating <u>lasting</u> colonic adaptation to small bowel re- section. At earlier times (2-4 weeks postoperatively) ileal re- section[18] jejunal resection[9,19,20] and mid-enterectomy[21,22] have all stimulated structural and cytokinetic adaptation of caecum and colon.

Enteric Bypass

Bypassed small bowel undergoes severe hypoplasia[20,22-24] whereas the segment remaining in continuity undergoes hyperplasia similar (though not identical) to that seen after equivalent re- section[20,23]. Changes in the colon after enteric bypass seem to depend on the amount of small bowel remaining in circuit; after 50 per cent small bowel bypass little or no adaptive colonic change is apparent[20] whereas indices of hyperplasia persist 30 weeks after sub-total (85 per cent) bypass[25]. The atrophic changes in the bypassed segment reverse promptly on restoration of normal intestinal continuity[26].

Pancreatobiliary Diversion

Pancreatobiliary secretions help to maintain normal mucosal mass and modulate adaptive changes in the shortened gut. Ligation of the pancreatobiliary duct and subsequent enteric resection still allows some post-resectional hyperplasia to occur, but the response is diminished[27]. By contrast, diverting these secretions into the ileum enhances the compensatory response to jejunectomy[28]. Pancreatobiliary diversion to mid-small bowel without concomitant resection produces intense ileal hyperplasia persisting for 30 weeks as well as a smaller and shorter colonic response[20,29]. Bile and pancreatic juice are independently tropic to the ileum[20]. Since they are just as effective when rats are given an elemental diet their effect is independent of any improved digestibility of food- stuffs increasing the availability of luminal nutrients[20,28]. The effect of deprivation of pancreatobiliary secretions on jejunal mucosa is unclear. Hyperplasia has been described[30] but we and others have found a tendency towards hypoplasia[20,31].

Colectomy

Sub-total colectomy provokes compensatory ileal hyperplasia in rats[32-34]. In man, after colectomy, ileostomy effluent appears to reduce in volume <u>pari passu</u> with increased villous height detectable in the terminal ileum[34,35]. Adaptive changes in the shortened colon are less pronounced. We have found modest hyperplasia in the right colon 8 months after caecal resection or left hemicolectomy in rats[36] whereas others have found left colonic hyperplasia 3 months after right hemicolectomy[33]. It is possible that the colonic response to partial colectomy is impaired in the presence of proximal intact small bowel which may itself be adapting and obviating the need for the colon to do so.

Colostomy

Diversion of faeces from the distal colon by a proximal defunctioning colostomy leads to lasting hypoplastic changes similar to those found in isolated loops of small bowel[23,37,38]. We have shown that mucosal contents of RNA, DNA and protein in the defunctioned colon decrease by 53-58 per cent 4 weeks after operation, and all these changes are reversed within one week of closing the colostomy[39]. The lack of overproduction during this restorative phase indicates that precise regulatory mechanisms are operating. Other studies confirm the hypoplastic effect of defunction on distal colon. The total number of epithelial cells per crypt is lower 6 weeks after the creation of a proximal colostomy, while the labelling index, relative size of the proliferative compartment, and life-span of epithelial cells are unchanged[40]. Our own preliminary data show that the crypt cell production rate is defunctioned colon is less than 20 per cent of normal values[41].

The operative procedures described produce marked hyper- or hypoplasia detectable in part or all of the remaining gut. These adaptive changes are generally thought of as a favorable sequence enabling the organism to adapt to loss of functioning tissue or other stress[1]. Increased cell proliferation could however predispose to cancer. For instance, in the two-stage process of malignant transformation, hyperplasia could stabilize any mutation by increasing the replication of abnormal DNA damaged during the initiation phase. Thus bile acids, bacteria, food and chromic inflammatory disease could promote intestinal neoplasia by stimulating epithelial cell renewal. Indeed, hyperproliferative changes can be detected in premalignant colonic mucosa, both in rodents exposed to chemical carcinogens and in patients with familial polyposis coil[45,46]. We and others have investigated the co-carcinogenic potential of intestinal operations known or expected to give rise to colonic hyperplasia, and these will now be reviewed.

EXPERIMENTALLY-INDUCED CARCINOGENESIS

Spontaneous intestinal neoplasms in animals, particularly the common laboratory rodents, are rare[47]. The serendipitous discovery by Laquer and colleagues in 1963 that cycad meal extracted from the seeds and roots of cycad plants, produced intestinal (and other) tumors when fed to rats[48] heralded the onset of an explosion of interest in chemically-induced bowel tumors. It was suggested that the active carcinogen in the cycad meal was cycasin or its aglycone methylazoxymethanol[48]. At about the same time Druckrey and co-workers demonstrated that the synthetic compounds dimethylhydrazine and azoxymethane, both metabolic precursors of methylazoxymethanol, were highly selective intestinal carcinogens[49] inducing tumors mainly in the large bowel. These compounds have found widespread use since then and have been used in most of the experiments described below.

Partial Enterectomy

The effect of 50 per cent proximal enterectomy on intestinal carcinogenesis was tested in adolescent Fischer rats following a 16-week course of azoxymethane[12]. The yield of large bowel tumors was increased by 83 per cent when assessed at sacrifice 30 weeks later, at which time there was patchy evidence of colonic mucosal hyperplasia. Ileal hyperplasia was convincing, but there was no change in the tumor yield in this part of the gut. In another experiment, Sprague-Dawley rats were given a 12-week course of 1,2-dimethylhydrazine after resection of the distal third of the small bowel[50]. Adaptive hyperplasia of the colonic mucosa was subsequently found, in association with a significant increase in colonic neoplasms. A further experiment with a more extensive (60 per cent) resection confirmed this result [16].

Enteric Bypass

Initial experiments suggested that this operation actually protected against the enhancement of experimentally-induced large bowel tumors[51]. Subsequent work, by ourselves and others, has not confirmed this and it seems that 50 per cent[52], 66 per cent[53], 85 per cent[25] and 95 per cent[54] enteric bypass all lead to increased numbers of colonic neoplasms induced by dimethylhydrazine[52,53] or azoxymethane[25,54]. The reason for this discrepancy is possibly due to the fact that in the first study, the carcinogen was given after the bypass had been performed, on a weight for weight basis. Since rats with a bypass had already begun to lose weight compared with their sham-operated controls, the total dose of carcinogen received was considerably less[51]. Ileal bypass also produces enhanced colonic neoplasia[55].

Pancreatobiliary Diversion

The effects on intestinal carcinogenesis of transposing a 2 cm segment of duodenum bearing the pancreatobiliary duct to the mid-small bowel was studied both before and after treatment with azoxymethane[29]. This operation more than doubled the yield of large bowel tumors, whether operation preceded or followed the azoxymethane injections. As previously indicated, these operations were also associated with patchy evidence of colonic hyperplasia.

Large Bowel Operations

Sub-total colectomy and ileoprotostomy produced modest enhancement of rectal neoplasia 30 weeks later[51]. The effects of partial colectomy were less marked, with any increase in tumor yields accounted for by their occurrence at or around the anastomosis[36]. This latter phenomenon is one common to most experiments in which colon or other susceptible mucosa is cut and resutued, and is currently under investigation in this department. Creation of a colostomy to defunction the distal colon leads to a reduction of tumors in the distal segment[41], but colostomy closure enhances the subsequent yield over that of sham-operated controls even though the carcinogen was given immediately after colostomy closure when the mucosa is still hypoplastic[39].

The evidence presented above indicates that operative manipulation of the intestine, by shortening, bypass or transportation of various segments, is a strong stimulus to adaptive hyperplasia in the remaining gut, particularly that immediately downstream from the anastomosis. Most of these procedures are also followed by enhanced experimentally-induced neoplasia, particularly in segments of bowel susceptible to the chemical carcinogens used. In practice the large bowel is the area most notably affected. It seems remarkable to suggest that the two phenomena are linked, and that the surgically-induced hyperplasia predisposes to neoplasia either by increasing the number of intestinal epithelial cells exposed to the carcinogen[42] or by 'fixing' any mutation by allowing rapid division of transformed cells and the establishment of a clone[43].

The mechanisms responsible for the adaptive changes are unclear. Both luminal and systemic factors have complementary roles, but luminal factors such as food and endogenous secretions are likely to predominate[1,56]. Of the naturally occurring secretions, bile and its constituent bile acids have received particular attention, especially in view of the hypothesis linking bile acids with large bowel cancer in man[57]. It has been known for some time that direct application of bile acids to the colorectal mucosa of rodents promotes carcinogenesis[58,59]. On the other hand, binding agents that increase fecal output of bile acids may or may not increase chemical carcinogenesis[60-62]. Given the strong circumstantial evidence cited above that intestinal operations producing adaptive mucosal hyperplasia promote carcinogenesis in the large bowel, we undertook two specific experiments to study the effect of bile acids on both adaptation and carcinogenesis.

In the first experiment[63], rats were given azoxymethane by s.c. injection for 6 weeks prior to surgery. At operation, the colon was isolated as a Thiry-Vella fistula (TVF) and large bowel continuity restored with a caeco-protostomy. Shams had transection and resuture at equivalent sites. For the next 12 weeks the fistulae

were irrigated thrice weekly with either 0.9 per cent saline, 0.12 M
sodium deoxycholate (SDC) or a 12.5 per cent w/v suspension of rat
faeces in N. saline. A further group with TVF had no irrigation.
Rats were sacrificed 3 weeks after the last irrigation. Crypt depth
and tumor yield were reduced in non-irrigated TVF's compared to
controls. Irrigation with faeces or saline completely restored crypt
depth and partly restored tumor yields to the level in controls. No
such adaptive effects were seen in TVF's irrigated with SDC, nor were
tumor yields restored to control levels (Table 2).

In this model the secondary bile acid sodium deoxycholate appears to be neither tropic nor co-carcinogenic to hypoplastic defunctioned colon. The previously cited experiment showing that bile and
pancreatic juice could stimulate adaptive mucosal hyperplasia and
carcinogenesis after surgical diversion involved distal gut remaining
in continuity with the faecal stream[29]. Thus any effect of bile
acids in promoting colorectal neoplasia or in maintaining mucosal
cell turnover is likely to depend in part on other luminal factors.
In the bile acid/colon cancer hypothesis, colonic microbial flora is
implicated as the key intermediary modulating the luminal effect of
bile acids[57,64]. In another experiment we therefore examined the
tropic and co-carcinogenic potential of sodium deoxycholate instilled
directly into rat large bowel after exposure to azoxymethane. We
further examined the effect of the anaerobicide metronidazole in
modifying this potential[65].

115 rats received a 6-week course of azoxymethane as before.
Two groups then received 3 x weekly intrarectal (i.r.) instillations
of 0.9 per cent saline or 0.12 M SDC, for 18 weeks. Another group
received SDC i.r. and metronidazole 22.5 mg/kg^{-1} daily in the drinking water. Controls had no instillations or metronidazole alone.
Sacrifice was 3 weeks after the last irrigation; oral metronidazole
was continued to the end of the experiment. The effects on colonic
adaptation and tumor yield are shown in Table 3.

Table 2. Crypt Depth and Tumor Yield (mean ± SEM) in Rat Colonic
Thiry-Vella Fistulae.

	Group	Colonic crypt depth (μm)	Colonic tumors
1.	Sham TVF	274 ± 4	3.6 ± 0.5
2.	TVF alone	242 ± 6**	2.4 ± 0.4*
3.	TVF + saline	276 ± 7	2.9 ± 0.4
4.	TVF + SDC	241 ± 6**	2.3 ± 0.4
5.	TVF + faeces	280 ± 6	3.1 ± 0.6

SDC = sodium deoxycholate
Significance versus shams * $p < 0.05$ ** $p < 0.001$

Table 3. Crypt Depth and Tumor Yield (mean ± SEM) in Rat Colorectum at Sacrifice (28 weeks).

Group	Crypt depth (μm)	Tumors
1. Controls (n = 20)	226 ± 3	2.4 ± 0.4
2. Controls + metronidazole (20)	211 ± 3*	2.2 ± 0.6
3. Intrarectal saline (25)	228 ± 4	2.8 ± 0.5
4. Intrarectal SDC (25)	246 ± 3*	6.4 ± 0.5+
5. Intrarectal SDC + metronidazole (25)	242 ± 3*	4.2 ± 0.5++

SDC = sodium deoxycholate
* p<0.001 vs group 1 (controls)
+ p<0.001 vs groups 1,2,3
++ p<0.01 vs groups 1,2,4
SDC increased mean colonic crypt depth by 9 per cent (p<0.001) and almost trebled colorectal tumor yield (p<0.001).

Tumor yields after SDC and metronidazole were still 75 per cent greater than in controls (p<0.01) but 33 per cent less than after SDC alone (p<0.01). The increased crypt depth was maintained at 7 per cent (p<0.001). Neither metronidazole alone nor intra-rectal saline affected tumor yield; metronidazole also reduced crypt depth by 9 per cent (p<0.001).

Together, these two experiments indicate that sodium deoxycholate is a potent promoter of experimental colorectal carcinogenesis and an inducer of colonic hyperplasia, in large bowel remaining in normal continuity. It is therefore possible that the hyperplasia is responsible for the enhanced carcinogenesis, as is suggested earlier following various operative manoeuvres. Bile acids possibly produce hyperplasia by causing chronic irritation and inflammation of the mucosa, as is the case in subjects with ulcerative colitis who develop colorectal cancer[66]. Clearly other agents are important for these effects to be apparent; the partial suppression of the co-carcinogenic effect of intrarectal SDC by metronidazole (but not that of azoxymethane alone) suggests that the faecal anaerobic flora have a role to play, as suggested by Hill[67]. Extrapolation of these results to man is not possible. However, they do suggest that further examination of cell turnover in humans at risk of colorectal cancer, particularly those undergoing major intestinal resection or bypass, would be a prudent avenue of investigation.

REFERENCES

1. R. C. N. Williamson, Intestinal adaptation: Structural, functional and cytokinetic changes, N.Engl.J.Med., 298:1393-1402 (1978).
2. J. B. Bristol and R. C. N. Williamson, Colonic growth, Scand.J. Gastroenterol., 19 suppl 73:25-34 (1984).

3. W. W. L. Chang and N. J. Nadler, Renewal of the Epithelium in the descending Colon of the Mouse. IV. Cell population Kinetics of vacuolated-columnar and mucous cells, Am.J.Anat., 144:39-56 (1975).

4. H. Cheng, Origin, differentiation and renewal of the four main epithelial cell types in the mouse small intestine. II. Mucous cells, Am.J.Anat., 141:481-502 (1974).

5. H. Cheng and C. P. Leblond, Origin, differentiation and renewal of the four main epithelial cell types in the mouse small intestine. III. Entero-endocrine cells, Am.J.Anat., 141:503-520 (1974).

6. G. L. Eastwood, Gastrointestinal cell renewal, Gastroenterol., 72:962-975 (1977).

7. M. Lipkin, Proliferation and differentiation of gastrointestinal cells, Physiol.Rev., 53:891-915 (1973).

8. W. R. Hanson, J. W. Osborne, and J. G. Sharp, Compensation by the residual intestine after intestinal resection in the rat. II. Influence of postoperative time interval, Gastroenterol., 72:701-705 (1977).

9. H. Obertop, S. Nundy, D. Malamud, and R. A. Malt, Onset of cell proliferation in the shortened gut: Rapid hyperplasia after jejunal resection, Gastroenterol., 72:267-270 (1977).

10. R. C. N. Williamson, T. W. Buchholtz, and R. A. Malt, Humoral stimulation of cell proliferation in small bowel after transection and resection, Gastroenterol., 75:249-254 (1978).

11. E. Weser, T. Tawil, Epithelial cell loss in remaining intestine after small bowel resection in the rat, Gastroenterol., 71:412-415 (1971).

12. R. C. N. Williamson, F. R. L. Bauer, J. E. A. Osacarson, J. S. Ross, and R. A. Malt, Promotion of Azoxymethane-induced colonic neoplasia by resection of the proximal small bowel, Cancer Res., 38:3212-3217 (1978).

13. W. R. Hanson, J. W. Osborne, and J. G. Sharp, Compensation by the residual intestine after intestinal resection in the rat: I. Influence of amount of tissue removed, Gastroenterol., 72:692-700 (1977).

14. R. C. N. Williamson, Hyperplasia and neoplasia of the intestinal tract, Ann.R.Coll.Surg.Engl., 61:341-348 (1979).

15. R. C. N. Williamson and F. L. R. Bauer, Evidence for an enterotropic hormone: Compensatory hyperplasia in defunctioned bowel, Br.J.Surg., 65:736-739 (1978).

16. R. C. N. Williamson, P. J. Lyndon, and A. J. C. Tudway, Effects of anticoagulation and ileal resection on the development and spread of experimental intestinal carcinomas, Br.J.Cancer, 42:85-94 (1980).

17. J. H. B. Sacrpello, B. A. Cary, and G. E. Sladen, Effects of ilea l and caecal resection on the colon of the rat, Clin. Sci.Mol.Med., 54:241-249 (1978).

18. S. Nundy, D. Malamud, H. Obertop, J. Sczerban, and R. A. Malt, Onset of cell proliferation in the shortened gut: Colonic

hyperplasia after ileal resection, <u>Gastroenterol.</u>, 72:263–266 (1977).

19. M. D. Tilson and E. M. Livstone, Early proliferative activity: Its occurrence of the crypts of small bowel and colon after partial small bowel resection, <u>Arch.Surg.</u>, 115:1481–1485 (1980).

20. R. C. N. Williamson, F. L. R. Bauer, J. S. Ross, and R. A. Malt, Proximal enterectomy stimulates distal hyperplasia more than bypass or pancreatobiliary diversion, <u>Gastroenterol.</u>, 74:16–23 (1978).

21. K. Loeschke, J. Fabritius, and H. Hatz, Electrolyte transport of the rat colon following proximal intestinal resection, <u>in</u>: "Mechanisms of Intestinal Adaptation," J.W.L. Robinson, R.H. Dowling, E.O. Riecken, eds., MTP Press Ltd., Lancaster (1982).

22. E. Urban, P. E. Starr, and A. M. Michel, Morphologic and functional adaptations of large bowel after small bowel resection in the rat, <u>Dig.Dis.Sci.</u>, 28:265–272 (1983).

23. M. H. Gleeson, J. Cullen, R. H. Dowling, Intestinal structure and function after small bowel bypass in the rat, <u>Clin.Sci.</u>, 43:731–742 (1972).

24. I. O. Olubuyide, R. C. N. Williamson, J. B. Bristol, and A. E. Read, Goblet cell hyperplasia is a feature of the adaptive response to jejunoileal bypass in rats, <u>Gut</u>, 25:62–68 (1984).

25. J. B. Bristol, M. Wells, and R. C. N. Williamson, Adaptation to jejunoileal bypass promotes experimental colorectal carcinogenesis, <u>Br.J.Surg.</u>, 71:123–126 (1984).

26. H. Menge, R. Bloch, E. Schaumloffel, and E. O. Riecken, Jejunal bypass and reconstitution, <u>in</u>: "Intestinal Adaptation," R. H. Dowling and E. O. Riecken, eds., Schattauer Verlag, Stuttgart 61–67 (1974).

27. P. C. Shellito, E. Peterson Dahl, O. T. Terpstra, and R. A. Malt, Post-resectional hyperplasia of the small intestine without bile and pancreatic juice, <u>Proc.Soc.Exp.Biol.Med.</u>, 158:101–104 (1978).

28. E. Weser, R. Heller, and T. Tawil, Stimulation of mucosal growth in the rat ileum by bile and pancreatic secretions after jejunal resection, <u>Gastroenterol.</u>, 73:524–529 (1977).

29. R. C. N. Williamson, F. L. R. Bauer, J. S. Ross, J. B. Watkins, and R. A. Malt, Enhanced colonic carcinogenesis with Azoxymethane in rats after pancreatobiliary diversion to mid-small bowel, <u>Gastroenterol.</u>, 76:1386–1392 (1979).

30. B. M. Miazza, H. Levan, S. Vaja, and R. H. Dowling, Pancreatobiliary diversion (PBD) by duodenal transposition: A new model for stimulating jejunal and pancreatic adaptation, <u>Gut</u>, 21:A917–A918 (1980).

31. M. D. Gelinas and C. L. Morin, Effects of bile and pancreatic secretions on intestinal mucosa after proximal small bowel resection in rats, <u>Can.J.Physiol.Pharmacol.</u>, 58:1117–1123 (1980).

32. T. W. Buchholtz, D. Malamud, J. S. Ross, and R. A. Malt, Onset of cell proliferation in the shortened gut: Growth after subtotal colectomy, Surgery, 80:601-607 (1976).

33. P. C. Masesa and J. M. Forrester, Consequences of partial and subtotal colectomy in the rat, Gut, 18:37-44 (1977).

34. H. K. Wright, T. Poskitt, J. C. Cleveland, and T. Herskovic, The effect of total colectomy on morphology and absorptive capacity of ileum in the rat, J.Surg.Res., 9:301-304 (1969).

35. L. Hulten, C. Holm, and J. Kerwenter, A comparison of ileostomy function in patients proctocolectomized for ulcerative colitis in Crohn's disease of the colon, Acta Chir.Scand., 137:689-691 (1971).

36. R. C. N. Williamson, P. W. Davies, J. B. Bristol, and M. Wells, Intestinal adaptation after partial colectomy: Increased tumor yields are confined to the anastomosis, Gut, 23:316-325 (1982).

37. G. G. Altmann and C. P. Leblond, Factors influencing villus size in the small intestine of adult rats as revealed by transposition of intestinal segments, Am.J.Anat., 127:15-36 (1970).

38. R. P. C. Rijke, H. M. Plaisier, H. de Ruitier, H. Galjaard, Influence of experimental bypass on cellular kinetics, Gastroenterol., 72:896-901 (1977).

39. O. T. Terpstra, E. Peterson Dahl, R. C. N. Williamson, J. S. Ross, and R. A. Malt, Colostomy closure promotes cell proliferation and dimethylhydrazine-induced carcinogenesis in rat distal colon, Gastroenterol., 81:475-480 (1981).

40. R. P. C. Rijke, R. Gart, and N. J. Langedoen, Epithelial cell kinetics in the descending colon of the rat. II. The effect of experimental bypass, Virchows Arch.(Cell Pathol.) 31:23-30 (1979).

41. J. B. Bristol, M. A. Ghatei, S. R. Bloom, and R. C. N. Williamson, The atrophy and impaired carcinogenesis of defunctioned colon are unaffected by postoperative evaluations of plasma enteroglucagon, Br.J.Surg., 69:677 (1982).

42. T. C. Richards, Early changes in the dynamics of crypt cell populations in mouse colon following administration of 1,2 dimethylhydrazine, Cancer Res., 37:1680-1685 (1977).

43. E. Cayama, H. Tsuda, D. S. R. Sarma, and E. Farber, Initiation of chemical carcinogenesis requires cell proliferation, Nature, 275:60 (1978).

44. I. B. Weinstein, Cell regulation and cancer differentiation, 13:65-66 (1979).

45. E. E. Deschner, Early proliferative defects induced by Six weekly injections of 1,2 dimethylhydrazine in epithelial cells of mouse distal colon, Z.Krebsforsch., 91:205-216 (1978).

46. M. Lipkin, E. E. Deschner, Early proliferative changes in intestinal cells, Cancer Res., 36:2665-2668 (1976).

47. C. H. Lingeman and F. M. Garner, Comparative study of intestinal
     adenocarcinomas of animals and man, J.Natl.Cancer Inst.,
     48:325-346 (1972).
48. G. L. Laquer, O. Mickelsen, M. G. Whiting, and L. T. Kurland,
     Carcinogenic properties of nuts from Cycas circinalis L.
     indigenous to Guam, J.Natl.Cancer Inst., 31:919-995 (1963).
49. R. Preussmann, H. Druckrey, S. Ivankovic, and A. von Hodenberg,
     Chemical structure and carcinogenicity of Aliphatic Hydrazo,
     Azo and Azoxy compounds and of Triazenes, potential in vivo
     alkylating agents, Ann.NY.Acad.Sci., 163:697-716 (1969).
50. J. E. A. Oskarson, H. F. Veen, J. S. Ross, and R. A. Malt, Ileal
     resection potentiates 1,2 dimethylhydrazine-induced colonic
     carcinogenesis, Ann.Surg., 189:503-508 (1979).
51. R. C. N. Williamson, F. L. R. Bauer, O. T. Terpstra, J. S. Ross,
     and R. A. Malt, Contrasting effects of subtotal enteric
     bypass enterectomy and colectomy on Azoxymethane-induced
     intestinal carcinogenesis, Cancer Res., 40:538-543 (1980).
52. C. H. Scudamore and H. J. Freeman, Effects of small bowel tran-
     section, resection or bypass in 1,2 dimethylhydrazine-induced
     rat intestinal neoplasia, Gastroenterol., 84:725-731 (1983).
53. R. M. Bell, D. L. Oschwald, B. A. Bivens, P. F. Hagihara, and W.
     O. Griffen, Increased potential for carcinoma of the colon in
     rats following jejunoileal bypass, Surg.Forum, 83:382-383
     (1982).
54. J. B. Bristol, P. W. Davies, and R. C. N. Williamson, Subtotal
     jejunoileal bypass enhances experimental colorectal carcino-
     genesis unless weight reduction is profound, in: "Colonic
     Carcinogenesis," R.A. Malt and R.C.N. Williamson, eds., MTP
     Press Ltd., Lancaster, 275-281 (1981).
55. J. B. Rainey, P. W. Davies, and R. C. N. Williamson, Relative
     effects of ileal resection and bypass on intestinal adap-
     tation and carcinogenesis, Br.J.Surg., 71:197-202 (1984).
56. R. H. Dowling, Small bowel adaptation and its regulation, Scand.
     J.Gastroenterol., 17 suppl. 74:53-74 (1982).
57. V. Aries, J. S. Crowther, B. S. Drasar, M. J. Hill, and R. E. O.
     Williams, Bacteria and the aetiology of cancer of the large
     bowel, Gut, 10:334-335 (1969).
58. T. Narisawa, N. E. Magadia, J. H. Weisburger, and E. L. Wynder,
     Promoting effect of bile acids on colon carcinogenesis after
     intrarectal instillation of N-methyl-N[1]-nitro-N-nitrosogua-
     nidine in rats, J.Natl.Cancer Inst., 53:1093-1097 (1974).
59. B. S. Reddy, K. Watanabe, J. B. Weisburger, and E. L. Wynder,
     Promoting effect of bile acids in colon carcinogenesis in
     germ-free and conventional rats, Cancer Res., 37:3238-3242
     (1977).
60. N. D. Nigro, N. Bhadrachari, C. Chomica, A rat model for study-
     ing colonic cancer: Effect of cholestyramine on induced
     tumors, Dis.Colon Rectum, 16:438-443 (1973).
61. T. Asano, M. Pollard, and D. C. Madsen, Effects of cholestyra-
     mine on 1,2 Dimethylhydrazine-induced enteric carcinoma in
     germ-free rats, Proc.Soc.Exp.Biol.Med., 150:780-785 (1975).

62. J. P. Cruse, M. R. Lewin, and C. G. Clark, Colon cancer, bile-salt binding, and aluminium hydroxider, *Lancet*, i:1261 (1978).

63. J. B. Rainey, P. W. Davies, J. B. Bristol, and R. C. N. Williamson, Adaptation and carcinogenesis in defunctioned rat colon: Divergent effects of faeces and bile acids, *Br.J. Cancer*, 48:477-484 (1983).

64. M. J. Hill, Roll of bacteria in human carcinogenesis, *J.Hum. Nutr.*, 33:416-426 (1979).

65. J. B. Rainey, M. Maeda, C. Williams, and R. C. N. Williamson, The cocarcinogenic effect of intrarectal deoxycholate in rats is reduced by oral metronidazole, *Br.J.Cancer*, 49:631-636 (1984).

66. J. A. Van Heerden and R. W. Beart, Carcinoma of the colon and rectum complicating chronic ulcerative colitis, *Dis.Colon Rectum*, 23:155-159 (1980).

67. M. J. Hill, Bacteria and the aetiology of colonic cancer, *Cancer*, 34:815-818 (1974).

SIMILARITIES AND DIFFERENCES BETWEEN PRIMARY BILIARY
CIRRHOSIS AND PRIMARY SCLEROSING CHOLANGITIS

D. H. Van Thiel, S. Lasky, J. S. Gavaler,
T. Whiteside* and R. R. Schade

Department of Medicine and Pathology*
University of Pittsburgh School of Medicine
Pittsburgh, PA 15261

Primary Biliary Cirrhosis (PBC) and Primary Sclerosing Cholangitis (PSC) are hepatic diseases of unknown etiology[1,2]. They
both affect the liver primarily but are associated also with a wide
range of nonhepatic organ dysfunctions that are commonly considered
to be "autoimmune" in origin. Moreover, they are quite similar in
terms of their clinical presentation and course. Thus, they both
usually present relatively early in life during the third or early
fourth decade and are slowly but steadily progressive thereafter.
Initial complaints are usually rather nonspecific and include
fatigue, malaise, right upper quadrant abdominal discomfort, pruritus
and arthralgia. Initial laboratory abnormalities include elevations
in the serum levels of alkaline phosphatase, aminotransferases, gamma
glutamyl transpeptidase and total as well as direct reacting bilirubin. Table 1 demonstrates the frequency with which these various
signs and symptoms were present in patients with the two conditions
seen at the University of Pittsburgh during the last decade.

Not only are the two conditions similar in their clinical presentations (signs and symptoms) as shown in Table 1 but they are
similar also in terms of their hystopathology and their metabolic
consequences experienced as a result of prolonged cholestasis (Figure
1-4). Thus a chronic portal inflammatory reaction characterizes both
disease conditions[3,4]. With time, the portal inflammatory reaction
in both conditions involves the biliary radicles with both small and
moderate-sized bile ducts demonstrating evidence of injury while the
smaller bile ductules progressively proliferate. At the same time,
the portal inflammatory reaction extends beyond the portal areas and
gradually but progressively involves the hepatic parenchyma. Ultimately, this type of histopathologic progression leads to biliary

185

Table 1. Frequency of Signs and Symptoms in 100 Consecutive Patients with PBC and 100 with PSC Seen at the University of Pittsburgh.

Sign/symptom	PBC	PSC
Abdominal pain	12	90
Weight loss	13	40
Anorexia	8	90
Nausea/vomiting	8	85
Pruritus	58	70
Malaise/fatigue	24	75
Hyperpigmentation	6	20
Xanthomas/xanthelomas	6	4
Variceal bleeding	1	10
Hyperbilirubinemia	23	65
Hyperalkaline phosphatemia	100	100
Hyper-α-glutamyltranspeptidasemia	100	100
Hypercholesterolemia	90	50
Increased plasma bile salt levels	90	85
Hepatomegaly	70	55

cirrhosis. As a result, hepatic retention of bilirubin, bile salts, cholesterol, and copper characterizes advanced disease in both conditions. Clinically, jaundice, pruritus, xanthoma, xanthelasma, hyperpigmentation, fat malabsorption and weight loss ensue as discussed earlier and shown in Table 1.

Immunologic phenomena are a common occurrence in both conditions and may be important pathophysiologically. Autoantibodies, circulating immune complexes, evidence of abnormal delayed or cellular immunity (anergy) a mononuclear inflammatory infiltrate and putative autoimmune disease manifestations such as Sjogren's syndrome, rheumatoid arthritis and hemolytic anemia are common coexistent occurrences in both diseases.

Despite these numerous similarities, several differences exist between the two disease conditions (Table 2) and these usually allow the thoughtful clinician to distinguish between the two diseases.

Because immune mechanisms of "disorders" of immune function appear to contribute importantly to both conditions, a review of immune effector mechanisms is in order when one considers these two uncommon diseases.

Lymphocytes are the long lived effector cells of the immune system[5,6]. They have the ability to leave and re-enter the circulation. Morphologically, they can not be separated from one

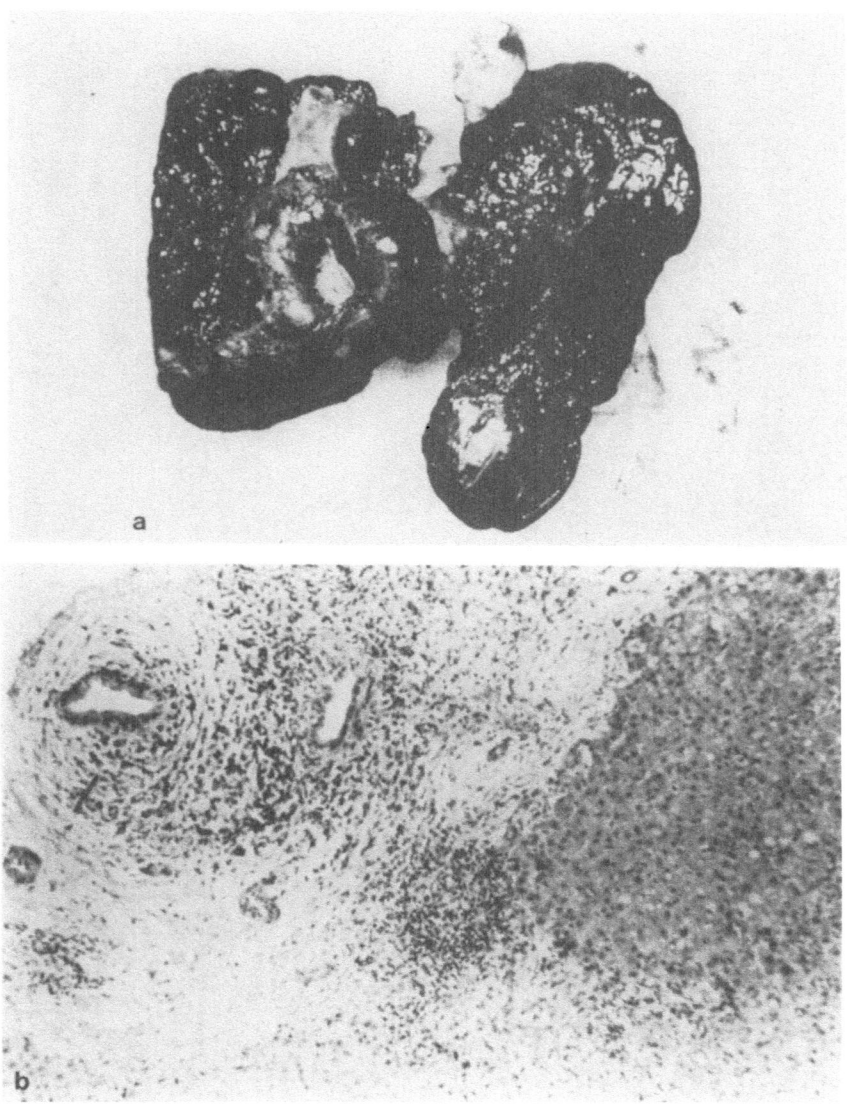

Fig. 1.   (a) Gross liver pathology in a patient with PBC.   (b) Low
power histopathology of a liver of a patient with early PBC
demonstrating a chronic portal inflammatory infiltrate and a
periductular granuloma.

another, however, using immunologic methods to detect cell surface
markers they can be distinguished and divided into 3 main types: T
cells, B cells and null cells.

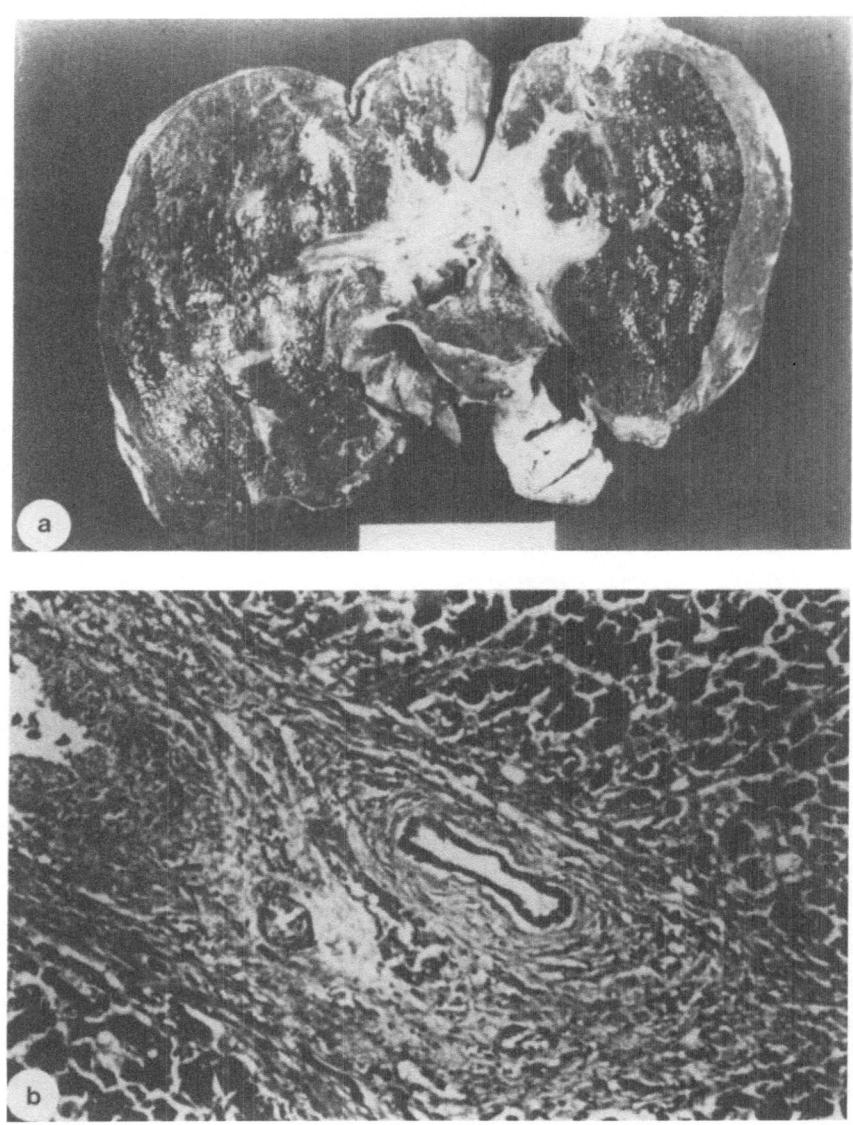

Fig. 2. (a) Gross liver pathology in a patient with PSC. (b) Low power histopathology in a liver of a patient with early PSC demonstrating periductular fibrosis and bile ductular proliferation.

The immunologic functions and characteristics of T cells are shown in Table 3. T helper cells function by interacting with other cells: both other T cells and B cells as well as macrophages,

188

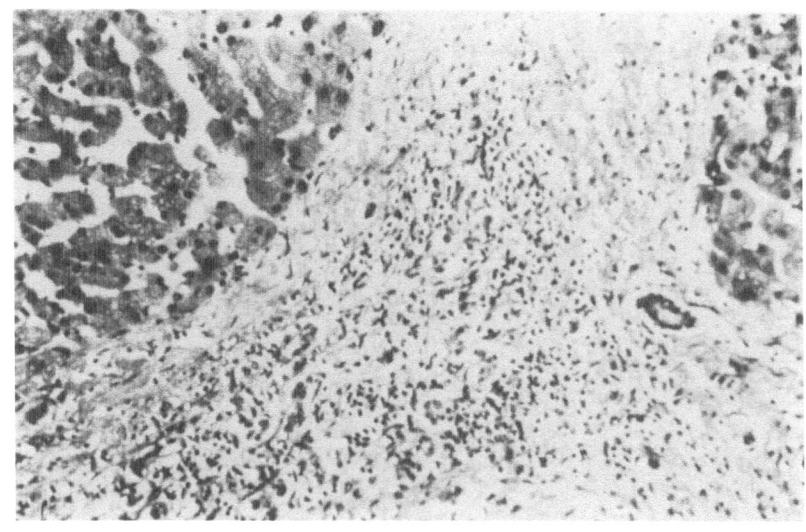

Fig. 3. Low power histopathology in a liver of a patient with advanced cirrhotic PBC demonstrating absence of bile ducts in large fibrous portal areas.

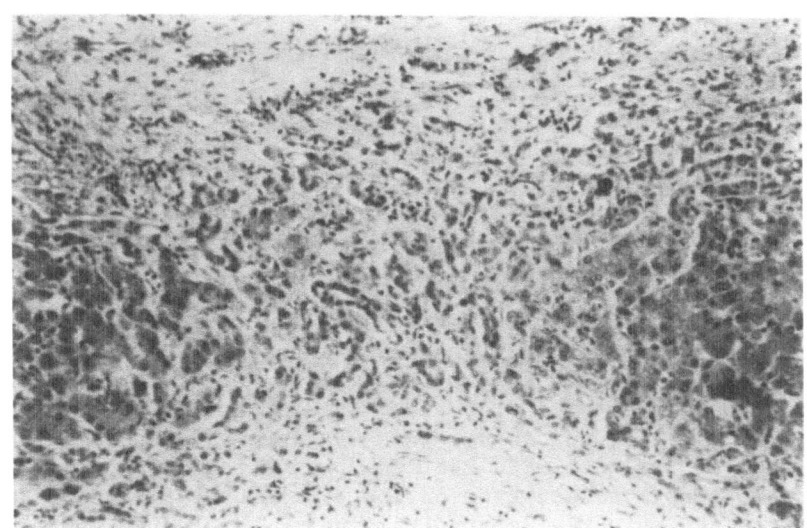

Fig. 4. Low power histopathology in a liver of a patient with advanced cirrhotic PSC demonstrating a marked proliferation of the biliary ductules.

Table 2. Differences Between PBC and PSC.

Sex	PBC	PSC
(males/females)	1:9	2:1
Autoantibodies	common (esp.AMA*) 90% of cases + for AMA	present but none specific or sensitive
HLA antigens associated with the disease condition	HLA B8	none
Inflammatory bowel disease	rare if ever	90%
Bile ducts present cirrhotic stage	absent	increased
Cholangiolar carcinoma	rare if ever	10-20% of advanced cases

* antimitochondrial antibody

hematopoietic precursors and fibroblasts. These instructions serve to initiate cell proliferation, antibody production, target cell lysis, and macrophage activation. In contrast, T suppressor cells function to regulate the magnitude of the immune response. Excessive suppressor cell activity is present in infectious mononucleosis and in various types of hypogammaglobulinemias. In contrast, reduced suppressor cell activity is seen in many, if not all, autoimmune disease conditions.

B cells are the effector cells for the humeral immune system. In response to antigenic challenge, they differentiate into plasma cells and synthesize specific antibody. Their characteristics and functions are shown in Table 4.

Because lymphocytes characterize the cellular inflammatory reaction in both PBC and PSC and because evidence of autoimmune dysfunction is common to both disease conditions, we have characterized the T and B cells present in the blood as well as in the portal areas of the liver in both conditions. This was accomplished utilizing 25 biopsies from 20 patients with PBC and 20 biopsies from patients with PSC. Ten biopsies obtained from patients without evidence of liver disease were used as normal control tissues. The technique utilized was the avidin-biotin-peroxidase complex method utilizing monoclonal antibodies for total T cells (OKT3), T helper-inducer cells (OKT4) and suppressor-cytotoxic cells (OKT8)[7,8]. The specific details of these techniques, as used in our laboratories, have been described in detail elsewhere[8,9,10].

Table 3. Immunologic Characteristics and Function of T Cells.

A. Characteristics
   Predominant lymphocyte in blood (60-80%)
   React with sheep erythrocytes
   React with OKT3 monoclonal antibody

B. Functions
   Protect against intracellular pathogens
   Tumor cell rejection
   Transplant rejection reactions
   Delayed hypersensitivity reactions
   Helper function for immunoglobulin synthesis
   Suppressor cell function
   Graft vs. host reactions
   Autoimmune disease effector cells

Table 4. Characteristics and Immunologic Functions of B Cells.

A. Characteristics
   Comprise only 5-10% of circulating lymphocytes
   Have cell surface immunoglobulins

B. Functions
   Mature into plasma cells
   Synthesize specific antibodies

The number of T cells present in the circulating blood of
patients with PBC and PSC are reduced compared to that present in
controls. The reduction was more apparent in the PBC patients than
it was in the PSC patients with the difference between the two being
significant ($p < 0.05$) (Figure 5A). The T4/T8 (helper/suppressor)
ratio of the peripheral blood lymphocytes in the patients studied is
shown in Figure 5B. The ratio was reduced ($p < 0.05$) in the PBC
patients as compared to that present in the blood of patients with
PSC and the normal controls. Thus, in addition to the differences
reported in Table 2, it may also be said that both the number of
circulating total T cells and the ratio of T4/T8 cells in peripheral
blood reduced in PBC patients as compared to PSC patients. Further,
both disease groups have reduced values for both of these parameters
when compared to normal controls ($p < 0.05$).

When the same comparisons are made for the cells present within
the portal areas of the liver tissue studied, both PBC and PSC patient
can be shown to have increased numbers of such cells compared to the
controls (Figure 6). The increase in total T cells and T helper
cells is more apparent in the livers of the PBC patients than it is

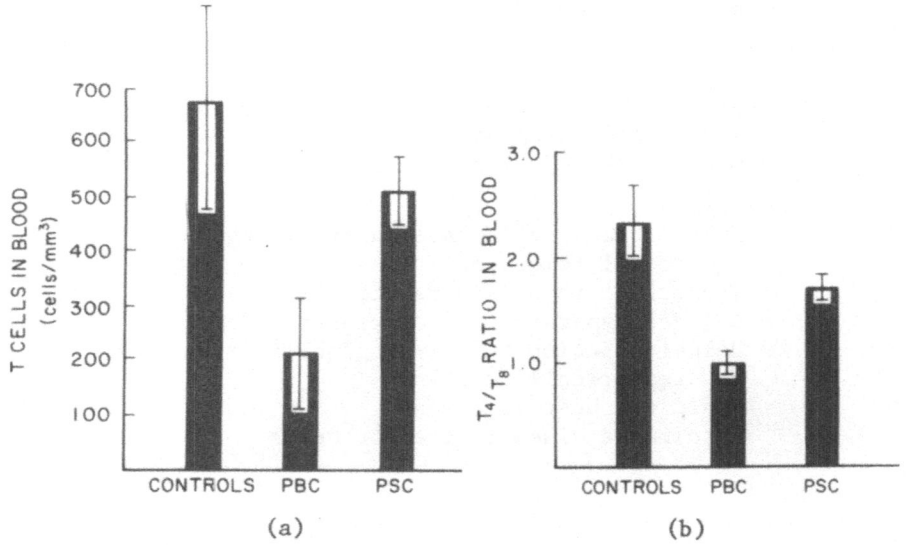

Fig. 5. (a) Number of total T cells present in the circulating blood of patients with PBC, PSC and normal controls. (b) Helper-inducer/suppressor-cytotoxic cell ratios in with PBC, PSC and controls. The bars represent mean values. The brackets represent SEM.

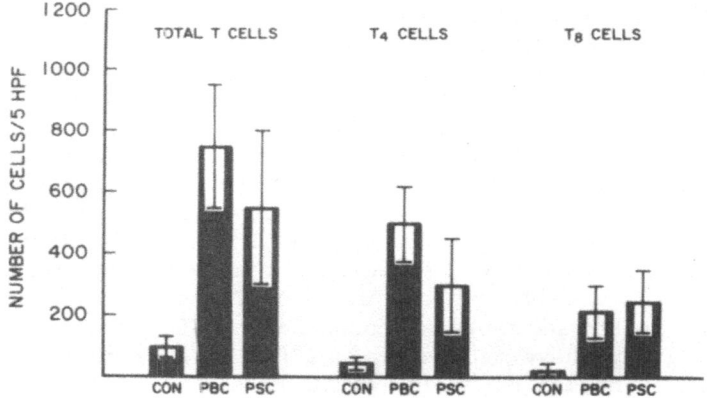

Fig. 6. Total T cells, helper-inducer and suppressor-cytotoxic cells present in five portal areas of each liver obtained from the patients with PBC, PSC and controls studied. The bars represent mean values and the brackets represent the SEM.

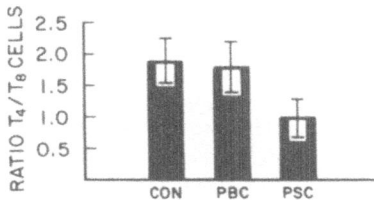

Fig. 7. Ratio of T4/T8 cells present in the portal areas of the
livers obtained and studied from the patients with PBC, PSC
and controls. The bars represents the mean values. The
brackets represent the SEM.

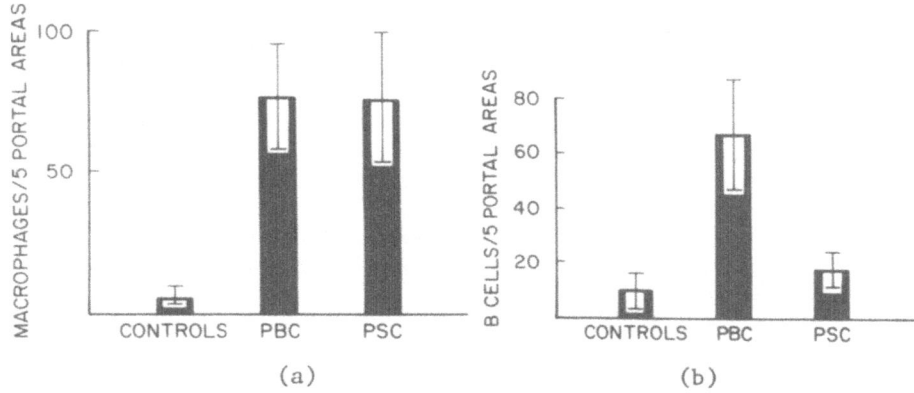

Fig. 8. Number of macrophages (a) and B cells (b) present within the
portal areas of the livers obtained from patients with PBC,
PSC and controls studied. The bars represent mean values.
The brackets represent SEM.

among those obtained from patients with PSC. No difference in the
number of T8 suppressor-cytotoxic cells is seen between the two
conditions. As a result, in comparison to normal control tissue the
ratio of T4/T8 cells in the portal areas of patients with PBC is
increased while the ratio in PSC is reduced (Figure 7). This
represents yet another difference between PBC and PSC which can be
added to those already known to exist and shown in Table 2.

Finally, when the number of macrophages (Figure 8a) and B cells
(Figure 8b) present in the portal area of the liver of patients with
PBC and PSC are counted yet another difference is noted between the
two conditions. Specifically, the number of B cells present in the
portal areas of livers obtained from patients with PBC is markedly
increased ($p < 0.01$) when compared to either that present in the portal
areas of liver tissue obtained from patients with PSC and/or the
normal controls.

193

Taken together, these data suggest that the immunologic factors that either initiate or perpetuate PBC and PSC probably differ. Moreover, these data demonstrate that PBC and PSC can be differentiated histopathologically from each other when the number of total T, T4 and T8 cells as well as the ratio of the T4/T8 cells are determined in hepatic tissue. These findings also suggest that the B cell or humeral immune system is an active participant in the pathogenesis of PBC but is not in PSC.

This work was supported in part by a grant from the Gastroenterology Medical Foundation of Southwestern Pennsylvania.

REFERENCES

1. J. M. Vierling, Primary biliary cirrhosis, in: "Hepatology," D. Zakim and T.D. Boyer, eds., W.B. Saunders Co., Philadelphia, pp.825-862 (1982).
2. J. M. Vierling, Hepatobiliary complications of ulcerative colitis and Crohn's disease, in: "Hepatology," D. Zakim and T.D. Boyer, eds., W.B. Saunders Co., Philadelphia, pp.797-824 (1982).
3. S. Sherlock, "Primary Bilary Cirrhosis in Disease of the Liver," L. Schiff and E.R. Schiff, eds., J.B. Lippincott, Philadelphia, pp.979-982 (1982).
4. E. C. C. Tan and K. W. Warren, Disease of the gallbladder and bile ducts, in: "Disease of the Liver," L. Schiff and E.R. Schiff, eds., J.B. Lippincott Co., Philadelphia, p.1533 (1982).
5. G. Janossy and H. G. Prentice, T cell subpopulations, monoclonal antibodies and their therapeutic applications, Clin.Haemat., 11:631-660 (1982).
6. S. D. Douglas and S. K. Ackerman, Anatomy of the immune system, Clin.Haemat., 6:299-330 (1977).
7. S. Hsu, L. Raine, and H. Fanger, Use of Abiden-Biotin-Peroxidase Complex (ASC) in immunoperoxidase techniques: A comparison between ABC and unlabeled antibody (PAP) procedures, J.Hist. Cytochem., 29:577-580 (1981).
8. L. Si, T. L. Whiteside, R. R. Schade, and D. H. Van Thiel, Lymphocyte subsets studied with monoclonal antibodies in liver tissues of patients with alcoholic liver disease, Alc.Clin.Exp.Res., in press.
9. I. L. Paradis, L. Si, B. S. Rabin, D. H. Van Thiel, T. E. Starzl, T. Rosenthal, M. Liebert, and T. Hakala, Effect of cyclosporine A on hepatic and Ren Allograft mononuclear cell infiltration, Transplantation Proceedings, in press.
10. L. Si, T. L. Whiteside, R. R. Schade, and D. H. Van Thiel, Studies on lymphocyte subpopulations in the liver tissue and blood of patients with chronic active hepatitis, J.Clin. Immunol., in press.

LIVER TRANSPLANTATION: AFTER 20 YEARS OF EXPERIENCE THE PROCEDURE

HAS COME OF AGE

David H. Van Thiel[1], Robert R. Schade[1], and
Thomas E. Starzl[2]

Departments of Medicine[1] and Surgery[2], University of
Pittsburgh School of Medicine, Pittsburgh,PA 15261

Abstract

The status of liver transplantation is reviewed with emphasis
upon the current survival statistics and the quality of life to
be expected in survivors. Present day indications and contraindications for the procedure are reviewed.The operative procedure
and the peri-operative problems which are to be expected following
a successful transplant are discussed.

The first orthotopic liver transplant performed in a human
was accomplished in March 1963[1]. Since that time, over 500 such
procedures have been performed worldwide[2]. The vast majority,
however, have been performed by a single surgical team headed
by Thomas E. Starzl at the University of Colorado and since 1981
at the University of Pittsburgh. Moreover,since relocating at the
University of Pittsburgh, the performance rate of the procedure
has accelerated such that Dr. Starzl's entire experience prior
to 1981 (extending over an 18-year period) has been duplicated in
less than 3 years[2].More important than the frequency of performance,
both to the patient and referring physician however,is the recent
dramatic improvement in survival figures achieved with liver transplantation[3]. Prior to 1980, the best survival figures ranged
from 20-30% at 1 year. Since 1980, survival has approached 80%
for all comers and averages between 80-90% for pediatric recipients
and 50-70% for adult recipients. The ranges cited for the survival
figures depend primarily upon the presence or absence of prior

195

surgery,co-existing hepatic or biliary sepsis,and disease severity as determined by the performance status of the patient at the time of the transplant surgery [2,4]. Specifically, those patients who are ICU bound prior to transplantation have the poorest prognosis with a 42% operating survival.In contrast,are patients who are ill with advanced to near fatal chronic liver disease but who are not hospital-bound (those who are admitted solely for the surgical procedure rather than necessary medical care and management of their hepatic disease prior to surgery) have a survival rate of 68% at 1 year. Those who do best, however, are those who are hospital-bound but not ICU-bound; they have a 1-year survival of 84%.

Equally important as survival, once it has been established that such heroic procedures can be performed with a reasonable chance of survival, is the quality of life which is to be expected after liver transplantation [5,6]. Pediatric recipients of a liver transplant would appear to be the most successfully rehabilitated patients.Thus,87.5% of pediatric survivors are fully rehabilitated and free of medical problems exclusive of those associated with routine postoperative follow-up care aimed at the recognition and control of the rejection process. Normal growth and physical as well as psychosocial development have occurred in most. Those who had demonstrated either growth or psychological developmental delays due to their liver disease prior to transplantation usually demonstrate a catch-up phenomenon following transplantation.

The quality of life data for adult liver transplant survivors are equally good with 85% of surviving adults returning to their pre-illness occupation on a full-time or regular basis following surgery.In addition,several younger adult recipients have returned to school, others have married,and two women have had three normal pregnancies between them since having been transplanted. Moreover, when careful evaluations of psychosocial and neuropsychiatric parameters have been performed pre- and post-transplantation, consistent improvement has been noted across a wide number of such variables in the adults so studied.

Now that this remarkable procedure can be shown to be accomplishable, and the quality of life experienced by survivors following the procedure has been shown to be considerably better than acceptable, the next question that arises is: who are the candidates for the procedure? Regardless of the nature of the primary liver disease mandating the procedure, several generalizations can be made concerning this issue [2,6]. These are first, that acceptable candidates should be between 1 year and 50 years of age, older individuals are less able to survive the rigors of the procedure and the various cardiopulmonary challenges that accompany the procedure. In contrast, infants less than 1 year of age frequently provide a surgical challenge that is unacceptably great and as a result immmediate surgical complications are greatest in this group. Secondly, regardless of the age of the subject, acceptable candidates should be free of infection. Thus, to guarantee success, all pulmonary,urinary tract and hepatobiliary bacterial and fungal infections must be eradicated or have resolved prior to the per-formance of the procedure. Similarly, all viral illnesses should be eradicated prior to transplantation. In the absence of the ability to eradicate such infections, as occurs with patients with sclerosing cholangitis, secondary biliary cirrhosis, and hepatitis B antigenemia, 1 year survival rates of greater than 30-40% are not to be expected [7].

Other conditions which mitigate against successful liver transplantation in patients with chronic liver disease are active drug or alcohol abuse, uncontrolled psychiatric disorder, primary extrahepatic or metastatic hepatobiliary malignancy, advanced mental retardation, portal vein thrombosis, and disabling cardiopulmonary or renal failure [6].These latter two situations,however,particularly the last, are only relative contraindications as multiple organ transplants are becoming a reasonable therapeutic option and may in the future be applied more broadly as success with individual organ transplantation continues to improve.

Acute fulminant hepatic failure has not been an important condi-tion which has been treated to date with liver transplantation [2,6,7]. This apparently paradoxical situation obtains because such patients rapidly deteriorate and consideration of transplantation as a thera-peutic option usually is initiated only after advanced coma has occurred. In such case, brain edema leading to herniation usually occurs before an appropriate donor can be identified and transplan-tation can be accomplished. Moreover, the likelihood of recurrent infection in cases of fulminant viral hepatitis would seem to be great and therefore not warrant the procedure.

The conditions for which hepatic transplantation has been applied differ in pediatric and adult cases and are shown in Tables 1 and 2. 50% of the pediatric cases have been transplanted for biliary atresia.The majority of the other pediatric recipients have been transplanted for alpha 1 antitrypsin deficiency or chronic liver disease of unknown ethiology. In contrast, the leading conditions for which hepatic transplantation has been applied in adult recipients are postnecrotic cirrhosis, primary biliary cirrhosis and primary hepatic malignancy.

Table 1.   INDICATIONS FOR TRANSPLANTATION IN
           PEDIATRIC PATIENTS   (< 18 YEARS)

Liver Pathology	%
Biliary atresia *	50%
Alpha-1-antitrypsin deficiency	15%
Chronic aggressive hepatitis	8%
Byler's disease	8%
Secondary biliary cirrhosis	2%
Budd-Chiari syndrome	2%
Neonatal hepatitis	2%
Subacute Wilson's disease	2%
Tyrosinemia	2%
Type 1 glycogen storage disease	2%
Sea-blue histiocyte syndrome	2%
Cellular inflammatory pseudotumor	2%

* Two had Alagille's syndrome

Table 2.   INDICATIONS FOR TRANSPLANTATION
            IN ADULT PATIENTS   (> 19 YEARS)

Liver Pathology	%
Postnecrotic cirrhosis	30%
Primary biliary cirrhosis	20%
Primary liver malignancy	18%
Sclerosing cholangitis	12%
Secondary biliary cirrhosis	7%
Budd-Chiari syndrome	5%
Alpha-1-antitrypsin deficiency	3%
Alcoholic cirrhosis	3%
Adenomatosis	1%

After the three main disease conditions described above, a wide variety of metabolic liver diseases make up the majority of the other conditions for which liver transplantation has been performed in pediatric patients[8]. In contrast, acquired liver diseases make up the majority of the other conditions for which liver transplantation has been applied in adult cases[2,6,7].

Factors that make surgery more difficult and as a consequence, extract a toll in terms of early survival are previous surgical procedures, particularly those in the right upper quadrant, such as prior attempts at biliary tract, reconstruction and portal caval shunting[7,9]. Such procedures make identification and dissection of the hilar structures more difficult and may have altered the anatomy further complicating the surgical dissection. Moreover, in attempts to take down a pre-existing portal caval shunt, the portal vein can be damaged, at times back to the confluence of the inferior mesenteric and splenic veins making the reestablishment of portal continuity difficult, if not impossible following graft insertion even with the use of an iliac vein graft.

Finally, portal hypertension, a common accompaniment of advanced chronic liver disease, results in the formation of fragile, but at times, massive venous collaterals within adhesions which have formed from prior surgical procedures. Such adhesions can lead to major problems in terms of obtaining hemostasis throughout the procedure from the point of host organ removal through attempts at obtaining hemostasis prior to closure following engraftment and completion of all of the vascular and biliary anastomoses necessitated as a result of the transplant procedure.

Each phase is associated with its own particular difficulties and technical procedures have been developed for each. The most recent surgical advances would seem to have been made during phase 3, when the patient is ahepatic and consists of the creation of femoral and portal venous bypasses to either the internal jugular or more commonly the axillary veins using a heparin-free system which has eliminated the need for systemic heparinization. This technical advance has markedly reduced the rate and severity of postoperative bleeding while allowing that fraction of the cardiac output delivered to the lower body below the diaphram during the procedure to be returned to the heart during the performance of the ahepatic phase of the operation. As a result, the organ engraftment can be accomplished in a careful determined way without the time restraints necessitated by systemic hypotension due to a declining central venous return and resultant reduction in cardiac output. Moreover, the immediate postoperative period also has been made more easy as a result of this advance. Specifically, as the volume of blood and colloid administered during the ahepatic phase of the procedure in an effort to maintain the cardiac output, has been reduced by this advance, the postengraftment volume overload experienced in terms of pulmonary edema has not been seen or has been reduced considerably. As a result, postoperative Intensive Care Unit time, problems with oxygenization and respiration usage have all been reduced.

Postoperatively, three different phases of potential graft failure can be identifiable. They are: 1) early (day 1 to 5) technical failures due to a vascular thrombosis or biliary anastomatic leak; 2) sepsis which occurs between day 3 through day 14; and 3) rejection which is a late cause of graft failure usually seen during the third and fourth weeks postoperatively. The presenting signs of each of these three postoperative problems are remarkably similar and include development of a large firm and tender liver, increasing jaundice and fever, with or without an accompanying leucocytosis. Early presentation of any of these signs necessitates evaluation of the grafts vascular and biliary anastomosis. After an initial period of little or no difficulty, a later change in the transplant patient's condition mandates a search for infection in or around the liver and biliary structures and finally consideration of rejection. Sonography and cholangiography should be attempted early when the patient's postoperative progress either halts or deteriorates.Early intervention directed at resolving the various differential possibilities that might exist in a given case are to be pursued actively[7,9]. Such procedures not only establish a specific diagnosis but also guide attempts at subsequent therapy such as surgical repair or drainage, antibiotic administration, or enhanced immunosuppression.

The infections that most plague patients postoperatively are those due to gram negative organisms and fungi that presumably leak into the surgical wound from the gut during the surgical procedure[10]. Acute CMV viral infection or its reactivation appear to occur universally in such patients also and can be demonstrated by buffy coat isolation or identification of the characteristic changes present in urinary sediment and liver tissue obtained by biopsy.

Infection with the herpes family of viruses also occurs commonly postoperatively and is usually manifested as either nasal labial genital or zoster-like lesions[11]. Rarely, herpetic hepatitis occurs and can be identified by isolation of the virus from hepatic tissue obtained at biopsy or by using specific immunohistologic techniques. Candida infection of the esophagus, stomach, and wound are seen less often. Finally, aspergillosis and mucor infections also occur and may necessitate treatment with Amphotericin.

As with all life extending advances in medicine ad surgery, new problems develop in patients so treated which are unique to either the procedure or the medical care necessitated by it. Thus, problems of chronic low grade rejection and the late development of recurrent hepatic failure in the transplanted organ and the need for a second transplant procedure should be kept in mind. To date, a single patient has been retransplanted late (after 5 years of survivorship with their original grafted organ). Similarly, problems occurring as a consequence of the necessary lifelong need for immunosuppression should be expected. These include those dependent upon cyclosporine administration such as nephrotoxicity, hepatotoxicity, tremor, hypertension, seizures, gingival hypertrophy, increased body hair and the various other problems shown in Table 3.

Table 3. RECOGNIZED CYCLOSPORINE TOXICITY

1. excessive immunosuppression
2. neuropathy
3. hypertension
4. hirsutism
5. gingival hypertrophy
6. tremor
7. cholestasis/hepatotoxicity
8. lymphoma (?pseudolymphoma)
9. pseudotumor cerebri
10. drug-drug interactions

The specific mechanisms responsible for the cyclosporine-associated postoperative problems are only slowly being identified. Thus the hypertension can be shown to be due, at least in part, to an enhanced activation of the renin angiotension aldosterone system as well as an apparent angiotension independent enhancement of systemic vascular resistance[12]. Similarly, the lymphomas that have been reported to occur with cyclosporine use would appear to be new or reactivated Epstein Barr virus infections that are associated with cyclosporine use and appear to be dose-dependent[13]. Thus their prevalence is greater in heart and renal transplantation situations which require greater immunosuppression than it is in liver transplant recipients. Moreover, on at least two occasions, the tumor has resolved when the cyclosporine dose has been reduced dramatically or replaced with Azathiaprine. It is clear that with advances in virology, hypertension, and tumor research which are to be expected in the future, these unique problems associated with cyclosporine use will become less and less of a problem for the transplant surgeon, his medical colleagues and their patients. Moreover, with steady refinements in surgical procedures, donor organ preservation and pretransplant assessment, immunotherapy and application of the procedure per se, success with orthotopic liver transplantation should improve even more. Even in the absence of such expected refinements it is clear that hepatic transplantation is here to stay, and that it has indeed, come of age.

REFERENCES

1. T.E. Starzl, T.L. Marchioro, K.N. Von Kaulla et al., Homo-transplantation of the liver in humans, Surg.Gynecol.Obstet., 117:659-679 (1963).
2. T.E. Starzl, S. Iwatsuki, D.H. Van Thiel, et al., Evaluation of liver transplantation, Hepatology, 2:614-636 (1982).
3. T.E. Starzl, G.B.G. Klintmalm; R. Weil III, et al., Liver transplantation with the use of cyclosporin A and prednisone, N. Eng. J. Med., 305:266-269 (1981).
4. T.E. Starzl, S. Iwatsuki, B.W. Shaw, Jr. et al., Consensus conference report on liver transplantation,Hepatology,in press.
5. D.H. Van Thiel, R.R. Schade, T.E. Starzl, After 20 years, liver transplantation comes of age, Ann. Int. Med., in press.

6. D.H. Van Thiel, R.R. Schade, J.S. Gavaler et al., Medical aspects of liver transplantation, Hepatology, in press.

7. S. Iwatsuki, B.W. Shaw Jr, T.E. Starzl, Current status of hepatic transplantation, Semin. Liver Dis., 3:173-180 (1983).

8. B.J. Zitelli, J.J. Malatack, J.C. Gartner, B.W. Shaw, S. Iwatsuki, T.E. Starzl, Orthotopic liver transplantation in children with hepatic based metabolic disease, Transplant. Proc., in press.

9. R.R. Schade, B.W. Shaw Jr, Liver transplantations:1984. Viewpoints in Digestive Diseases, in press.

10. M. Ho, C.P. Wajszczak, A. Hardy, J.S. Drummer, T.E. Starzl, T.R. Hakala, H.T. Bahnson, Infections in kidney, heart, and liver transplant recipients on cyclosporine, Transplant. Proc., in press.

11. D.H. Van Thiel, R.R. Schade, T.E. Starzl, et al., Liver transplantation in adults, Hepatology, 2:637-640 (1982).

12. M.E. Thompson, E.H. Ginchereou, R.A. Reeves, J.M. Itzkoff, A.P. Shapiro, R. McDonald Jr, B.P. Griffith, H.T. Bahnson, Hypertension following cardiac transplantation. First International Congress on Cyclosporine, Houston TX, May 16-19, 1983 (abstract).

13. Unpublished data in preparation.

EFFECTS OF INHIBITORS OF CHOLESTEROL BIOSYNTHESIS IN ISOLATED RAT HEPATOCYTES

Giuliana Cighetti, Giovanni Galli[*], Rita Paroni and
Marzia Galli Kienle

Department of Medical Chemistry and Biochemistry and
*Institute of Pharmacology and Pharmacognosy
University of Milan, Italy

INTRODUCTION

3-Hydroxy-3-methylglutaryl CoA reductase (HMG-CoA R), the microsomal enzyme catalyzing the synthesis of mevalonate from 3-hydroxy-3-methylglutaryl CoA, is known as one of the key enzymes in the regulation of cholesterol biosynthesis.[1] Many authors have demonstrated that the enzyme activity is modulated by a phosphorylation-dephosphorylation reaction.[1] The equilibrium between the two forms of the enzyme has been proposed as a rapid mechanism for the regulation of cholesterol synthesis. Studies in vitro for testing the inhibitory effects of oxygenated sterols and drugs have been mainly carried out using hepatocyte cultures[2,3]. However in these cell cultures, the HMG-CoA R was reported to be only in its dephosphorylated active form, whereas in the rat liver, the enzyme is present mainly as the inactive form (80%)[4].

To study the effect of some inhibitors on cholesterol synthesis we have developed a model where freshly isolated hepatocytes were used[5]. Differently from cultured cells hepatocytes isolated and incubated under our conditions show a dephosphorylated phosphorylated ratio as that found in the rat liver.

EXPERIMENTAL

Rat hepatocytes were isolated by the perfusion procedure, washing the liver with buffer containing collagenase (0,05%). The cells were homogenized in buffer containing NaF (50 mM) which prevents the activation of the enzyme during liver fractionation.

For the determination of the active form, the microsomes were incubated 30 min with cofactors and substrate. For the total form, microsomes were preincubated with a partially purified rat liver phosphatase[6] and then incubated. The mevalonate formed during the microsomal incubation was evaluated by the selected ion monitoring technique using $\left[^2H_4 \right]$ mevalonolactone as the internal standard[7].

RESULTS AND DISCUSSION

In the isolated hepatocytes, the active form of HMGCoA R was 20% of the total (Table 1), as reported to be in the rat liver. Moreover, the ratio of the two forms remained unchanged during 3 hours incubation. This experimental model was used to test the effect of inhibitors of cholesterol synthesis such as 25-hydroxycholesterol and pantethine.

Table 1. CELL VIABILITY AND HMGCoA REDUCTASE ACTIVITY OF HEPATOCYTES AFTER INCUBATION[a]

Incubation Time hr	Cell Viability[b] %	HMGCoA Reductase Activity[c]	
		Total	Dephosphorylated % of the total
0	96 $\pm$ 3	1560 $\pm$ 131	21.1
1	92 $\pm$ 2	1360 $\pm$ 99	22.0
2	87 $\pm$ 2	1480 $\pm$ 231	23.0
3	77 $\pm$ 5	1466 $\pm$ 78	22.0

a) Two flasks containing 4×10^7 cells in 10 ml final volume were incubated for each indicated time.
b) Values are means $\pm$ SD of the viability found by the trypan blue exclusion text after quadruplicate evaluation in one aliquot of the cell suspension at each incubation time.
c) HMGCoA R activity of the microsomes obtained from the cells either before or after the incubation was evaluated measuring mevalonate formed from HMGCoA by selected ion monitoring. Values represent means $\pm$ SD of $pmol \times min^{-1} \times mg \ protein^{-1}$ for the total enzyme and the percent of the total for the dephosphorylated form.

The mechanism of inhibition of HMGCoA R by 25-hydroxycholesterol is still controversial: some authors reported that the sterol inhibits the enzyme synthesis[4,8] but it was also suggested that the effect is modulated by the phosphorylation-dephosphorylation mechanism[9]. In our experiments the hepatocyte suspensions (4×10^7 cells) were incubated for one hour in the presence of 25-hydroxycholesterol (50 μM). The oxygenated sterol induced about 50% inhibition of total HMG-CoA R activity but the relative amount of the two forms was not modified (Table 2).Because the reduced total activity was not compensated for by dephosphorylation, the results seem to confirm the action of the oxygenated sterol on the enzyme synthesis.

Table 2. HMGCoA REDUCTASE ACTIVITY IN HEPATOCYTES BEFORE (to) AND AFTER (t1) ONE HOUR INCUBATION EITHER IN THE PRESENCE OR ABSENCE OF 25-HYDROXYCHOLESTEROL (25OH)[a].

| | HMGCoA REDUCTASE ACTIVITY | |
	Total	Dephosphorylated
to activity	1538 ± 985	330 ± 252
t1 activity	1196 ± 660*	349 ± 229*
t1 activity with 25OH	562 ± 148*	178 ± 54*

a) Values (pmolxmin^{-1}xmg protein^{-1}) are means $\pm$ SD of ten cell preparations each obtained from the liver of one rat. In each experiment with one cell preparation the enzyme activity was evaluated in microsomes before (to) and after one hr incubation either in the absence (t1) or in the presence of 25-hydroxycholesterol (t1 with 25OH). Significance of the differences was evaluated by the the t test for paired comparisons after control of variance homogeneity by the Bartlett test.
* $p < 0.05$ vs t1 activity.

Pantethine deriving from the oxidation of pantetheine, was shown to be a precursor of CoA. Moreover, pantethine was shown to reduce plasma cholesterol levels in hypercholesterolemic patients[10] but the mechanism of its action is still not clarified. Studies "in vitro" on fibroblast cultures demonstrated an inhibitory effect of the drug on cholesterol synthesis from mevalonate associated with the accumulation of methyl sterols.[11] In order to check whether pantethine induces the same effect in the liver, isolated hepatocytes (2x10[7] cells) were preincubated with pantethine (1 mM) for 1 hour and then incubated 1 hour in the presence of [2-^{14}C]mevalonolactone. Effects similar to those described in fibroblasts were observed only when the mevalonolactone added to the incubation medium was high enough to modify the rate of cholesterol synthesis also in control samples which were preincubated in the absence of pantethine. When the concentration of the precursor was low, cholesterol levels and the rate of cholesterol synthesis, as determined from the incorporation of mevalonate into cholesterol, did not differ from those of control samples. Moreover, no effects of pantethine were observed on the activity of HMGCoA R, cholesterol 7α–hydroxylase and acylCoA cholesterol acyl transferase (ACAT).

Preliminary data on the distribution of the radioactivity of ^{14}C acetate in lipids suggest that pantethine modifies fatty acid turnover in hepatocytes. The mechanism of this effect is under investigation.

REFERENCES

1. Rodwell, V. W., Nordstrom, J. L. & Mitschelen, J, J., 1976, Regulation of HMGCoA–reductase, Adv. Lipid Res., 14: 1.
2. Havel, C., Hansbury, E., Scallen, T. J. & Watson, J. A., 1979, Regulation of cholesterol synthesis in primary rat hepatocyte culture cells, J. Biol. Chem., 254: 9573.
3. Gibbons, G. F., Pullinger, C. R., Chen, H. W., Cavenee, W. K. & Kandutsch, A. A., 1980, Regulation of cholesterol biosynthesis in cultured cells by probable natural precursor sterols, J. Biol. Chem., 255: 395.
4. Brown, M. S., Goldstein, J. L. & Dietschy, J. M., 1979, Active and inactive forms of 3-hydroxy-3-methylglutaryl coenzyme A reductase in the liver of the rat, J. Biol. Chem., 254: 5144.
5. Cighetti, G., Galli, G. & Galli Kienle, M., 1983, A simple model for studies on the regulation of cholesterol synthesis using freshly isolated hepatocytes, Eur.J.Biochem., 133: 573.
6. Brandt, H., Capulong, Z. L. & Lee, E. Y. C., 1975, Purification and properties of rabbit liver phosphorylase phosphatase, J. Biol. Chem., 250: 8038.
7. Cighetti, G., Santaniello, E. & Galli, G., 1981, Evaluation of 3-hydroxy-3-methylglutaryl-CoA reductase activity by multiple- selected ion monitoring Anal. Biochem., 110: 153.
8. Beirne, O.R., Heller, R. & Watson, J. A., 1977, Regulation of 3-hydroxy-3methylglutaryl coenzyme A reductase in minimal deviation hepatoma 7288 C, J. Biol. Chem. 252: 950.
9. Erickson, S. K., Matsui, S. M., Shrewsbury, M. A., Cooper, A. D., & Gould, R. G., 1978, Effects of 25-hydroxycholesterol on rat hepatic 3-hydroxy-3-methylglutaryl coenzyme A reductase activity in vivo, in perfused liver and in hepatocytes, J. Biol. Chem., 253: 4159.
10. Goto, Y., Hata, Y., Kumagai, A. & Saito, Y., 1980, A double blind study on the effects of pantethine on hyperlipidemias, Abstracts of the 7th International Symposium on Drugs Affecting Lipid Metabolism, p.2, Milan, Italy
11. Ranganathan, S., Jackson, R.L. & Harmony, J.A.K., 1982, Effect of pantethine on the biosynthesis of cholesterol in human skin fibroblasts, Atherosclerosis, 44: 261.

BILE ACID SYNTHESIS BY CULTURED HEPATOCYTES REGULATION BY CHOLESTEROL AVAILABILITY

Haya Herscovitz and Alisa Tietz

Department of Biochemistry
Tel Aviv University
Tel Aviv, Israel

INTRODUCTION

The liver is the major organ for both synthesis and degradation of plasma cholesterol. These processes are carried out by the parenchymal cells. These cells have at least two distinct surfaces, sinusoidal and canalicular. The interaction with the plasma occurs on the sinusoidal surface; biliary lipids: cholesterol, bile acids and phosphatidylcholine are secreted through the canalicular surface. The rate of bile acid synthesis in vivo is determined by the efficiency of the enterohepatic circulation and the cholesterol content of the diet. Bile acid synthesis is stimulated when a high-cholesterol diet is fed or when the enterohepatic circulation is interrupted by feeding cholestyramine - a bile acid sequestrant.

There are at least three different sources for biliary cholesterol and bile acids. 1) De-novo synthesis; 2) Dietary cholesterol, delivered to the liver as chylomicron remnants; 3) Body or plasma - cholesterol carried to the liver as LDL or HDL.

Mitropoulos et al.[1] showed that newly synthesized cholesterol is preferentially converted to bile acids. On the other hand Schwarz et al. and Portman et al. showed the preferential conversion of HDL-cholesterol to bile acids[2,3] in man and squirrel-monkeys. Although many anatomical features present in vivo are altered when parenchymal cells are cultured, these hepatocytes afford a direct approach to examining how bile acid synthesis is regulated.

We used chick-embryo hepatocytes to examine the availability of different cholesterol sources as precursors for bile acids. Our results suggest that HDL is the preferential source for bile acid synthesis <u>in vitro</u>.

EXPERIMENTAL PROCEDURES

Preparation of Hepatocytes

Hepatocytes were prepared from livers of 14 day old chick-embryos[4]. The livers were cut into small pieces with scissors and incubated for 30 min at 37°C in Ca^{++} and Mg^{++} free Krebs-Hanselit buffer at pH 7.6. This was followed by a second 30 min. incubation in the presence of collagenase (0.5mg/ml) and hyaluronidase (1mg/ml). At the end of the incubation period 3 volumes of M-199 medium were added and the free cells collected by centrifugation. The isolated cells were washed 3 times with M-199. They were finally suspended in M-199 in presence of 10% new-born calf serum and plated (Nunc 9 cm diameter plates; 1.5 livers per plate). After 18 hr the medium and unattached cells were removed. The adherent cells were washed and incubated in fresh M-199 medium. C^{14} or H^3 labelled precursors were added as indicated in the text. To eliminate contamination, penicillin (10,000 u/ml) streptomycin (10mg/ml) and mycostatin (1 250 u/ml) were added to all media. Incubations were done at 37°C in a controlled CO_2 enriched atmosphere. At the end of the incubation period the medium was collected and kept separately for lipid and bile acid analysis. The cells were removed from the plates with EDTA-trypsin (0.25%) and were washed twice with phosphate buffered saline. The washed cells were homogenized with a small volume of H_2O. An aliquot was removed for protein determination[5] and the rest kept for lipid analysis.

Preparation of Liposomes

Cholesterol and egg yolk-phosphatidycholine were mixed at a molar ratio of 1 to 10. The organic solvent was removed, medium M-199 was added to yield a concentration of 3mM phosphatidycholine and the mixture was sonicated for 10 min. at room temperature.

Preparation of HDL Labelled with H^3 or C^{14} Cholesterol

HDL was isolated from the serum of young roosters according to Havel et al. It was first precipitated from serum plus NaBr at a solvent density of 1.065g/ml and was then floated on top of a NaBr solution of density 1.21g/ml. The lipoprotein was dialyzed extensively against several changes of phosphate buffered saline. HDL was labelled with $(4-C^{14})$ or $(1,2(n)-H^3)$-cholesterol (Amersham, UK), according to the procedure of Spector and Hoak[7]. Approximately 30% of the cholesterol initially added onto the celite was incorporated into HDL.

Cholesterol and Bile Acids Analysis

Lipids were extracted from cells or incubation media with chloroform-methanol according to Bligh and Dyer[8]. After phase separation cholesterol (Ch) and cholesterol ester (CH) were concentrated in the chloroform layer; the conjugated bile acids were contained in the methanol-water layer. Ch and CE were separated by chromatography on thin layers of silica gel G (Merck, Darmstadt, FRG) employing hexane: diethylether: acetic acid: methanol (90:20:2:3, by vol.) as solvent. The isolated lipids were located under UV light after spraying the plates with a 0.1% solution of 2,7 dichlorofluorescein in 50% ethanol. To determine the amount of radioactivity associated with the different lipids, the corresponding spots were scraped directly into scintillation vials and the radioactivity determined in a Prias liquid scintillation spectrometer (Packard, USA) after addition of Hydroluma (Lumac Sys. Inc., The Netherlands). To determine the amounts of Ch and CE present, the lipids were eluted from the gel. CE was saponified with 1 M KOH in methanol for 1 hr at 60°. Quantitative determinations were done according to Zlatkis and Zak[9].

BA were isolated from the methanol-water extract on lipidex-100 (Packard, USA) columns by ion-pairing with decyltrimethylammonium bromide according to Sjovall[10]. The BA were then separated on thin layers of silica gel G employing butanol: acetic acid:water (10:1:1, by vol.) as solvent. BA were located under UV light after spraying the plates with dichlorofluorescein. Radioactivity was determined as described above. All counts were corrected for quenching using an external standard. H^3-glycocholic acid served as an internal standard to calculate the overall efficiency of the methods employed.

Recently we developed a method for separation and quantitative estimation of BA employing high-pressure liquid chromatography. BA were extracted from the culture media according to DeMark et al.[11] using SepPak C-18 cartridges (Waters, Milford, Mass. USA). The BA were then separated on a column of Lichrosorb RP-18 of 7 μm (Merck, FRG) using methanol: water: acetic acid (340:180:0:58 by vol; the mixture was adjusted to pH 5.2 with 10N NaOH). The BA were detected spectrophotometrically at 207nm and the amounts eluted were calculated from the areas under the peaks using a Spectra-Physics model SP-4100 Computing Integrator. The relationship between area and μg BA were determined for each of the known BA. To determine the radioactivity associated with the separated BA the eluates were collected directly into scintillation vials using an LKB (LKB, Denmark) fraction collector, and counted as described above. All results are expressed as nmol product formed per mg protein assuming that 5 mol of $(2-C^{14})$ MVA yield 1 mol CH and 4 mol yield 1 mol of BA.

RESULTS

Incorporation of (2-C^{14}) Mevalonolactone into Cholesterol and Bile Acids

When (2-C^{14}) mevalonolactone (MVA) was added to the incubation medium the labelled precursor was taken up by the cultured hepatocytes and incorporated into Ch, CE and BA. The uptake of MVA by the cells seems to be rate limiting, since when increasing concentration of MVA were added Ch, CE and BA synthesis increased also (Figure 1). We did not try to saturate the system and generally 0.5 mM MVA was added. Figure 2 shows the time course of Ch, CE and BA synthesis during the first 25 hr. of incubation. On longer incubation periods, the amounts of products formed increased at a nearly linear rate for 5 days. At all times approximately 75% of the newly synthesized Ch and over 95% of the CE were found inside the cells; 25% Ch were secreted into the medium. The BA were found exclusively in the medium. Only conjugated BA were isolated; free BA were not detected. From the results shown in Figure 1 it can be calculated

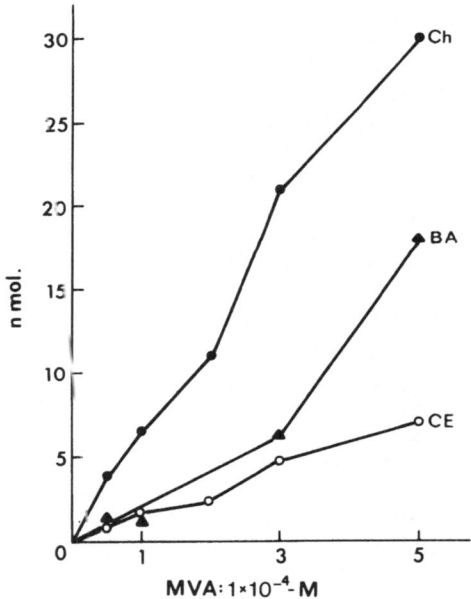

Fig. 1. The effect of increasing concentrations on mevalonolactone on cholesterol and bile acid synthesis. Hepatocytes were incubated for 5 days in the presence of different concentrations of (2-C^{14})-mevalonolactone (MVA). To attain the desired concentration MVA was mixed with "cold" substrate. Ch – cholesterol; CE – cholesterol ester; BA – conjugated bile acids.

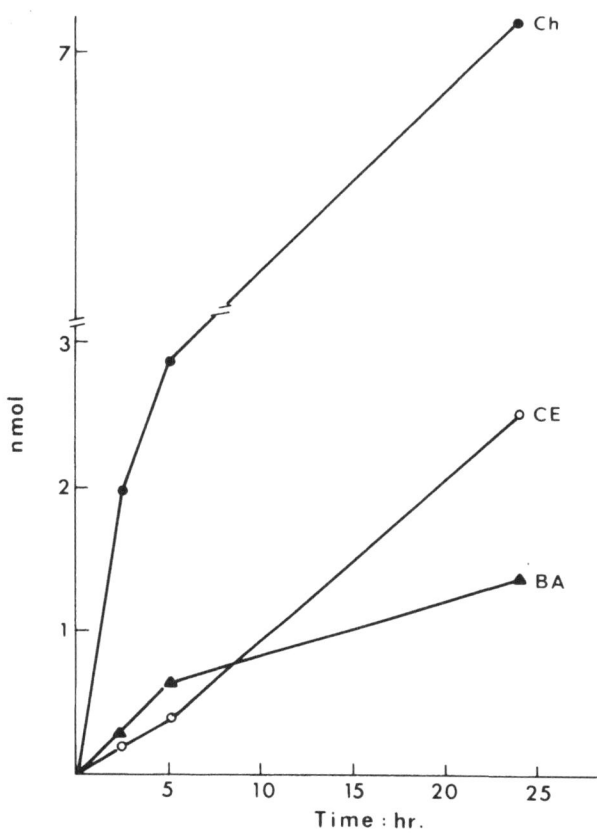

Fig. 2. Time course of cholesterol and bile acid synthesis.
$(2-C^{14})$MVA, $5\times10^{-4}\underline{M}$ was added to the incubation medium.

that approximately 30% of the newly synthesized cholesterol was
converted into BA. The major BA formed were taurocholic and taurochenodeoxycholic acid; small amounts of glycocholic acid were
isolated in some experiments (Table 1).

Conversion of Externally Added Cholesterol to Bile Acids

When cultured hepatocytes were incubated with phosphatidycholine
liposomes containing $(4-C^{14})$-cholesterol, Ch was taken up by the
cells and converted to BA (Figure 3). When increasing amounts of
liposomes were added, more Ch was incorporated into the cells and
converted into BA. Approximately 30% of the Ch taken up by the cells
was converted to BA.

To compare the efficiency of cholesterol-liposomes and MVA as
source for BA synthesis, liposomes containing (H^3)-Ch and $(2-C^{14})$-MVA

Table 1. The effect of increasing amounts of HDL on bile acid synthesis.

| HDL added | | BA synthesized; nmol/mg protein | | | | |
| Ch | Protein | Total synthesis | | | From C^{14}-Ch | |
nmol/ml	µg/ml		TC	TCDC	TC	TCDC
9.3	47	5.5	3.9	1.6	0.7	0.4
27.8	141	5.2	1.9	3.3	1.9	1.3
55.6	282	6.0	2.5	3.5	3.2	2.4

Hepatocytes were cultured in F-10 medium for 2 days in 4 cm plates. HDL was added as indicated. Cells (3mg protein) and media from 2 plates were pooled. BA were separated by HPLC as described in the methods. Total synthesis was calculated from the area under the corresponding peaks. The amount of BA synthesized from C^{14}-Ch was calculated from the radioactivity recovered in each peak and the specific radioactivity of the C^{14}-Ch in HDL.
TC – taurocholic acid; TCDC – taurochenodeoxycholic acid.

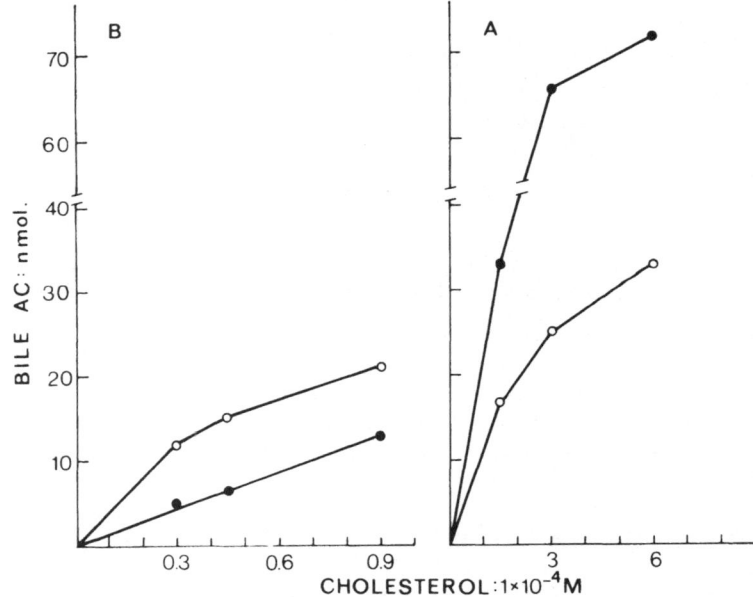

Fig. 3. Utilization of C^{14}-cholesterol incorporated into liposomes or HDL, for bile acid synthesis. (A) Mixed liposomes of egg phosphatidycholine and $(4-C^{14})$-cholesterol (molar ratio 10:1), were added to the medium. (B) $(4-C^{14})$-cholesterol was incorporated into HDL as described in the methods[7]. The concentrations of ^{14}C-Ch in HDL was determined assuming complete mixing of added C^{14}-Ch and HDL-Ch. The corresponding amounts of HDL protein were: 150, 225 and 450 µg. Ch uptake ●——● ; BA secreted ○——○ .

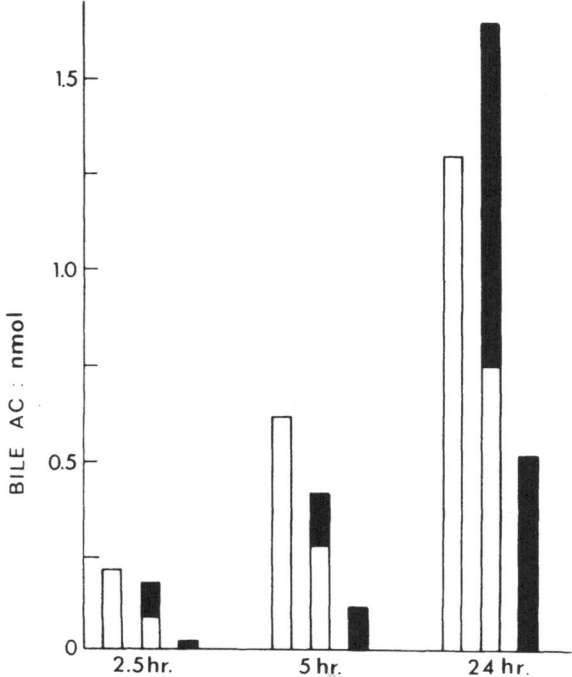

Fig. 4. A comparison of the availability of liposomal cholesterol and mevalonolactone for bile acid synthesis. $(2-C^{14})$-MVA 4×10^{-4} and/or lipsomes containing H^3-Ch 1.5×10^{-4} were added as indicated. White bars: BA synthesis from C^{14}-MVA; black bars: from H^3-Ch.

were added to the cultures either alone or simultaneously. As can be seen from Figure 4, addition of Ch inhibited the conversion of MVA to BA by approximately 50%; the conversion of MVA to Ch was inhibited by 35% only. In contrast, the conversion of H^3-Ch to BA was slightly stimulated by the simultaneous addition of MVA.

Conversion of HDL-cholesterol to Bile Acids

$(4-C^{14})$-Ch incorporated into HDL was a better source for BA synthesis than liposomal-Ch. As can be seen from Figure 3 approximately similar amounts of BA were synthesized by cultured hepatocytes from 0.3 mM liposomal-Ch or 0.09mM HDL-Ch. Furthermore, in most experiments in which HDL-Ch were added, very little "new" cholesterol accumulated inside the cells. Approximately 70% of the HDL-Ch taken up by the cells was converted to BA.

Conversion of Endogenous Cholesterol to Bile Acids

To compare the availability of endogenous substrate to that added externally (MVA or Ch) we attempted to label the endogenous Ch pool. Cultures were incubated for 2 days with liposomes containing $(1,2(n)-H^3)$-Ch. The cells were then washed and new medium containing C^{14}-Ch or MVA added. As can be seen from Figure 5, BA formation from the H^3- prelabeled pool continued throughout the second incubation period (3 days) and was not effected by the addition of MVA or Ch. Different results were obtained when the secretion of BA was followed using HPLC. As can be seen from Table 1, only small changes were noted in the total amounts of BA synthesized during 2 days of incubation. This amount was not dependent on the concentration of HDL. In the presence of HDL, taurocholic (TC) and taurochenodeoxycholic acid (TCDC) were synthesized from HDL-Ch. The synthesis of TC and TCDC from HDL-Ch increased when higher concentrations of HDL were added, suppressing the utilization of endogenous cholesterol. In the presence of large amounts of HDL, HDL cholesterol was preferentially used and the endogenous cholesterol was no longer available.

DISCUSSION

Several studies on BA synthesis by isolated rat hepatocytes have been reported in the past[12-14]. These studies indicated that hepatocytes isolated from cholestyramine fed rats maintained a much higher rate of BA synthesis than hepatocytes isolated from control rats. The BA formed were identified as taurine conjugates of cholic and muricholic acid. The viability of free hepatocytes rapidly deteriorated, therefore in order to conduct long term experiments cultivated hepatocytes seem preferable. In the present study we used cultured chick-embryo hepatocytes.

The two major BA formed from the endogenous Ch pools were taurocholic and taurochenodeoxycholic acid. In some preparations small amounts of glycholic acid were also formed. Approximately 5 nmoles of conjugated BA per mg protein were synthesized and secreted during 2 days of incubation. Unconjugated BA were not detected, neither were BA found inside the cells. In a recent publication Davis et al.[15,16] studied BA synthesis by cultured rat hepatocytes. Cholic and muricholic acid were isolated from these cultures. The rate of synthesis by normal cells were only 0.8 nmol/mg protein/48 hr. incubation. However, when hepatocytes were isolated from rats previously fed a fat containing diet, BA synthesis increased 5 fold reaching a rate comparable to that found in chick embryo hepatocytes. Since the procedure adapted by Davis et al. for the isolation of BA required hydrolysis of the conjugated acids, it was not stated whether glyco or tauro conjugates were formed.

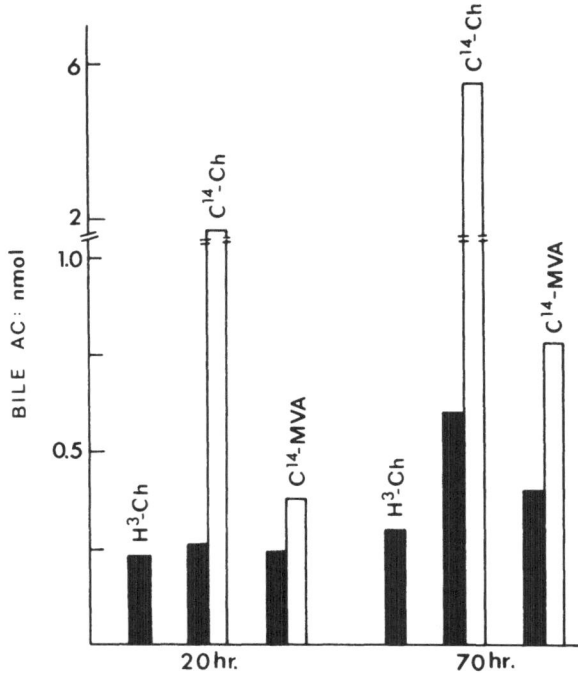

Fig. 5. Biosynthesis of bile acids from different sources of
cholesterol. Hepatocytes were incubated for 2 days with
liposomes containing 1.5×10^{-4}M $(1,2(n)-H^3)$-Ch. The medium
was removed, cells were washed and fresh medium to which
$(2-C^{14})$MVA 4×10^{-4}M or liposomes containing $(4-C^{14})$Ch $1.5 \times$
10^{-4}M was added. The secretion of H^3 and C^{14}-labeled BA was
measured after 3 additional days of incubation.

To investigate the ultimation of different cholesterol sources,
MVA or Ch were added to the incubation medium. The rate of BA synthesis from MVA (0.5mM) was of the order of 0.5-1.0 nmole/mg protein
per day. Approximately 30% of the Ch synthesized from MVA were
converted to BA; 25% were secreted unchanged, most likely as VLDL
[17,18]. When the cells were incubated with homologous HDL labelled
with C^{14}-Ch, the C^{14}-Ch was taken up by the cells and metabolized to
BA. Approximately 20% of the HDL-Ch added were converted to BA,
suppressing the utilization of endogenous cholesterol. Davis et
al.[15] also studied the effect of MVA and lipoproteins on BA synthesis. In the presence of 10 mM MVA, BA synthesis was increased by
approximately 40%. When various lipoprotein fractions were added
only VLDL + LDL stimulated BA synthesis; LDL and HDL had no effect.
These results seem to contradict our findings. However, since a
different method was employed the results cannot be readily compared.
Using C^{14}-labelled HDL we could measure simultaneously BA formation

from endogenous Ch pools and from HDL and show that although total BA synthesis was unchanged (as has also been shown by Davis et al.), HDL-Ch provided a most efficient source for BA synthesis. These results are in agreement with the in vivo observations of Schwarz and Portman and their associates[2,3]. The mechanism of Ch delivery from HDL to the liver is under investigation.

REFERENCES

1. K. A. Mitropoulos, N. B. Myant, G. F. Gibbons, S. Balasubramaniam, and B. E. A. Reeves, J.Biol.Chem., 249:6052-6061 (1974).
2. O. W. Portman, M. Alexander, and J. P. O'Malley, Biochim. Biophys.Acta., 619:545-558 (1980).
3. C. C. Schwarz, C. R. Vlahcevick, L. G. Halloran, and L. Swell, Biochim.Biophys.Acta., 663:143-162 (1981).
4. P. Belleman, R. Gelhardt, and D. Mecke, Anal.Biochem., 81:408-415 (1977).
5. O. H. Lowry, W. J. Rosebrough, A. L. Farr, and R. J. Randall, J.Biol.Chem., 193:265-275 (1951).
6. R. J. Havel, H. A. Eder, and J. H. Bragdon, J.Clin.Invest., 34:1345-1353 (1955).
7. A. A. Spector and J. C. Hoak, Anal.Biochem., 32:297-302 (1969).
8. E. G. Bligh and W. C. Dyer, Can.J.Biochem.Physiol., 37:911-917 (1959).
9. A. Zlatkis and B. Zak, Anal.Biochem., 29:143-148 (1969).
10. A. Dyverman and J. Sjovall, "Biological Effects of Bile Acids," G. Paumgartner, A. Stiehl, and W. Gerok, eds., MTP Press Ltd., p.281-286 (1979).
11. B. R. DeMark, G. T. Everson, P. D. Klein, R. B. Showalter, and F. Kern, jr., J.Lipid Res., 23:204-210 (1982).
12. M. J. Whiting and A. M. Edwards, J.Lipid Res., 20:914-918 (1979).
13. K. M. Botham, G. J. Beckett, I. W. Percy-Robb, and G. S. Boyd, Eur.J.Biochem., 103:299-305 (1980).
14. H. J. M. Kempen, M. P. M. Vos-Van Holstein, and J. de Lange, J.Lipid Res., 23:823-830 (1982).
15. R. A. Davis, P. M. Hyde, J. W. Kuan, M. Malone-McNeal, and J. Archambault-Schexnayder, J.Biol.Chem., 258:3661-3667 (1983).
16. R. A. Davis, W. E. Highsmith, M. Malone-McNeal, J. Archambault-Schexnayder, and J. W. Kuan, J.Biol.Chem., 258:4078-4082 (1983).
17. R. A. Davis, S. C. Engehorn, S. H. Pangburn, D. B. Weinstein, D. Steinberg, J.Biol.Chem., 254:2010-2016 (1979).
18. P. Siuta-Mangano, D. R. Janero, and M. D. Lane, J.Biol.Chem., 251:11463-11467 (1982).

Key Words: Chick-embryo hepatocytes, Cholesterol, HDL, Tauro-Cholic acid, Taurochenodeoxycholic acid.

MATURATION OF BILE ACID UPTAKE IN FRESHLY ISOLATED HEPATOCYTES

FROM FETAL AND NEWBORN RABBITS

M.A. Evans, R. Bhat, M.S. Bernstein, R.J. Anderson and
D. Vidyasagar
Departments of Pediatrics, Pharmacology and
Epidemiology – Biometry Program University of
Illinois Health Sciences Center Chicago, IL 60612

INTRODUCTION

Previous studies have demonstrated that hepatic uptake of bilirubin and bile acids show the characteristic features of a carrier-mediated transport and have suggested that maturation of this system may in part account for the developmental immaturity of the hepatic excretory system (Scharschmidt et al, 1975; Iga and Klaassen, 1982; Suchy and Balistreri, 1982). Clinically, impaired uptake of bile acids is supported by the finding of elevated serum concentrations of cholylglycine and conjugates of chenodeoxycholate during the first months of life (Barbara et al, 1980). This elevation in serum bile acid concentration is considered especially striking in light of the probable inefficiency of intestinal bile acid reabsorption in the first months of life, which would tend to blunt the increase in serum bile acids. In animal studies Belknap et al (1981) have demonstrated that serum concentrations of total cholate conjugates are markedly elevated in the serum of suckling and weaning rats.

A number of recent studies have shown that the use of freshly isolated hepatocytes system allows the study of functions specific to this cell type without the variability of blood flow and the interference of supporting tissue (Suchy and Balistreri, 1982; Klassen et al. 1981). Additionally, the use of isolated hepatocytes facilitates kinetic determination at various substrate concentrations and a more precise examination of the various processes and factors involved in hepatic disposition of chemicals. Eaton and Klassen (1978) have recently demonstrated that chemically induced changes in the adult sinusoidal transport system reflect the observed in vivo changes in disposition of selected drugs and physiological compounds.

These studies were designed to examine the age-related development of bile acid uptake in freshly isolated rabbit hepatocytes.

RESULTS

The cellular uptake process for taurocholate was found to be linear for at least the first four min for all substrate concentrations examined. The initial rate of uptake (V_0) was determined from linear regression analysis of the increase in taurocholate concentrations in the cell pellet with time (1-4 min). The regression correlation coefficient in all cases was greater than 0.95. Extrapolation of the V_0 line to zero time yielded a positive intercept indicative of nonsaturable nonspecific binding such as adherence to the outer cell membrane. The derived values for V_0 were combined within each age-group and substrate concentration. These values were then analyzed according to Michaelis-Menten kinetics using Lineweaver-Burk or Eadie-Hofstee plots to obtain K_m and V_{max} (Dixon and Webb, 1964).

The uptake of sodium taurocholic acid into the isolated rabbit hepatocytes was found to increase with incubation time on a per unit of protein basis. As shown in Figure 1, individual flasks containing hepatocytes isolated from the newborn group (5 days-old) and neonate (15 days old) incubated with various taurocholate concentrations demonstrated increasing bile acid concentration in the hepatocytes with time. The concentration of taurocholate remaining in the incubation media after 30 min was found to be unchanged from that measured at a time point of 1 min. Therefore, the relative plateau in the cell concentration at 30 min was probably not due to decreased bile salt availability in the media but rather to equilibration of cellular flux. At 30 min the concentration of taurocholate in the hepatocytes was 6 to 28 times greater than that present in the incubation media. A comparison of the hepatocyte/media concentration gradient of taurocholate (75 μm) showed a significant age dependant concentration gradient of taurocholate in the isolated hepatocytes at 30 min with cells from fetal rabbit showing the highest cell/media gradient (Fig. 2). No significant difference between the three age groups was observed in the hepatocyte/media concentration gradient after 1 min of incubation.

The initial uptake velocity (V_0) increased with increasing concentration of taurocholate, and an approach to a maximal V_0 with increasing substrate concentration was observed for each age group. The V_0 values within a given age-group were plotted

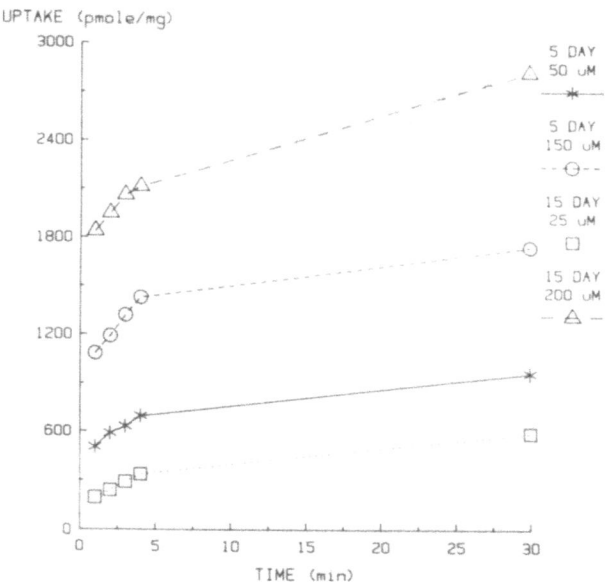

Fig. 1.   Uptake of taurocholate into freshly isolated
           hepatocytes from newborn (5 day old) and neonatal (15
           day old) rabbit.

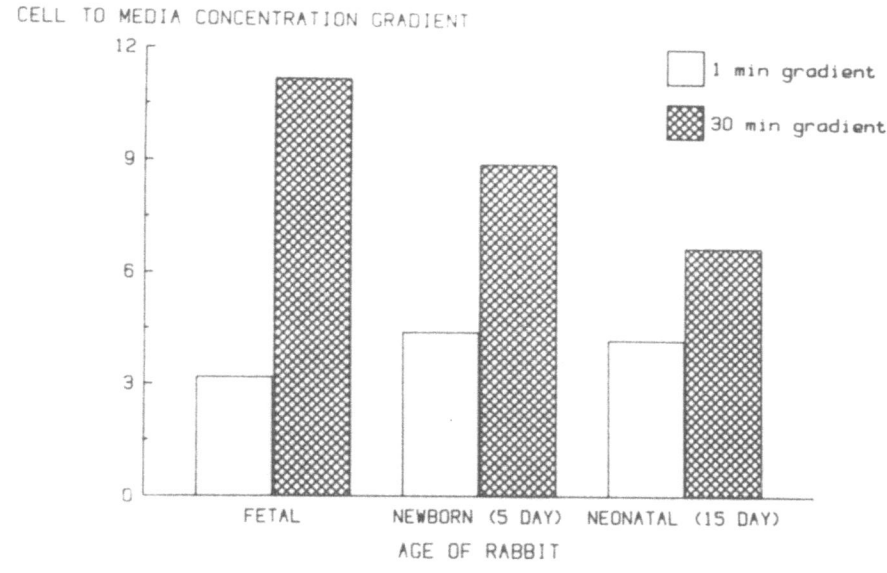

Fig. 2.   Maturation of the hepatocyte to media concentration
           gradient for taurocholate.

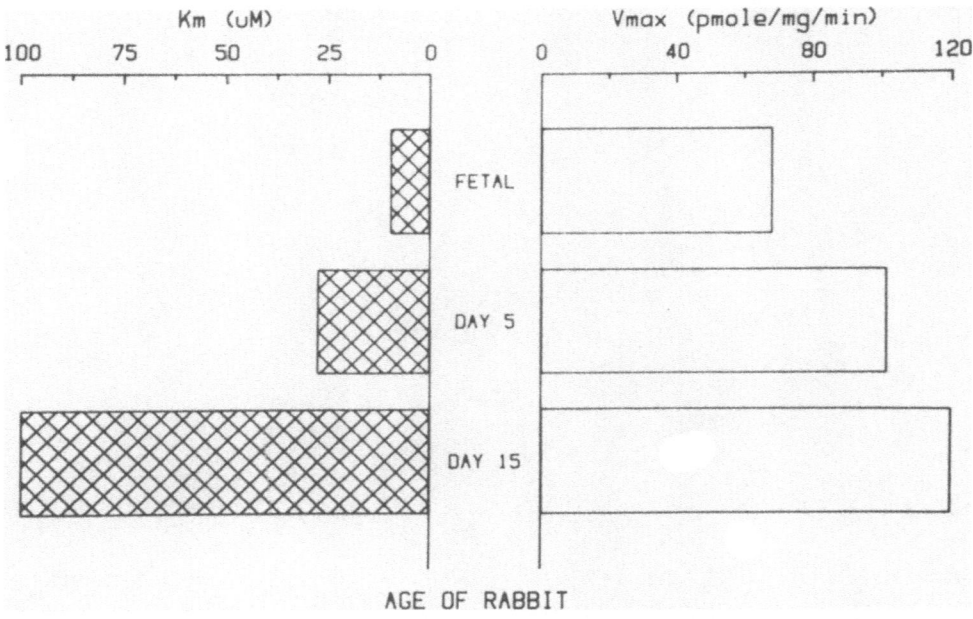

Fig. 3.   Calculated K_m and V_{max} for uptake of taurocholate by freshly isolated hepatocytes from fetal, newborn and neonatal rabbits.

against the incubation concentration and yielded results typical of Michaelis-Menton kinetics. Calculated K_m and V_{max} for uptake of taurocholate by hepatocytes from fetal, newborn and neonatal rabbits are shown in Fig. 3. Analysis of covariance applied to the data of the three age-groups revealed equality of $1/V_0$-intercepts and distinct slopes (p<0.0001). Therefore, the differences in K_m values between the age-groups were statistically significant but this did not hold three for the age related changes observed in the V_{max} values.

DISCUSSION

Conceptually, carrier-mediated transport across a membrane involves 3 steps (Anwer, 1976), 1) Initial binding of substrate to carrier at the outer membrane surface; 2) Rotation or trans-lation of carrier-substrate complex within the membrane; and 3) Dissociation of carrier-substrate complex at inner membrane sur-face. Thus, K_m or the rate constant of translocation involves more than the affinity of a substrate(s) for its carrier and is in fact inversely proportional to the overall efficiency of carrier-mediated transport of a given compound across a membrane.

The findings of the present investigation indicate that the K_m value for hepatic taurocholate uptake significantly increases at birth in the rabbit. This observed increase in K_m indicates that the overall efficiency of hepatic uptake of taurocholate decreases at birth. Conceptually, this observed change in K_m can be attributed to two factors (a) alterations in the hepatocyte membrane to affect carrier conformation and mobility; (b) structural modifications in the carrier protein. Recent studies by Benz et al. (1977) on the influence of membrane structure on carrier-mediated transport demonstrated that the translocation rate constant or K_m is strongly dependent on the nature of the membrane structure.

The observed increase in K_m values for hepatic uptake of taurocholate at birth therefore implies a developmentally related decrease in efficiency of uptake for bile acid and may be relevant to the development of clinical neonatal cholestasis.

REFERENCES

Anwer, M.S., Kroker, R. and Hegner, D.: Cholic acid uptake into isolated rat hepatocytes. Hoppe-Seyler's Z. Physiol. Chem. 357: 1477 (1976).

Barbara, L., Lazzari, R., Roda, A., Aldini, R., Festi, D., Sam, C., Morselli, A.M., Collina, A., Bazzoli, F., Mazzella, G. and Roda, E.: Serum bile acids in newborns and children. Pediatr. Res. 14: 1222 (1980).

Belknap. W.M. Balistreri, W.F., Suchy, F.J. and Miller, P.: Physiologic cholestasis. II: Serum bile acids reflect the development of the enterohepatic circulation in rats. Hepatology J. 613 (1981).

Benz, R., Frohlich, O. and Lauger, P.: Influence of membrane structure on the kinetics of carrier-mediated ion transport through lipid bilayers. Biochem Biophys Acta 464:465-481, 1977.

Dixon, M. and Webb, E.C.: Enzymes, 2nd ed. London, Longmans, 1964. Eaton, D.L. and Klaassen, C.D.: Carrier-mediated transport of the organic cation procaine amide ethobromide by isolated rat liver parenchymal cells. J. Pharmacol. Exp. Ther. 206:595, (1978).

Iga, T. and Klaassen, C.D.: Uptake of bile acids by isolated rat hepatocytes. Biochem. Pharmacol. 31: 211 (1982).

Klaassen, C.D., Eaton, D.L. and Cagen, S.Z.: Hepatobiliary disposition of xenobiotics. In, Progress in Drug Metabolism, eds, J.W. Bridges and L.F. Chasseaud, Vol. 6, pp. 1-76. New York, John Wiley a Sons, 1981.

Scharschmidt, B.F., Waggoner, J.G. and Berk, P.D.: Hepatic organic anion uptake in the rat. J. Clin Invest. 56: 1280 (1975).

Suchy, F.G. and Balistreri, W.F.: Uptake of taurocholate by hepatocytes isolated from developing rats. <u>Pediatr. Res.</u> 16:
282 (1982).

SULFATED LITHOCHOLIC ACID CONJUGATES AND CHOLESTASIS:

CLINICAL IMPLICATIONS AND PROTECTING FACTORS

Folkert Kuipers, Charles M. A. Bijleveld,
C. M. Frank Kneepkens, John Fernandes
and Roel J. Vonk

Department of Pediatrics
University Hospital of Groningen
Groningen, The Netherlands

INTRODUCTION

The cholestatic properties of monohydroxy bile acids, especially of lithocholic acid, are well established in experimental animals. Intravenous administration of lithocholic acid and its taurine or glycerine conjugate to rats or hamsters causes a dose dependent reduction in bile flow[1,2,3,4], associated with specific ultra-structural and biochemical changes in the bile canalicular membrane and pericanalicular region[5,6,7]. Lithocholic acid is a normal albeit only a minor constituent of normal human bile and serum[8]. It originates mainly from bacterial 7α-dehydroxylation of chenode-oxycholic acid in the intestine, but can also be formed in the liver by an alternative pathway involving 26-hydroxylation of choles-terol[9]. Little is known about the significance of lithocholic acid in the pathogenesis of cholestasis in man. It has been claimed that the human liver is protected from lithocholic acid-hepatoxicity by the efficient sulfation of the 3α-hydroxy group[10], which increases the bile acids' polarity. Sulfated bile acids are poorly absorbed from the intestine[11,12] and their renal clearance is relatively high[13]. Therefore, sulfation of lithocholic acid should promote its elimination from the body[14].

However, the effectiveness of sulfation as a protecting mechan-ism against monohydroxy bile acid-induced cholestasis has recently been questioned by Yousef and co-workers[15], who showed that sulfated lithocholic acid conjugated with glycine (SGLC) is still cholestatic in rats, in contrast to its taurine conjugated analogue (STLC). This may be related to the fact that despite sulfation, SGLC remains relatively water insoluble at body temperature[16]. Similarly, cholestatic effects have been described recently for the sulfate ester of isollolithocholic acid[17] and for sulfated tauro-3-β-hydroxy-5-cholenoic acid[18], another major monohydrate bile acid in man. These findings implicate that sulfation of monohydroxy bile acids is not a general detoxifying mechanism. This has been shown previously for various xenobiotics[19].

CLINICAL IMPLICATIONS

To evaluate the possible role of sulfated lithocholic acid conjugates in human liver disease, we studied the prevalence of these potentially toxic bile acids in pediatric patients with various hepatic and gastro-intestinal disorders. The concentrations of sulfated lithocholic acid conjugates and glycocholic acid (GC) were estimated by radioimmuno-assay (RIA SGLC and RIA CG, Abbott Laboratories, Chicago, Ill). The SGLC-assay measures both the taurine and glycine conjugates of sulfated lithocholic acid, but does not show significant cross-reactivity with unsulfated lithocholic acid conjugates, sulfated allolithocholic acid and sulfated 3β-hydroxy-5-cholenic acid (unpublished results). Concentrations of 3α-hydroxy bile acids were determined by an enzymatic method (Sterognost-Flu®, Nyegaard & Co, Oslo, Norway).

Sera of 266 patients, ranging in age from 0 to 14 years, were screened. In 88 patients the SGLC concentration exceeded 1.0 μmol/l, which was considered the upper limit of normal values. Twenty nine of these patients suffered from liver disease with a distinct cholestatic component, as characterized by high serum bile acid levels (SGLC = 2.7 ± 0.4, GC = 40.9 ± 6.7, 3α-hydroxy bile acids = 128.2 ± 21.6, mean in μmol/l ± SEM).

The remaining 59 patients, with relatively low serum bile acid concentrations (SGLC = 2.2 ± 0.3, GC = 2.2 ± 0.3, 3α-hydroxy bile acids = 10.3 ± 0.9), included patients with mild liver disease, intestinal dysfunctions such as Crohn's disease, coeliac disease and gastroenteritis, acute lymphatic leukemia treated with methotrexate, contaminated small bowel syndrome and three patients with benign recurrent intrahepatic cholestasis (BRIC).

In two patients with BRIC, brothers born in 1969 and 1972 respectively, we studied the prevalence and origin of the elevated SGLC levels in more detail. BRIC is a syndrome that has been described in a familial[20,21] and a nonfamilial form[22]. The clinical features of the syndrome include episodes of jaundice with biochemical signs of cholestasis alternating with symptoms-free intervals of several months or years. The etiology remains obscure; although Van Berge-Henegouwen et al.[23] have suggested that a selective defect in bile acid transport might be responsible, a casual factor initiating a cholestatic attack has never been described. The younger patient had one attack at the age of eight, the older one had a number of cholestatic attacks, characterized by very high serum bile acid concentrations (> 400 µmol/l) preceeding the rise in serum bilirubin levels. The same pattern was reported by other groups[23,24]. During symptom-free intervals, in which clinically or biochemically abnormalities could be detected, the serum concentration of SGLC were elevated[25].

Over the past two years, the general condition of these patients was monitored by regularly measuring the urinary bile acid concentration. Samples of morning urine were collected at home and screened on the presence of 3α-hydroxy bile acids. Measurements were performed directly on 0.1 ml of urine, without prior extraction. No solvolysis step was included, although it has been reported that in normal urine up to 80 per cent of the bile acids is sulfated, a percentage that may be even higher in cholestatic urine[13,26]. However, the urinary concentration bile acids measured in this way was found to correlate well with the degree of liver dysfunction in these patients (Figure 1). The concentration varies between 15 and 35 µmol/l when clinical symptoms of liver dysfunction were absent, but increased rapidly during periods of malaise, before clinical signs of cholestasis were observed. The latter periods probably represent so-called pre-icteric phase that proceed the onset of cholestasis[21]. By measuring urinary bile acid concentrations, we are able to trace the onset of cholestasis in these patients in a very early stage. Treatment can be started immediately after the initiation of a cholestatic attack, which might reduce its severity and duration.

To investigate the origin of the elevated serum levels of SGLC in these two BRIC patients, the postprandial response of serum SGLC was measured after a testmeal of 1 g fat/kg body weight. Serum SGLC concentrations were determined at 0, 60, 120 and 180 minutes after the testmeal. In addition, serum concentration of GC were measured to ascertain gallbladder-contraction. The response was expressed as maximal increase towards fasting values (Δ, in µmol/l). In the group of patients with basal SGLC levels below 1.0 µmol/l, the SGLC response was small or absent (0.2 ± 0.05, mean $\pm$ SEM, $\underline{n}$ = 26). In contrast, when the test was performed in the pediatric BRIC patients during anicteric interval, in a period with low urinary bile acid excretion and a good general condition, the mean ΔSGLC was 2.8 ± 0.20, $\underline{n}$ = 7 (Figure 2A). In these tests, the mean ΔGC was 4.2 ± 0.47, which was higher than in the control group (ΔGC was 2.1 ± 0.26, $\underline{n}$ = 26), but much lower than in patients with cholestatic liver disease: ΔGC = 18.4 ± 2.8, $\underline{n}$ = 6. No correlation was found between the magnitude of ΔSGLC and ΔGC in the total group of patients studied, which indicates that the observed ΔSGLC is not caused by a decreased hepatic clearance of bile acids. When cholestyramine (4 g.) was added to the testmeal during the same interval, a post-

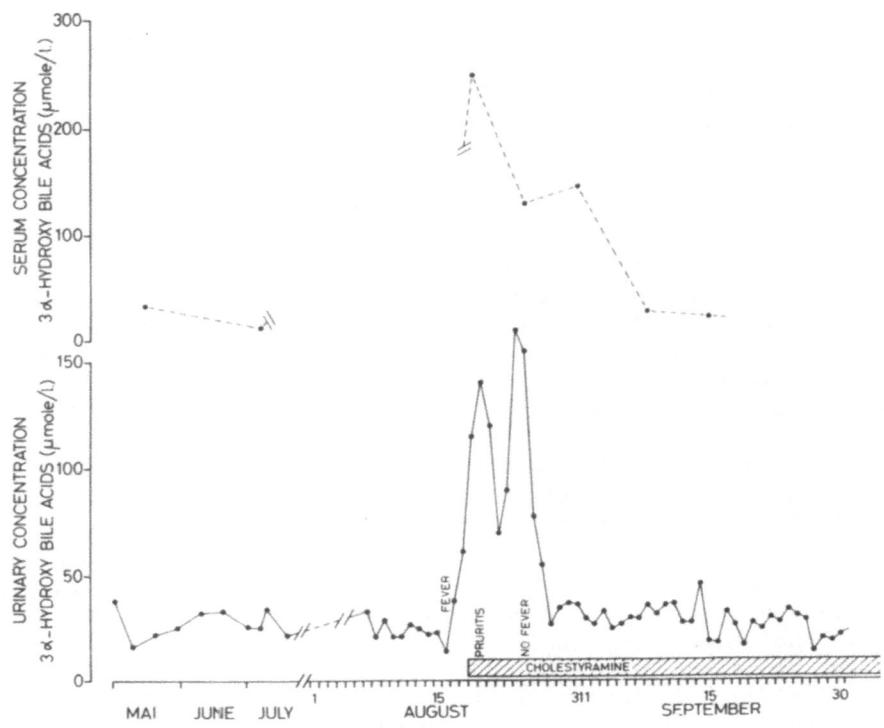

Fig. 1. Concentration of 3α-hydroxy bile acids in urine and serum of
a pediatric patient with benign recurrent intrahepatic
colestasis.

prandial decrease in SGLC levels was found, and the GC response was
strongly reduced (Figure 2B). During periods of malaise and an
increased urinary bile acid excretion, the test resulted in a very
strong postprandial increase both in SGLC and GC concentrations
(Figure 2C). Fasting levels of SGLC were high in these tests and GC
concentrations were also elevated.

     The results presented suggest that the elevated serum levels of
SGLC found in BRIC patients might be caused by an increased influx of
these sulfated bile acids from the intestine. The postprandial rise
in serum SGLC is possibly a reflection of an altered net intestinal
transport in these patients that may be related to the occurrence of
cholestasis. The small increase in ΔGC in the BRIC patients during
the anicteric phase suggests a diminished overall hepatic clearance
of this bile acid. Van Berge-Henegouwen et al.[27] reported a
reduced hepatic clearance capacity for intravenously injected GC in
one out of four patients with a familial form of BRIC during
anicteric phases. Hepatic bile acid clearance appears to become more

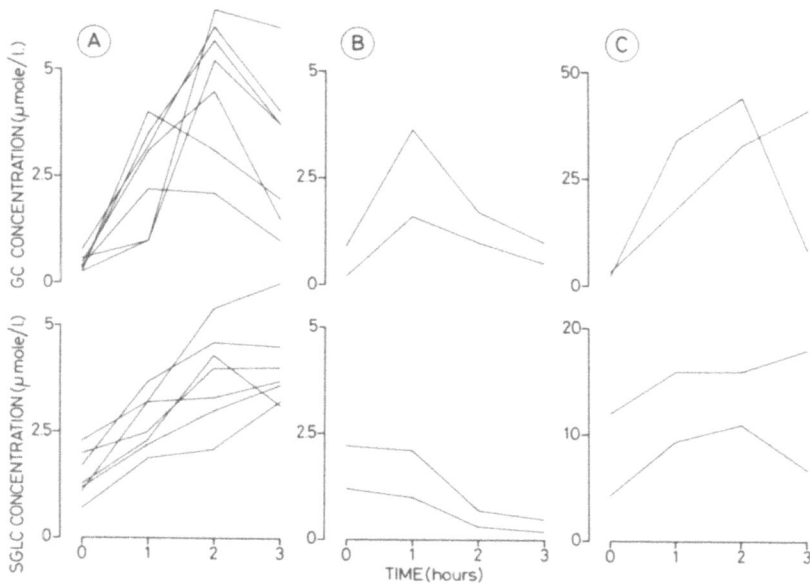

Fig. 2.   Serum concentration of sulfated lithocholic acid conjugates
(SGLC) and glycocholic acid (GC) in two brothers with benign
recurrent intrahepatic cholestasis after oral fat loading at
t = 0 hours: A. during a symptom-free period;   B. as A,
cholestyramine added;   C. during a pre-icteric period.

defective in the period just before a cholesterol attack, which
confirms the hypothesis of Van Berge-Henegouwen et al.[23].

PROTECTING MECHANISMS

Because SGLC is hepatotoxic in experimental animals and may
participate in the initiation and/or perpetuation of human liver
diseases, it is of interest to know factors that protect the liver
from the cholestatic action of this bile acid. As mentioned before,
Yousef et al.[15] showed that SGLC is cholestatic in rats, while STLC
administered in an equimolar dose is not. In man[28] and in most
animals[29] bile acids are conjugated preferentially with taurine,
and the proportion of bile acids conjugated with glycine or taurine
is dependent upon the availability of taurine[30]. Recently, Dorvil
et al.[31] showed that increasing the availability of taurine by
dietary means protects the liver against cholestasis induced by
sulfated lithocholic acid. In this study the cholestatic effects of
unconjugated, sulfated lithocholic acid (SLC) was investigated in
guinea pigs, an animal species which normally conjugates its bile
acids almost exclusively with glycine. Taurine administration at a
concentration of 0.5% in the drinking water for 3 days prevented

cholestasis after injection of 18 µmol/100 g body weight of SLC. The injected SLC was largely recovered from bile as the tauro-conjugate. In contrast, control animals that did develop severe cholestasis after injection of the same dose of SLC, formed predominantly glyco-conjugates. The protective effect of taurine in the BRIC patients mentioned before is currently under investigation.

Protection of the liver may furthermore be accomplished by facilitating or accelerating the elimination of the toxic compound. It has been shown that simultaneous infusion of taurocholic acid overcomes the cholestatic effect of lithocholic and taurolithocholic acid[2,32,33], possibly by micellar solubilization of the toxic molecules and promotion of their excretion into bile. Therefore, in situations that are characterized by low biliary bile acid output rates, the liver may be more susceptible to the hepatoxic action of monohydroxy bile acids. We studied the effects of endogenous bile acids on the cholestatic action of SGLC in rats. For this purpose we used an animal model in which the enterohepatic circulation (EHC) can be interrupted and restored without direct surgical intervention. Rats are equipped with permanent catheters in the bile duct and the duodenum. Both catheters are attached on top of the skull. There, the bile duct catheter can be connected to the duodenum catheter (intact EHC), or to a tubing which drains the bile (interrupted EHC). In the latter case, exhaustion of the bile acid pool takes place within 3-4 hours[34]. The rats are furthermore provided with a permanent catheter in the heart[35], which allows intracardial admin-istration of compounds and sampling of blood without disturbing the animal. Rats are used in experiments only after complete recovery from the operation. Details of the technique are described else-where[34]. This model was used to investigate the cholestatic effect of SGLC in two situations: firstly, immediately after interruption of the EHC, in the presence of endogenous bile acids and secondly, after 24 h of bile diversion, i.e. after exhaustion of the bile acid pool, when only newly synthetized bile acids are excreted.

Intravenous administration of SGLC (8 µmol/100 g body weight) in the presence of circulating endogenous bile acids did not induce cholestasis (Figure 3, solid lines). Only in the first 15 min. interval after the injection a significant reduction in bile flow was observed, when compared with controls injected with the vehicle alone (4% albumin in saline). In SGLC-treated and in control rats bile production decreased after 2 hours which is due to exhaustion of the bile acid pool[34]. In contrast, when injected after depletion of the bile acid pool by 24 h bile diversion, the same dose of SGLC caused a complete cessation of bile flow that lasted for more than 6 hours (Figure 3, broken lines).

The protective effect of endogenous bile acids is presumably accomplished by a faster excretion of SGLC. When a small, non-cholestatic dose of radiolabeled SGLC was injected in both situ-

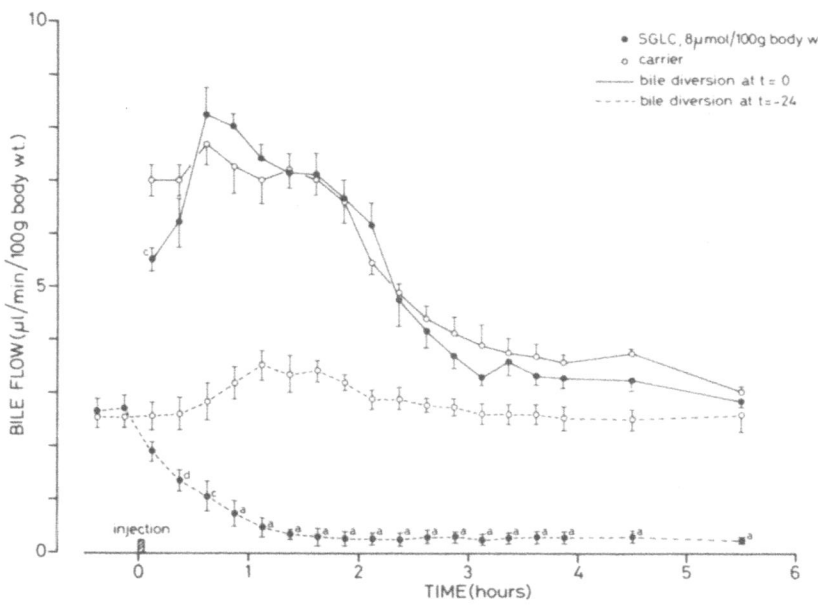

Fig. 3. Bile production of rats after injection of SGLC (●) or the vehicle alone (○), in the presence (----) and in the absence (---) of the endogenous bile acid pool ($\bar{X}$ ± SEM, $\underline{n}$ = 5 in all groups).

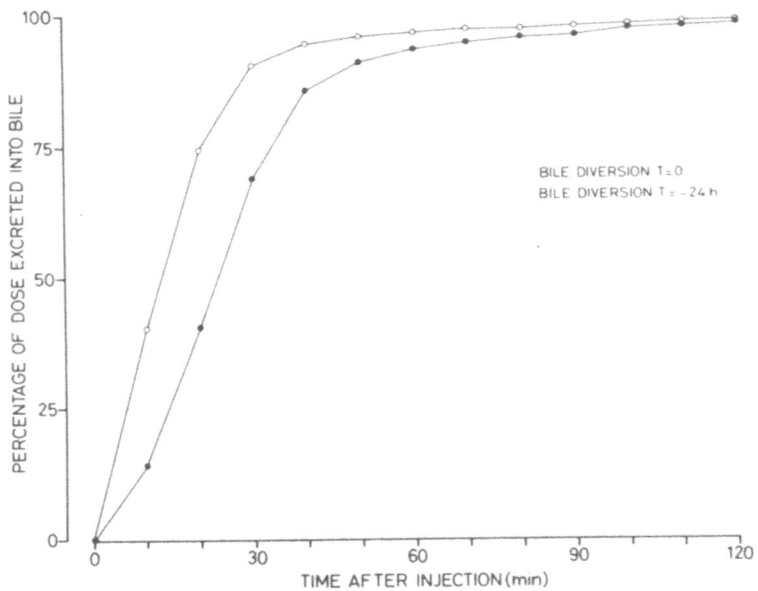

Fig. 4. Biliary excretion of [^{14}C]-SGLC in the presence (○) and in the absence (●) of the endogenous bile acid pool.

ations, the biliary excretion was much faster in the rats with an intact pool (Figure 4). In both situations the recovery of injected radioactivity in bile was almost complete after two hours. Urinary excretion of SGLC was negligible: less than 0.2% of the injected dose was recovered from 24-hours urine collections.

SUMMARY

The data presented show that evaluated serum concentrations of the hepatoxic bile acid SGLC in patients with benign recurrent intrahepatic cholestasis may be caused by an altered intestinal transport, and suggest a possible role of SGLC in the pathogenesis observed in these patients. Furthermore, it was shown in the rat that the liver is more susceptible to the cholestatic action of SGLC in the absence of circulating endogenous bile acids, which is possibly due to the slower biliary excretion of the toxic compound in this situation.

REFERENCES

1. N. B. Javitt, Cholestasis in rats induced by taurolithocholate, Nature, 210:1262 (1966).
2. N. B. Javitt and S. Emerman, Effect of sodium taurolithocholate on bile flow and bile acid excretion, J.Clin.Invest., 47:1002 (1968).
3. G. Kakis and I. M. Yousef, Pathogenesis of lithocholate- and taurolithocholate induced intrahepatic cholestasis in rats, Gastroenterol., 75:595 (1978).
4. J. E. King and L. Schoenfield, Cholestasis induced by sodium taurolithocholate in isolated hamster liver, J.Clin.Invest., 50:2305 (1971).
5. G. Kakis, M. J. Phillips and I. M. Yousef, The respective role of membrane cholesterol and of sodium potassium adenosine triphosphatase in the pathogenesis of lithocholate induced cholestasis, Lab.Invest., 43:73 (1980).
6. T. J. Layden, J. Schwartz and J. L. Boyer, Scanning electron microscopy of the rat liver. Studies on the effect of tauro-lithocholate and other models of cholestasis, Gastroenterol., 69:724 (1975).
7. K. Miyai, A. L. Richardson, W. Mayr and N. B. Javitt, Subcellu-lar pathology of rat liver in cholestasis and choleresis induced by bile salts. 1. Effects of lithocholic, 3β-hydroxy-5-cholenoic, cholic, and dehydrocholic acids, Lab.Invest., 36:249 (1977).
8. G. P. Van Berge-Henegouwen, A. Ruben and K. H. Brandt, Quanti-tative analysis of bile acids in serum and bile, using gas-liquid chomatography, Clin.Chim.Acta, 54:249 (1974).
9. K. Anderson, E. Kok and N. B. Javitt, Bile acid synthesis in man: metabolism of 7α-hydroxycholesterol-^{14}C and 26-hydroxy-cholesterol-^{3}H, J.Clin.Invest., 51:112 (1972).

10. R. H. Palmer and M. G. Bolt, Bile acid sulfates. I. Synthesis of lithocholic acid sulfates and their identification in human bile, J.Lipid Res., 12:671 (1971).
11. E. H. DeWitt and L. Lack, Effects of sulfation patterns on intestinal transport of bile salt sulfate esters, Am.J. Physiol., 238:34 (1980).
12. T. S. Low-Beer, M. P. Tyor and L. Lack, Effects of sulfation of taurolithocholic and glycolithocholic acids on their intestinal transport, Gastroenterol., 56:721 (1969).
13. I. Makino, H. Hashimoto, K. Shinozaki, K. Yoshino and S. Nakagawa, Sulfated and nonsulfated bile acids in urine, serum, and bile of patients with hepatobiliary diseases, Gastroenterol., 68:545 (1975).
14. A. E. Cowen, M. G. Korman, A. F. Hofmann, O. W. Cass and S. B. Coffin, Metabolism of lithocholate in healthy man. II. Enterohepatic circulation, Gastroenterol., 69:67 (1975).
15. I. M. Yousef, B. Tuchweber, R. J. Vonk, D. Massé, M. Audet and C. C. Roy, Lithocholate cholestasis- sulfated glycolithocholate induced intrahepatic cholestasis in rats, Gastroenterol., 80:233 (1981).
16. M. C. Carey, S. F. J. Wu and J. B. Watkins, Solution properties of sulfated monohydroxy bile salts. Relative insolubility of the disodium salt of glycolithocholate sulfate, Biochim. Biophys Acta, 575:16 (1979).
17. R. J. Vonk, B. Tuchweber, D. Massé, A. Perea, M. Audet, C. C. Roy and I. M. Yousef, Intrahepatic cholestasis induced by allomonohydroxy bile acids in rats, Gastroenterol., 80:242 (1981).
18. U. Mathis, G. Karlaganis and R. Preisig, Monohydroxy bile salt sulfates: tauro-3β-hydroxy-5-cholenoate-3-sulfate induces intrahepatic cholestasis in rats, Gastroenterol., 85:674 (1983).
19. G. J. Mulder, "Sulfation of Drugs and Related Compounds," CRC Press Boca Raton (1981).
20. A. G. F. de Pagter, G. P. Van Berge-Henegouwen, J. A. Ten Bokkel Huinink and K. H. Brandt, Familial benign recurrent intrahepatic cholestasis: Interrelation with intrahepatic cholestasis of pregnancy and from oral contraceptives, Gastroenterol., 71:202 (1976).
21. N. Tygstrup and B. Jensen, Intermittent intrahepatic cholestasis of unknown etiology in five young males from the Faroe Islands, Acta Med.Scand., 185:523 (1969).
22. W. H. J. Summerskill and J. M. Walshe, Benign recurrent intrahepatic 'obstructive' jaundice, Lancet, 2:686 (1959).
23. G. P. Van Berge-Henegouwen, K. H. Brandt and A. G. F. de Pagter, Is an acute disturbance in hepatic transport of bile acids the primary cause of cholestasis in benign recurrent cholestasis? Lancet, 1:1249 (1974).
24. J. A. Summerfield, A. P. Kirk, A. Chitranukroh and B. H. Billing, A distinctive pattern of serum bile acid and

bilirubin concentrations in benign recurrent intrahepatic cholestasis, Hepato-gastroenterol., 28:139 (1981).

25. R. J. Vonk, C. A. M. Bijleveld, C. Jousma, R. Havinga, J. Fernandes and A. van Zanten, Cholestatic effects of sulfated bile acids in: "Sulfate Metabolism and Sulfate Conjugation," G.J. Mulder, J. Caldwell, G.M.J. van Kempen and R.J. Vonk, eds., Taylor & Francis, London (1982).

26. B. Almé, A. Bremmelgaard, J. Sjövall and P. Thomassen, Analysis of metabolic profiles of bile acids in urine using a lipophilic anion exchanger and computerized gas-liquid chromatography-mass spectrometry, J.Lipid Res., 18:339 (1977).

27. G. P. Van Berge-Henegouwen, D. R. Ferguson, A. F. Hofmann and A. G. F. de Pagter, Familial and nonfamilial benign recurrent cholestasis distinguished by plasma disappearance of indocyanine green but not cholyglycerine, Gut, 19:345 (1978).

28. L. R. Haber, V. Vaupshas, B. B. Vitullo, T. A. Seemayer and R. C. DeBelle, Bile acid conjugation in organ culture of human fetal liver, Gastroenterol., 74:1214 (1978).

29. D. A. Vessey, The biochemical basis for the conjugation of bile acids with either glycine or taurine, Biochem.J., 174:621 (1978).

30. W. G. M. Hardison and J. H. Proffitt, Influence of hepatic taurine concentration on bile acid conjugation with taurine, Am.J.Physiol., 232:75 (1977).

31. N. P. Dorvil, I. M. Yousef, B. Tuchweber and C. C. Roy, Taurine prevents cholestasis induced by lithocholic acid sulfate in guinea pigs, Am.J.Clin.Nutr., 37:221 (1983).

32. G. Kakis and I. M. Yousef, Mechanism of cholic acid protection in lithocholate-induced intrahepatic cholestasis in rats, Gastroenterol., 78:1402 (1980).

33. T. L. Layden and J. L. Boyer, Taurolithocholate-induced cholestatis: taurocholate, but not dehydrocholate, reverses cholestasis and bile canalicular membrane injury, Gastroenterol., 73:120 (1977).

34. F. Kuipers, R. Havinga, H. Bosschieter, G. P. Toorop, F. R. Hindriks and R. J. Vonk, The enterohepatic circulation in the rat, Gastroenterol., accepted for publication.

35. A. B. Steffens, A method for frequent sampling of blood and continuous infusion of fluids in the rat without disturbing the animal, Physiol.Behav., 12:317 (1969).

ABNORMAL FECAL BILE ACID EXCRETION IN CYSTIC FIBROSIS:

PHYSIOPATHOLOGICAL MECHANISM AND CLINICAL IMPLICATIONS

Carla Colombo and Annamaria Giunta

Department of Pediatrics
University of Milan
Italy

Cystic Fibrosis (CF) is the most common genetic disorder of the Caucasian population it is estimated to occur in 1:2000 live births and it is inherited as an autosomal recessive trait.

Life expectancy of the patient with CF has improved over the last two decades, due to aggressive management of pulmonary infections and to pancreatic enzyme supplementation to improve nutrition. Eighty to ninety per cent of children with CF have exocrine pancreatic insufficiency[1]: substitutive therapy with pancreatic enzymes can improve fat and nitrogen absorption in the majority of the patients, but in a consistent number, even massive doses fail to normalize digestion. It is extremely important to achieve as normal a fat balance as possible in CF patients, since they have been reported to shown an improved respiratory prognosis as compared to patients with persistent steatorrhea[2].

The incapacity of pancreatic enzymes to completely normalize nutrient absorption in CF has been attributed to inactivation of the exogenous enzymes occurring not only in the stomach, but also at the reduced pH of the small intestine, as a result of low pancreatic bicarbonate secretion[3].

Moreover, intraluminal bile acid (BA) concentration can be lower than normal in patients with CF[4], as a consequence of persistent BA malabsorption, further abetting their maldigestion. In fact, increased fecal BA losses have been repeatedly reported to occur in CF patients with pancreatic insufficiency[5,6,7] and can produce other important clinical consequences. There may be a contraction of bile acid pool size, as the capacity of the liver to compensate these losses becomes insufficient[8]. Biliary bile acid concentration

235

decreases and bile becomes lithogenic[9]. As a matter of fact, an
increased incidence of cholelithiasis has been observed in CF (4-12%
of the patients)[10].

Finally, it has been postulated that the increased loss of BA
may cause or exacerbate the characteristic form of liver disease in
CF, as it has been observed in other conditions where a BA wastage
occurs[11]; actually, liver involvement has been observed only in
patients with pancreatic insufficiency.

So, there are a lot of clinical implications to reduce the
abnormal BA loss in CF. However, its physiopathological mechanisms
have not yet been definitively established.

A lot of studies have been carried out and several hypothesis
have been formulated: it is possible that more than one factor may
contribute to BA malabsorption in CF, but delineation of the exact
defect(s) is extremely important to prevent its often serious clinical consequences and to improve nutrition in CF patients.

Several studies have suggested that BA absorption is disturbed
in CF, owing to the interference of intraluminal factors due to
pancreatic insufficiency.

The role of undigested nutrients has been postulated, following
the observation that, when pancreatic enzyme supplementation was
withdrawn, CF patients showed a fecal BA output which was comparable
to that observed in children with ileal resection[5]. Substitutive
therapy was followed by a partial but consistent amelioration in BA
loss. In basal conditions, a positive and significant correlation
between fecal BA and fecal fat excretion was found and unhydrolyzed
triglycerides and/or free fatty acids have been considered as the
most responsible factors inhibiting BA absorption in CF.

This finding has not been confirmed by later investigations.
Smalley, for example, found that fecal BA excretion in CF patients
with pancreatic insufficiency was higher than in controls, but widely
variable, showing no significant correlation with fecal fat levels
[12]. However, also in these patients, substitutive therapy with
pancreatic enzymes resulted in a significant reduction of both fecal
fat and fecal BA excretion. This suggested that steatorrhea is
certainly a contributing factor in determining BA malabsorption in
CF, but the role of other endoluminal factors must not be under-
estimated. This speculation is supported by the results of bile acid
kinetics by means of stable isotope dilution technique in 6 CF
patients off and on pancreatic enzyme therapy[8]. Enzyme replacement
brought about a net increase of BA pool-size and a reduction of
fractional turnover rate of the BA pool; conversely, BA synthesis
changed little with therapy, and fecal BA excretion remained high,

despite a marked reduction of fat excretion. Therefore, fecal losses of BA persist when substitutive therapy is instituted and steatorrhea is at least in part corrected. It is possible that other undigested nutrients, such as protein, polysaccharide, fiber or carbohydrate may interfere with BA absorption by means of binding or competition mechanisms. Also the investigators, who studied CF patients while they were assuming pancreatic enzymes, could not find a significant correlation between fecal BA and fecal fats. Goodchild examined 29 CF patients, who were older than those studied by Weber and were on enzymatic therapy: fecal BA excretion showed a tendency to decrease with age, as a probable result of progressive liver involvement, which is likely to be more significant among the older patients, and which leads to insufficient compensatory synthesis of BA and contraction of BA pool.

We have recently used multivariate analysis of variance to evaluate the influence of different clinical and biochemical parameters on fecal BA excretion[13] and we have found that fecal BA losses in 76 CF patients on enzymatic therapy, are significantly correlated with the coefficient of fat absorption (and therefore with fecal fat excretion), a finding which is in agreement with the results of Weber[5]. We also found that enzymatic therapy has a different efficacy in reducing BA losses, depending on the degree of pancreatic insufficiency of each patient. Also this finding suggests that steatorrhea is one of the factor responsible for BA malabsorption in CF, especially in those patients who present severe pancreatic insufficiency, but it must not be the only one. Other physiopathological mechanisms must be considered.

Endoluminal pH is lower than normal in CF, as a result of low pancreatic bicarbonate secretion. At an acid pH, there may be an alteration of the physical state of BA, with precipitation, particularly of free and glycoconjugated BA, which have a pK of approximately 4. It has been recently demonstrated that cimetidine improves lipid digestion and solubilization in CF patients, just by reducing BA precipitation and hence increasing the solubilization of lipids.

Indirect evidence of the physiopathological role of reduced endoluminal pH seems to be suggested from the results obtained after ursodeoxycholic acid oral load in CF patients: serum levels, after a standard dose of this BA, were significantly different from controls and were inversely correlated with total fecal BA, but not with fecal fats[15]. Since ursodeoxycholic acid shows particular physical-chemical properties (being far less soluble than other BA), the reduced serum levels of this exogenous BA may be due to its endoluminal precipitation at a reduced pH value. As a matter of fact, different studies have reported the usefulness of the adjunct of cimetidine or bicarbonate in reducing steatorrhea azotorrhea, stool weight and fecal BA[16,17,18].

It is our opinion that this kind of therapy can prove to be very effective in a restricted and selected number of patients, who persist to show increased fecal BA and fat excretion, despite large dosing of pancreatic supplements.

There are other factors, which have been considered as potential responsible of BA malabsorption in CF.

The presence of a layer of thick surface mucus, covering intestinal mucosa, has been postulated to constitute a mechanical barrier, preventing normal BA absorption; absorption of BA to the abnormal intestinal mucus may occur, as it has been demonstrated to occur in vitro[19]. The addition of N-Acetyl-Cysteine to pancreatic enzymes resulted in an improvement of fat absorption in CF patients with steatorrhea[20], but this finding must be confirmed by clinical studies on larger patients' population.

Alterations of the intestinal microflora, due to frequent antibiotics administration accounts for the modification in qualitative fecal BA pattern, described for CF patients (increased percentage of primary BA)[6]. Moreover, a relationship between the anaerobic flora and BA loss in CF has been described[21]: intravenous antibiotics therapy resulted in a reduction of anaerobic bacteria, decreased biotransformation of BA and improvement of BA absorption, with normalization of fecal BA losses. These results suggest that the reciprocal interactions between microbial flora and BA may also be of importance in determining BA malabsorption in CF.

Finally, the existence in CF of a primary ileal mucosal defect for BA absorption has been recently investigated. The ileal mucosal uptake of taurocholate in vitro was found to be reduced in CF patients and comparable to those for passive jejunal taurocholic acid uptake in controls. An incapacity of the ileus to actively transport BA in CF has therefore been suggested, similarly to other small bowel mucosal dysfunctions previously described in this disease.

We have recently evaluated total and fractional fecal bile acid excretion in CF patients with and without pancreatic insufficiency and have compared these data with the serum postprandial curves of the two primary BA (conjugated cholic and chenodeoxycholic acids). We have found that patients without pancreatic insufficiency show a significantly increased fecal excretion of cholic acid, despite a total BA excretion similar to controls. Moreover, in these patients the postprandial levels of cholic acid were decreased, while those of chenodeoxycholic acid (which is absorbed not only by active transport mechanism in the terminal ileus, but also passively throughout the intestine) were normal.

In patients with pancreatic insufficiency, we confirmed the presence of BA malabsorption, which appears generalized, involving cholic, chenodeoxycholic and secondary BA; the postprandial concentrations of both primary BA were reduced. These data are consistent with a selective malabsorption of cholic acid in CF, independently from the presence of pancreatic insufficiency. In the presence of pancreatic insufficiency, the intraluminal factors mentioned above, seem to prevent also the absorption of other BA all along the intestine.

REFERENCES

1. R. W. Park and R. J. Grand, Gastrointestinal manifestations of cystic fibrosis: A review, Gastroenterology, 81:1143 (1981).
2. K. Gaskin, D. Gurwitz, P. Durie, M. Corey, H. Levison, and G. Forstner, Improved respiratory prognosis in patients with cystic fibrosis with normal fat absorption, J.Pediatr., 100:857 (1982).
3. B. Hadorn, G. Zoppi, and D. H. Shmerling, Quantitative assessment of exocrine pancreatic function in infants and children, J.Pediatr., 73:39 (1968).
4. J. T. Harries, P. R. Muller, J. P. K. McCollum, A. Lipson, E. Roma, and A. P. Norman, Intestinal bile salts in cystic fibrosis: Studies in the patient and experimental animal, Archs.Dis.Childh., 54:19 (1979).
5. A. M. Webern, C. C. Roy, C. L. Morin, and R. Lasalle, Malabsorption of bile acids in children with cystic fibrosis, New Engl.J.Med., 289:1001 (1973).
6. A. M. Weber, C. C. Roy, L. Chartrand, G. Lepage, L. Dufour, C. L. Morin, and R. Lasalle, Relationship between bile acid malabsorption and pancreatic insufficiency in cystic fibrosis, Gut, 17:295 (1976).
7. M. C. Goodchild, G. M. Murphy, A. M. Howell, S. A. Nutter, and C. M. Anderson, Aspects of bile acid metabolism in cystic fibrosis, Archs.Dis.Childh., 50:769 (1975).
8. J. B. Watkins, A. M. Tercyak, P. Szczepanik, and P. D. Klein, Bile salt kinetics in cycstic fibrosis: Influence of pancreatic enzyme replacement, Gastroenterology, 73:1023 (1977).
9. C. C. Roy, A. M. Weber, C. L. Morin, J. C. Combes, D. Nusslé, A. Mégevand, and R. Lasalle, Abnormal biliary lipid composition in cystic fibrosis: Effect of pancreatic enzymes, New Engl. J.Med., 297:1301 (1977).
10. J. Isenberg, P. L'Heureaux, W. Warwick, H. Sharp, Clinical observations on the biliary system in cystic fibrosis, Am.J. Gastroenterology, 65:134 (1976).
11. S. A. Bagheri, T. L. Barbato, D. J. Ferguson, and J. L. Boyer, The development of Laennec cirrhosis in asymptomatic patients with small bowel bypass for massive obesity (Abstr.), Gastroenterology, 66:878 (1974).
12. C. A. Smalley, G. A. Brown, M. E. Parkes, H. Tease, V. Brookes, and C. M. Anderson, Reduction of bile acid loss in cystic fibrosis by dietary means, Archs.Dis.Childh., 53:477 (1978).

13. C. Colombo, A. M. Morselli, P. Rucci, R. Maiavacca, M. Ronchi, and A. Giunta, Fecal bile acid excretion in patients with cystic fibrosis: Correlation with clinical and biochemical parameters (Abstr.) 115/B5, Proceedings of the 9th International Cystic Fibrosis Congress, Brighton 9-15 June (1984).

14. P. L. Munro Zentler, D. R. Fine, J. C. Batten, and T. C. Northfield, How cimetidine improves lipid digestion and solubilization in cystic fibrosis, in: "Current Problems and New Trends in Cystic Fibrosis," M. Shöni and R. Kraemer, eds., p.175 (1981).

15. C. Colombo, A. Roda, E. Roda, L. Piceni Sereni, and D. Maspero, Evaluation of an oral ursodeoxycholic acid load in the assessment of bile acid malabsorption in cystic fibrosis, Dig.Dis.Sci., 28:306 (1983).

16. K. L. Cox, J. N. Isenberg, A. B. Osher, and R. R. Dooley, The effect of cimetidine in cystic fibrosis, J.Pediatr., 94:488 (1979).

17. P. R. Durie, L. Bell, W. Linton, M. L. Corey, and G. Forstner, Effect of cimetidine and sodium bicarbonate on pancreatic replacement therapy in cystic fibrosis, Gut, 21:778 (1980).

18. B. J. Boyle, W. B. Long, W. F. Balistreri, S. J. Widzer, and N. Huang, Effect of cimetidine and pancreatic enzymes on serum and fecal bile acids and fat absorption in cystic fibrosis, Gastroenterology, 78:950 (1980).

19. R. S. Dubois, M. L. Selley, and J. M. Brown, In vitro adsorption of bile salts (BS) to mucus in cystic fibrosis (CF) (Abstr.), Gastroenterology, 72:1052 (1977).

20. H. J. Neijens, J. Bouquet, M. Sinoasappel, K. F. Kerrebijn, W. F. A. Grose, Comparison of the effects of pancreatic enzyme as acid resistent microspheres to granules and of the addition of N-Acetyl-Cysteine on the malabsorption in CF, Proceedings of the 11th Meeting of the European Working Group for Cystic Fibrosis, Bruxelles (1982).

21. C. C. Roy, G. Delage, A. Fontaine, L. Robitaille, L. Chartrand, A. Weber, and C. Morin, The fecal microflora and bile acids in children with cystic fibrosis, Am.J.Clin.Nutr., 32:2404 (1979).

22. J. D. Fondacaro, J. E. Henbi, and F. W. Kellog, Intestinal bile acid malabsorption in cystic fibrosis: A primary mucosal cell defect, Pediatr.Res., 16:494 (1982).

23. C. Colombo, A. Roda, E. Roda, L. Piceni Sereni, A. Brega, R. Fugazza, and A. Giunta, Bile acid malabsorption in cystic fibrosis with and without pancreatic insufficiency, J.Pediatr.Gastroenterol.Nutr., 3 (1984) in press.

EFFECT OF CHENODEOXYCHOLIC AND URSODEOXYCHOLIC ACID TREATMENT ON INTESTINAL MICROFLORA OF PATIENTS WITH CHOLESTEROL GALLSTONES

Annamaria Ferrari, Novella Pacini and Enrica Canzi

Institute of Agrarian and Technical Microbiology
University of Milan
Via Celoria, 2, 20133 Milan, Italy

INTRODUCTION

The positive results of treatment of cholesterol gallstones with chenodeoxycholic acid ($3\alpha,7\alpha$-dihydroxy-5β-cholan-24-oic acid) (CDA) and its epimer ursodeoxycholic acid ($3\alpha,7\beta$-dihydroxy-5β-cholan-24-oic acid) (UDA) are well known. In the colon these bile acids are mainly 7α-dehydroxylated by intestinal microflora into lithocholic acid (3α-monohydroxy-5β-cholan-24-oic acid) (LCA), whose toxicity at the hepatic level has been demonstrated in different higher animals.

The aim of our study was to verify whether, with respect to healthy subjects, patients affected by cholesterol gallstones and treated for different times with different quantities of CDA and UDA had alterations of the intestinal microflora composition and in vitro activity on the same bile acids.

METHODS

The study was carried out on fecal material from 5 treated patients (AD, BD, FC, GM, AC) (Table 1) and from 5 healthy subjects (controls) (AF, AG, GB, GV, FB). The bile acids treatment did not induce gastrointestinal side effects in any patients. The feces, within 2 h of collection, were placed in an anaerobic cabinet ($N_2:H_2:CO_2$ atmosphere, 85:10:5), subjected to bacteriological examination and to tests for biochemical activity on CDA and UDA[1]. The microbial groups examined were anaerobic bacteria, Bacteroidaceae, bifidobacteria, clostridia, anaerobic cocci, lactobacilli, coliform bacteria, aerobic bacteria. Different media were used[2] and the characterization of isolated strains was performed taking into con-

Table 1. Treatment of Patients with CDA and UDA.

Patients	UDA/pro die	CDA/pro die	Time of treatment
AD	300 mg	250 mg	1 month
BD	600 mg	150 mg	6 years
FC	450 mg		3 months
GM	750 mg		5 months
AC	450 mg		22 months

sideration the main morphological, cultural and physiological properties.

For the study of the behavior of the transformation of CDA and UDA, the fecal cultures in Marcus-Talalay medium[3], to which 0.01% CDA and UDA had been added, were examined at different times by thin layer chromatography[1] as well as by gaschromatography[4].

RESULTS AND DISCUSSION

Comparison of the data on the qualitative and quantitative composition of the fecal microflora of the two groups of subjects showed a significant increase on the number of bifidobacteria, Gram-positive anaerobic cocci, coliforms and total aerobes in the feces of the treated patients (Figure 1). However, these alterations do not represent a substantial modification of the intestinal microflora composition.

As regard the in vitro activity of the fecal microflora on the bile acids, the number of microorganisms capable of producing LCA from CDA as well as UDA was significantly higher in treated patients than in controls (Figure 2). Moreover both in patients and in control subjects the number of CDA and UDA transforming microorganisms was about of the same order.

In Figure 3 and 4, is shown the formation of different intervals of time of LCA from CDA and UDA in groups of homogeneous subjects as to the curve of transformation.

The transformation rate of CDA to LCA, although the total amount of LCA accumulated after 72 h of incubation remained almost the same was slower in control than in treated subjects (Figure 3). Of the latter group, 4 patients (AD, BD, FC, GM) transformed CDA almost completely into LCA after only 24 h of incubation, whereas the fifth patient (AC) (Figure 5) transformed CDA more slowly and not completely (70%). The transformation of UDA to LCA was also faster in

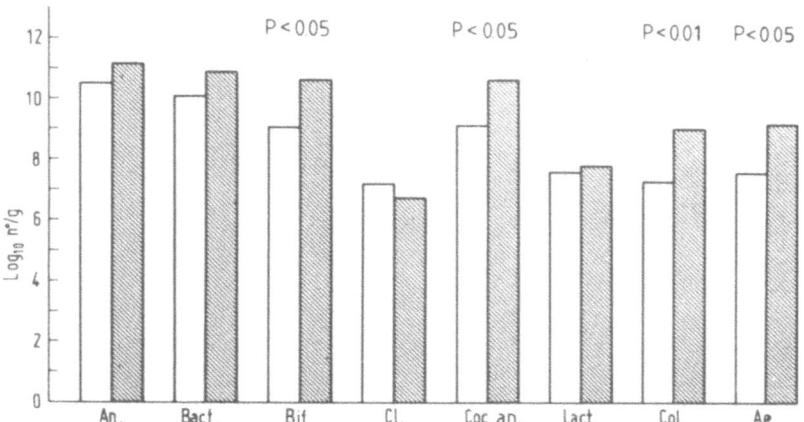

Fig. 1. Mean values of microbial counts/g dry weight in treated
patients (□) and controls (□).

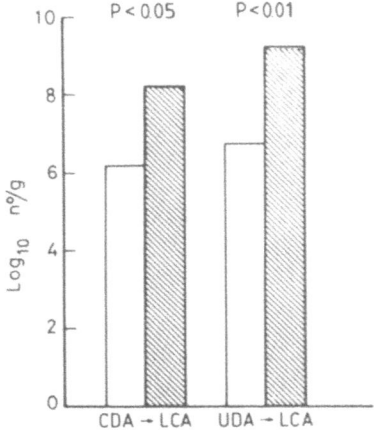

Fig. 2. Mean values of CDA and UDA 7α-dehydroxylating micro-
organisms/g of dry weight in treated patients (□) and
controls (□).

treated subjects than in controls (Figure 4). Only patient AC
(Figure 6) and controls AG and FB (Figure 7,8) transformed UDA to LCA
more slowly and incompletely. The lower ability to transform UDA we
found in controls AG and FB was found also by Hirano[5] in some
healthy subjects. In all controls and treated patients, with the
aforementioned exceptions, the transformation rate of UDA was similar
to that of CDA, in agreement with that reported by Bazzoli et al[6]
for healthy subjects and untreated subjects affected cholesterol
gallstones. Moreover in spite of the great heterogeneity in treatments (different bile acids, different doses and times), the intes-

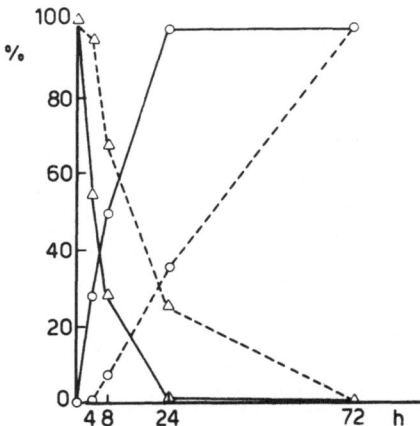

Fig. 3. Mean percentages of bile acids observed at different intervals of time during the transformation of CDA (△) to LCA (○) by intestinal microflora of 4 treated patients (AD,BD,FC,GM) (——) and of the 5 controls (---).

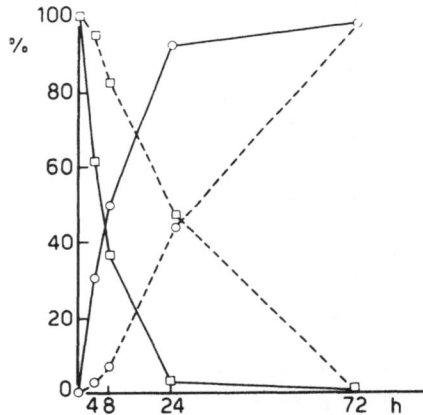

Fig. 4. Mean percentages of bile acids observed at different intervals of time during the transformation of UDA (□) to LCA (○) by intestinal microflora of 4 treated patients (AD,BD,FC,GM) (——) and of 3 controls (AF,GB,GV) (---).

tinal microflora composition and its activity on bile acids resulted similar in all tested patients.

In conclusion, on the basis of these preliminary results, the transformation of the bile acids examined, which was generally faster in treated patients, appears to be correlated to the number of micro-

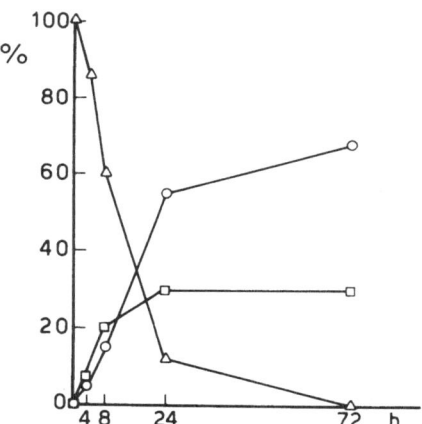

Fig. 5. Percentages of bile acids observed at different intervals of time during the transformation of CDA (△) to LCA (○) by intestinal microflora of patient AC.

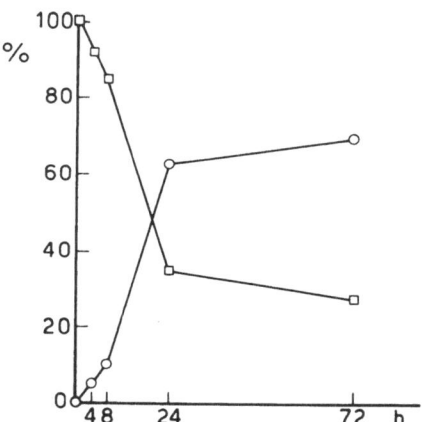

Fig. 6. Percentages of bile acids observed at different intervals of time during the transformation of UDA (□) to LCA (○) by intestinal microflora of patient AC.

organisms able to produce LCA from CDA and UDA. As a matter of fact that number is greater in treated subjects. Both from our preliminary controls and from what shown by Bazzoli et al[6] significant differences of microflora activity on CDA and UDA in untreated subjects affected by cholesterol gallstones compared with healthy subjects may be excluded. Thus, since it is not possible to state that

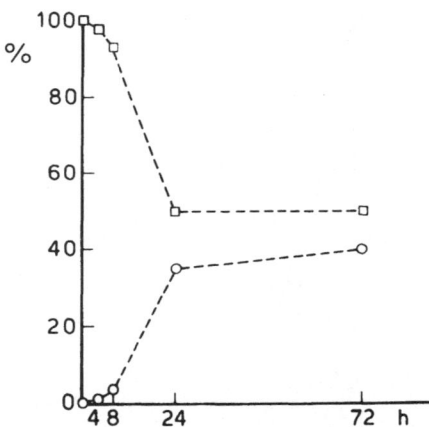

Fig. 7. Percentages of bile acids observed at different intervals of time during the transformation of UDA (□) to LCA (○) by intestinal microflora of control AG.

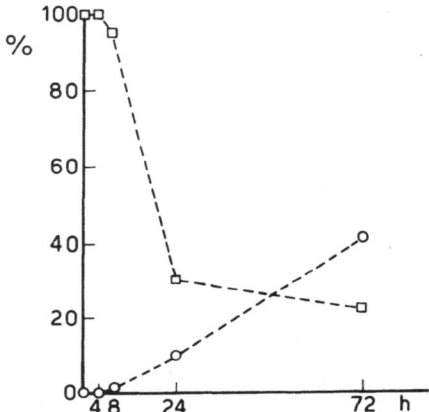

Fig. 8. Percentages of bile acids observed at different intervals of time during the transformation of UDA (□) to LCA (○) by intestinal microflora of control FB.

the general picture of the microflora in treated patients underwent alterations that affected its equilibrium, the faster transformation rate could be explained by an adaptation acquired by the microflora to a different bile acids situation in the intestinal lumen which occurred during the therapy.

REFERENCES

1. A. Ferrari, N. Pacini, E. Canzi, and F. Bruno, Prevalence of oxygen – intolerant microorganisms in primary bile acids 7α-dehydroxylating mouse intestinal microflora, Current Microbiol., 4:257 (1980).

2. N. Pacini, C. Calvi, and G. F. Greppi, Microflora intestinale nel coniglio a vario tenore proteico nella dieta, Atti della Società Italiana di Scienze Veterinarie n. 36, San Remo (1982).

3. P. I. Marcus and P. Talalay, Induction and purification of α- and β-hydroxysteroid dehydrogenases, J.Biol.Chem., 218:661 (1956).

4. E. Albini, G. Marca, and G. Mellerio, Further observations on the in vitro metabolism of chenodeoxycholic acid and ursodeoxycholic acid, Arzneim.Forsch., 12:1554 (1982).

5. S. Hirano, N. Masuda, and H. Oda, In vitro transformation of chenodeoxycholic acid and ursodeoxycholic acid by human intestinal flora, with particular reference to the mutual conversion between the two bile acids, J.Lipid Res., 22:735 (1981).

6. F. Bazzoli, H. Fromm, R. P. Sarva, R. F. Sembrat, and S. Ceryak, Comparative formation of lithocholic acid from chenodeoxycholic and ursodeoxycholic acids in the colon, Gastroenterology, 83:753 (1982).

THE INFLUENCE OF A LACTOVEGETARIAN, A VEGAN AND A MIXED

DIET ON COLONIC FUNCTION OF MAN: PRELIMINARY RESULTS

A. van Faassen, W. van Dokkum, N. A. Pikaar
and R. J. J. Hermus

Institute CIVO-Toxicology and Nutrition TNO
Zeist, The Netherlands

INTRODUCTION

In correlation studies a positive association has been found between the consumption of meat and/or animal protein and the incidence of colonic cancer[1]. Case-control studies, however, do not consistently reveal this association[2,3].

Fecal characteristics like a low bulk, high pH and a high concentration of (secondary) bile acids observed in correlation studies, are also related to a high incidence of colonic cancer[4-7]. For this reason we studied the effects on fecal bulk, defecation frequency, fecal pH and fecal bile acids of diets with different amounts and types of animal protein. The diets were chosen not only on account of differences in origin of protein, but also in order to provide customary diets containing meat, plant foods and milk-based products (lactovegetarian) or plant foods only (vegan).

MATERIALS AND METHODS

Twelve apparently healthy male Caucasian volunteers (students, age 20-25 years) were carefully selected for trustworthiness. They consumed the three different diets for 20 days each in randomized order. They were housed in the Institute's controlled metabolic ward for the duration of the study, i.e. 60 days, but continued their normal daily activities. All meals were served and consumed in the Institute. The diets consisted of constant and standardized meals and drinks. The mixed diet (M) was composed of normal Dutch foods like bread, vegetables, potatoes and different kinds of meat. The lactovegetarian diet (L) was similarly composed, except for all meat being replaced by milk- and soy-based products. The vegan diet (V) differed from the other two in that all foods of animal origin were replaced by vegetable products derived from soy beans or by nuts and yeast. The diets have been analyzed according to the description by van Dokkum et al.[8], also stating the method of measuring fecal bulk, defecation frequency, fecal bile acids and of statistical analysis. Collection of the stools took place at -20°C using deep-freeze toilets[9]. Fecal pH was measured as described by van Dokkum et al.[10].

RESULTS

Diet characteristics are shown in Table 1. Since the diets had to be essentially vegan, lactovegetarian and of a mixed composition, they did not only differ in origin of the protein. The mixed diet contained more fat and less dietary fiber than the other ones. The vegan diet contained the lowest amount of saturated fat and the highest amount of dietary fiber. The lactovegetarian and the vegan diet differed in the amount of linoleic acid, saturated fat and dietary fiber. Results with respect to colonic function are given in Table 2. Fecal bulk and defecation frequency were lower in the M diet period than in the L and V periods. Fecal pH was lower on the V diet than on the L and M diets. Excretion of bile acids was lowest on the V diet compared with the L and the M diet. Bile acid concentration increased in the sequence V - L - M.

DISCUSSION

The fecal characteristics observed in correlation studies to be associated with a lower incidence of colonic cancer (i.e. a high

Table 1. Chemical Analysis of the Characteristics of the 3 Diets.

	Mixed diet	Lactovegetarian diet	Vegan diet
Metabolizable energy (MJ)	12	13	13
Protein (energy%)	17	16	17
Fat (energy%)	38	32	33
Available carbohydrates (energy%)	45	52	50
Linoleic acid (energy%)	15	11	17
Saturated fat (energy%)	13	14	8
Dietary fiber (g/d)	22	28	40
Protein composition (%)			
Meat protein	46	0	0
Milk protein	28	54	0
Vegetable protein	26	46	100

Table 2. Mean Values ± s.d. of Colonic Function of Twelve Healthy Male Volunteers Consuming 3 Different Diets for a Period of 20 days each.

	Mixed diet	Lactovegetarian diet	Vegan diet
Fecal bulk (g/d)	101±34[b]	160±39[a]	160±36[a]
Defecation frequency (no. of stools/d)	0.9±0.2[b]	1.1±0.3[a]	1.1±0.3[a]
Fecal pH	7.2±0.3[a]	7.1±0.3[a]	6.7±0.2[b]
Fecal bile acids			
(μmol/d)	740±310[a]	730±340[a]	530±250[c]
(μmol/g wet feces)	7.4±3.0[a]	4.5±2.1[a]	3.3±1.5[c]

Non-matching superscripts denote a significant difference
a-b $p < 0.001$
a-c $p < 0.05$

bulk, a low concentration of bile acids and a low pH), were found in this study on the vegan diet. The greater amount of dietary fiber in this diet may be responsible for these results. Dietary fiber has been reported to increase the volume of the feces[11] and to lower fecal pH[12]. It is considered to influence the fecal pH, because it is metabolized by the colonic bacteria[13]. Meat does not influence fecal bulk, defecation frequency and has only a slight effect on the fecal concentration of bile acids[14]. These facts lead to the hypothesis that a low consumption of dietary fiber connected with a high consumption of meat and/or animal protein will account for the statistical association between the consumption of meat and/or animal protein and the incidence of colonic cancer.

In order to establish whether this type of diet and its fecal characteristics are really associated with carcinogenesis of the colon, a prospective investigation has to be carried out. Such a study is in preparation.

Acknowledgements

The authors wish to thank Miss A. Wesstra, Miss F. Schippers, Mrs. H. van Steenbrugge, Mr. B. C. J. de Boer and Mr. L. van Ginkel for their technical assistance and the volunteers for their cooperation. The Koningin Wilhelmina Fonds (Netherlands Cancer Foundation) granted a fellowship to Miss A. van Faassen.

REFERENCES

1. P. Correa, Epidemiological correlations between diet and cancer frequency, <u>Cancer Res.</u>, 41:3685 (1981).
2. W. Haenszel, J. W. Berg, M. Segi et al., Large-bowel cancer in Hawaiian Japanese, <u>J.Natl.Cancer Inst.</u>, 51:1765 (1973).
3. W. Haenzxel, F. B. Locke, and M. Segi, A case-control study of large bowel cancer, <u>J.Natl.Cancer Inst.</u>, 64:17 (1980).
4. O. M. Jensen, R. MacLennan, and J. Wahrendorf, Diet, bowel function, fecal characteristics, and large bowel cancer in Denmark and Finland, <u>Nutr.Cancer</u>, 4:5 (1982).
5. S. L. Malhotra, Fecal urobilinogen levels and pH of stools in population groups with different incidence of cancer of the colon, and their possible role in its etiology, <u>J.R.Soc.Med.</u>, 75:709 (1982).
6. B. S. Reddy, A. R. Hedges, K. Laakso, and E. L. Wynder, Metabolic epidemiology of large bowel cancer: Fecal bulk and constituents of high-risk North American and low-risk Finnish population, <u>Cancer</u>, 42:2832 (1978).
7. M. J. Hill, A. J. Taylor, M. H. Thompson, and R. Wait, Fecal steroids and urinary volatile phenols in four Scandinavian populations, <u>Nutr.Cancer</u>, 4:67 (1982).
8. W. van Dokkum, N. A. Pikaar, and J. T. N. M. Thissen, Physiological effects of fiber-rich types of bread 2. Dietary fiber from bread: digestibility by the intestinal microflora and water-holding capacity in the colon of human subjects, <u>Brit.J.Nutr.</u>, 50:61 (1983).
9. Y. Ghoos and G. van Trappen, Clean collection and manipulation of stools, <u>Lancet</u>, i:884 (1977).
10. W. van Dokkum, B. C. J. de Boer, and A. van Faassen, Diet fecal pH and colorectal cancer, <u>Br.J.Cancer</u>, 48:109 (1983).
11. M. A. Eastwood, W. G. Brydon, and K. Tadesse, Effect of fiber on colon function, <u>in</u>: "Medical Aspects of Dietary Fiber," G.A. Spiller and R.M. Kay, eds., Plenum Medical Book, New York (1980).
12. A. R. P. Walker, B. F. Walker, and I. Segal, Fecal pH value and its modification by dietary means in South African black and white school children, <u>S.A.Medical J.</u>, 55:495 (1979).
13. J. H. Cummings, A. M. Stephen, and W. J. Branch, Implications of dietary fiber breakdown in the human colon, <u>in</u>: "Branbury Report 7: Gastrointestinal Cancer: Endogenous Factors," W.R. Bruce, P. Correa, M. Lipkin, S.R. Tannenbaum, T.D. Wilkins, eds., Cold Spring Harbor Laboratory, Cold Spring Harbor, New York (1981).
14. J. H. Cummings, M. J. Hill, T. Jivraj et al., The effect of meat protein and dietary fiber on colonic function and metabolism. I. Changes in bowel habit, bile acid excretion, and calcium absorption, <u>Am.J.Clin.Nutr.</u>, 32:2086 (1979).

INDEX